Family Practice Review

A PROBLEM ORIENTED APPROACH

Family Practice Review

A PROBLEM ORIENTED APPROACH

SIX HUNDRED AND SIXTY-TWO BOARD-TYPE
MULTIPLE-CHOICE QUESTIONS WITH ANSWERS,
EXPLANATIONS, AND CURRENT REFERENCES

RICHARD W. SWANSON, B.Sc., M.D., C.C.F.P. (C)

Associate Professor of Family Medicine
University of Saskatchewan
Saskatoon, Saskatchewan

1987

B.C. Decker Inc • Toronto • Philadelphia

Publisher

B.C. Decker Inc
3228 South Service Road
Burlington, Ontario   L7N 3H8

B.C. Decker Inc
P.O. Box 30246
Philadelphia, Pennsylvania   19103

Sales and Distribution

United States and Possessions	**The C.V. Mosby Company** 11830 Westline Industrial Drive Saint Louis, Missouri 63146
Canada	**The C.V. Mosby Company, Ltd.** 5240 Finch Avenue East, Unit No. 1 Scarborough, Ontario M1S 4P2
United Kingdom, Europe and the Middle East	**Blackwell Scientific Publications, Ltd.** Osney Mead, Oxford OX2 OEL, England
Australia	**CBS Publishing Australia Pty. Limited** 9 Waltham Street Artarmon, N.S.W. 2064 Australia
Japan	**Igaku-Shoin Ltd.** Tokyo International P.O. Box 5063 1-28-36 Hongo, Bunkyo-ku, Tokyo 113, Japan
Asia	**CBS Publishing Asia Limited** 10/F, Inter-Continental Plaza Tsim Sha Tsui East Kowloon, Hong Kong

Family Practice Review

ISBN 1–55009–019–4

Library of Congress catalog card number: 86-72328

10 9 8 7 6 5 4 3 2

To my wife Stella and my children Heidi, Eric, and Jason.

To two special people, Tim and Carol Posyluzny,
who have taught us the true meaning of friendship.

To my parents, for everything.

To family practice residents everywhere,
who have chosen family medicine as their life's work.

Preface

This book is written as a review of problems commonly occurring in family medicine. The problems that are presented in this book are not esoteric, rare, or complicated, but rather are important problems seen by family physicians every day.

Each problem is followed by a set of multiple-choice questions that include both a single and multiple answer format. In addition, matching exercises and true and false questions are occasionally included. The questions relate either directly to the brief description of the given patient or to the topic in general. The answers, complete with explanations and practical considerations, follow on the next page. A current reference is included for each problem.

This book is intended for senior medical students, family practice residents, and practicing family physicians. It should serve as a solid review for board certification examinations.

It is the hope of the author that the physicians who read this book and work through the problems enjoy and find it a stimulating, challenging, and useful learning experience.

Richard W. Swanson, M.D.

Acknowledgements

I wish to acknowledge the following persons who supported me during the publication of this book.

First, Mr. Walter Bailey, of B.C. Decker Inc, who expressed a keen interest in the book from the beginning. It was his enthusiasm that provided me with the needed incentive to complete what grew into a very large project.

Second, my reviewers, Dr. Stanley Smith, Professor and Head of the Department of Family Medicine, University Hospital, Saskatoon, Saskatchewan; Dr. Vivian Walker, former chief resident, Department of Family Medicine, University Hospital, Saskatoon; Dr. Brian Berger, senior resident, Department of Family Medicine, University Hospital, Saskatoon; Dr. Peter Butt, family physician, Meadow Lake, Saskatchewan; and Dr. Marilyn Basinger, family physician, Saskatoon.

Third, all of the family medicine residents at the University of Saskatchewan in Saskatoon, for their words of encouragement and their confidence, which increased as the book progressed.

Fourth, Dr. Gordon Johnson, for reviewing the drug dosages in this book.

Last, my wife, Dr. Stella Swanson, for the editing of the manuscript.

Contents

Obstetrics and Gynecology

Pediatrics

Internal Medicine

PROBLEM #1: AN 18 YEAR OLD MALE WITH SHORTNESS OF BREATH AND WHEEZING

1. An 18-year-old male presents to your office with shortness of breath and wheezing following the onset of a respiratory tract infection. He has a history of similar episodes. On careful questioning you also discover that he becomes short of breath on exertion. On examination expiratory rhonchi are heard in all lobes. You conclude that he has reactive airways disease or "asthma". Which of the following medications is the agent of first choice for this patient?

   a) an oral theophylline preparation
   b) an inhaled beta-2 agonist
   c) an oral beta-2 agonist
   d) inhaled sodium cromoglycate
   e) an inhaled corticosteroid

2. The patient described in question #1 is begun on therapy. However, after 2 weeks he is still wheezing. The treatment of choice at this time is the addition of which of the following medications?

   a) an oral theophylline preparation
   b) an inhaled beta-2 agonist
   c) an oral beta-2 agonist
   d) inhaled sodium cromoglycate
   e) an inhaled corticosteroid

3. Asthmatic patients can be divided into two types: extrinsic and intrinsic. Which of the following IS NOT a characteristic of intrinsic asthma?

   a) age of onset greater than 35 years
   b) a family history of allergies

1

    c) normal IgE values
    d) nonspecific skin tests
    e) a normal blood eosinophil count

4. Which of the following IS NOT a characteristic of chronic obstructive bronchitis?

    a) daily cough and sputum production
    b) shortness of breath
    c) expiratory wheezing
    d) development of right-sided heart failure
    e) characterization as a "pink puffer"

For question 5-9 match the appropriate lettered drug action to the numbered drug. Each lettered action may be used once, more than once, or not at all.

5) theophylline

6) beta-2-agonist

7) sodium cromoglycate

8) corticosteroids

9) atropine

    a) decreases cyclic GMP
    b) stabilizes lysosomal membranes
    c) increases formation of cyclic AMP directly
    d) decreases destruction of cyclic AMP by phosphodiesterase inhibition
    e) prevents mast cell degranulation

ANSWERS

1. b)
2. a) For the patient with mild to moderate symptoms of reactive airways disease, an inhaled beta-2 agonist will frequently suffice. This may be taken regularly or as needed (for example, prior to vigorous exercise). For patients with moderately severe or severe symptoms, or those who cannot be controlled on a single agent, a long-acting theophylline preparation should be added. Usually, a 12-hour sustained release tablet is preferable. Bedtime dosing may prevent nocturnal shortness of breath. The combination of an oral theophylline and an inhaled beta-agonist should be sufficient to control approximately 80% of patients with chronic obstructive airways disease.

When an oral theophylline preparation is used therapy should be guided by serum theophylline levels, drawn approximately 4 hours after the last dose.

Additional therapy can be initiated for those patients who still have symptoms and in whom no other precipitating factors such as infection or allergy have been defined. For outpatients, this usually consists of the addition of an oral beta agonist or aerosol atropine. Another option is the initiation of an inhaled corticosteroid.

If allergy is a factor, inhaled sodium cromoglycate may be extremely effective.

3. b) Asthmatic patients can be divided into two types, extrinsic and intrinsic. The patients in the extrinsic category have the following characteristics:

1) they are young (usually less than 20 years).
2) they have a history of allergies allergens such as ragweed.
3) there is a family history of allergies.
4) immunoglobulin E (IgE) levels are elevated.
5) they usually have both blood and sputum eosinophils.
6) they frequently have positive immediate skin tests to allergens.
7) their disease is usually seasonal.
8) they are usually responsive to treatment and frequently outgrow their disease. However, some develop persistent problems that may become chronic. As these patients grow older, their disease becomes less responsive to therapy, and irreversible changes develop.

Patients with intrinsic asthma are characterized by the following:

1) they are older (usually older than 35 years).
2) they do not have a history of allergies.
3) there is no family history of allergies.
4) IgE levels are normal.
5) skin tests are non-specific.
6) they may have sputum eosinophils but blood eosinophils are unusual.
7) they are difficult to treat, frequently requiring prolonged therapy.

4. e) Chronic obstructive pulmonary disease is characterized by daily productive cough and sputum, shortness of breath (initially with exercise and later at rest), and chest tightness. The patients are usually well nourished and may be obese. Auscultation primarily reveals expiratory wheezing, but there may also be inspiratory wheezing. Later, signs of right-sided heart failure, pedal edema and cyanosis may develop. These patients are commonly referred to as "blue bloaters" because of obesity, plethora, cyanosis and somnolence. They tend to develop severe hypoxemia, and as a result polycythemia, as the disease progresses.

"Pink puffers" is a term used to refer to patients with emphysema. They usually present with a chief complaint of shortness of breath with exertion, usually denying any significant cough, sputum production or wheezing. They will, however, complain of chest tightness or chest pain. These patients usually have a thin habitus and a barrel chest. Breath sounds are difficult to hear. The heart sounds are also distant and are best heard in the middle of the chest. The patient maintains low arterial carbon dioxide levels and relatively normal arterial oxygen pressures. They are, therefore, not cyanotic, and therefore the origin of the term "pink puffers".

5. d) Theophyllines decrease the destruction of cyclic AMP by inhibiting the enzyme phosphodiesterase. The increased concentration of cyclic AMP results in bronchodilatation. The usual oral dose is 300 mg. q12h, preferably in a sustained release preparation. However, dosage should be individualized and should be guided by serum theophylline levels.

6. c) Beta-2-agonists such as salbutamol and terbutaline increase the formation of cyclic AMP directly via beta-receptor stimulation. This results in bronchodilatation. Given in a metered form the usual dose is 1-2 puffs up to 4 times daily. In an oral form, 2-4 mg. 4 times per day is the usual dose.

7. e) Sodium cromoglycate prevents mast cell degranulation. This agent is useful in asthma that has an allergic basis. The usual dose is 2 inhalations q.i.d.

8. b) Corticosteroids work by stabilizing the mast cell membrane. Steroids, preferrably by inhalation, are indicated in asthma that has not responded to other therapeutic modalities. The usual initial dose of inhaled corticosteroid is 2 inhalations 3-4 times daily. If this dose is not sufficient it can be doubled. The daily dose should not exceed 1 mg. (20 puffs).

9. a) Atropine derivatives such as ipratropium bromide decrease cyclic GMP levels. This results in bronchodilatation. The usual dose is 2 inhalations (40 micrograms) 3 or 4 times daily. The maximum daily dose is 8 inhalations.

References

Telles C. Clinical Presentations of Chronic Obstructive Pulmonary Disease. Primary Care 1985; 12(2): 227-237.

Beck B. Pharmacologic Approaches to Obstructive Airway Disease. Primary Care 1985; 12(2): 239-252

PROBLEM #2: AN 80 YEAR OLD FEMALE WITH DYSPNEA AND FATIGUE

10. An 80 year old woman presents with a 3 week history of fatigue and shortness of breath, especially on exertion. She mentions having to get up at night because of acute shortness of breath to "open the window to get some air". She denies edema, weight gain or other symptoms. Physical examination reveals rales in both lung bases. Based on this history and these physical findings the most likely diagnosis is:

    a) left ventricular heart failure
    b) right ventricular heart failure
    c) biventricular heart failure
    d) cor pulmonale
    e) asthma

11. The patient described in question #10 is treated with bed rest and appropriate medication. She returns 1 month later complaining of dyspnea and fatigue as before, but now has developed dependant edema. She has gained ten pounds in weight since her last visit. On examination, her jugular venous pressure is elevated. At this time, the most likely diagnosis is:

    a) left ventricular heart failure
    b) right ventricular heart failure
    c) biventricular heart failure
    d) cor pulmonale
    e) asthma

12. The vasodilator of choice in the treatment of congestive cardiac failure is:

    a) prazosin
    b) hydralazine
    c) clonidine
    d) isosorbide dinitrate
    e) captopril

CODE: (a:1, 2 and 3; b: 1 and 3; c: 2 and 4; d: 4 only; e: all of the above)

13. The patient described in question #10 is begun on medical therapy. Which of the following drug(s) is/are indicated as first line therapy?

    1) digoxin
    2) hydralazine
    3) prazosin
    4) furosemide

14. Which of the following drugs is/are potassium sparing diuretics?

    1) chlorthalidone
    2) spironolactone
    3) ethacrynic acid
    4) triamterene

ANSWERS

10. a) This patient described a typical case of left ventricular heart failure. Dyspnea is the most common symptom of congestive cardiac failure. Initially, the dyspnea is present only with moderate amounts of exertion, but as the severity of the heart failure increases, the shortness of breath may occur with only minimal exertion or even at rest. Other fairly universal complaints are fatigue and lethargy. With left-sided heart failure, lying flat is often followed by increasing shortness of breath. Such positional dyspnea is produced by redistribution of blood flow to more central vascular structures, with the loss of gravitational pooling in the lower extremities that is present during normal activity. Paroxysms of nocturnal dyspnea (PND) are the hallmark of severe left ventricular failure. These bouts are characterized by marked breathlessness, which borders on suffocation, and are accompanied by severe anxiety. The patient has to sit upright or even stand to breathe and may have the urge to rush to an open window to relieve his breathlessness. Many patients find that sleeping on extra pillows will reduce the number and severity of attacks, and some patients resort to sleeping in reclining chairs in order to obtain needed rest. In severe cases, any type of semirecumbent position is intolerable. In such cases, pulmonary edema is usually severe and the shortness of breath is accompanied by cough, sometimes productive of frothy, blood-tinged secretions, and wheezing. Occasionally, an isolated nocturnal cough may be the first sign of heart failure.

    In this patient signs of right-sided heart failure have not yet developed. Asthma is not associated with the PND picture described in this question although left ventricular failure is sometimes referred to as "cardiac asthma".

11. c) At this time, the patient has developed signs of right ventricular heart failure as well. Chronic left ventricular failure usually leads to right ventricular failure. As the right ventricle fails, left ventricular end diastolic and pulmonary pressures may decrease and symptoms of left-sided failure may become less prominent, giving way to the signs of right heart failure. However, fatigue and dyspnea on exertion remain constant complaints.

    Right ventricular failure is manifested more by signs than by symptoms, although the pitting edema and weight gain may produce discomfort. In addition, enlargement of the liver and elevated jugular venous pressure occur.

If right atrial pressure is markedly elevated, splanchnic engorgement may accompany ascites, resulting in anorexia, nausea, vomiting and eventually cachexia.

12. e) Vasodilators can be very beneficial in the treatment of refractory cases of congestive cardiac failure, although they are not the agents of first choice. The best vasodilator is probably an angiotensin converting enzyme inhibitor such as captopril. With angiotensin converting enzyme inhibition, secondary sodium and fluid retension are uncommon, and the addition of anti-aldosterone agents is not required. During maintenance therapy, the dose of diuretic used can frequently be reduced. Furthermore, hyponatremia, if present, is corrected in the majority of patients. Decreased circulating norepinephrine levels found with angiotensin converting enzyme inhibitors are likely to be beneficial because of the prevention of the potential deleterious effects of excess catecholamines on organ function.

Captopril is usually begun in a dose of 12.5-25 mg. t.i.d.

13. d) The drug of first choice for the treatment of congestive cardiac failure is furosemide (or another diuretic). Furosemide is usually begun in a dose of 20 mg.-40 mg. b.i.d. The two strict indications for digoxin are: (1) atrial fibrillation, especially with ventricular rates over 90 beats per minute, and (2) congestive heart failure manifested by a dilated left ventricle and an S3 gallop rhythm. It is generally acknowledged that patients with normal-sized hearts and normal sinus rhythm derive little benefit from digoxin. Digoxin is usually begun as a loading dose of 1.0 milligram over 24 hours and given in a maintenance dose of 0.125-0.25 mg./day. In addition to diuretics other important first line measures include bed rest, restriction of daily sodium intake to 3-4 grams/day and oxygen therapy.

Vasodilator therapy, such as hydralazine or prazosin is not yet indicated as first line therapy. Of the vasodilators available, captopril is the agent of choice.

14. c) Hypokalemia is a significant problem with the use of potent loop diuretics like furosemide and ethacrynic acid and with the thiazide diuretics like hydrochlorothiazide. Hypokalemia increases the rate of firing of ectopic foci from the ventricles, with subsequent increases in ventricular tachycardia, ventricular fibrillation and sudden cardiac death. Therefore, prevention of hypokalemia is critical.

Prevention options include the use of potassium supplements with the potent diuretics or the addition of potassium-sparing agents such as spirono-lactone or triamterene. Spironolactone is usually begun in a dose of 50 mg. b.i.d. and triamterene as 100 mg. b.i.d.

References

Castle C. Cardiovascular Problems. Textbook of Family Practice 3rd edition; Rakel R, editor. W.B. Saunders Co., Philadelphia: 1984; pages 617-624.

Chatterjee K. Recent Advances in the Management of Chronic Heart Failure. Primary Care 1985; 12(1): 117-142.

PROBLEM #3: A 31 YEAR OLD MALE WITH DIARRHEA

A 31 year old male presents to the office with a 3 week history of diarrhea. He has just returned from Mexico.

Listed below are descriptions of several diarrheal syndromes. Match the lettered organism to the numbered description that best describes it. Each lettered item may be used once, more than once, or not at all.

15. Most common cause of diarrhea developing in a young male who has just returned from Mexico

16. Most common cause of bloody diarrhea associated with fever, crampy abdominal pain and tenesmus in adults

17. Most common cause of diarrhea in adults

18. A common cause of diarrhea often associated with home pets (from dogs to turtles) and with poultry and egg products

19. Most common cause of fever and bloody diarrhea in a young child

    a) Campylobacter
    b) Toxigenic E. coli
    c) Norwalk agent
    d) Shigella
    e) Salmonella
    f) Rotavirus

ANSWERS

15. b) Traveller's diarrhea is a conglomerate of illnesses acquired by travelers to tropical or semitropical countries. Toxigenic E. coli is the most common isolate, although viruses, Shigella, Salmonella, Entamoeba, and Giardia are all seen in this setting. Toxigenic E. coli produces a watery diarrhea of sudden onset, with abdominal cramps but no fever and no tenesmus. Stools are watery and are free of fecal leukocytes and blood. The treatment is symptomatic. Prophylaxis with bismuth subsalicylate and doxycycline (100 mg. b.i.d.) has been found useful, but the latter may predispose to infection with resistant organisms, particularly Shigella.

16. a) Campylobacter is a short gram-negative bacillus, recently recognized as a major cause of bacterial diarrhea in man. Campylobacter is usually transmitted by the oral-fecal route. The illness is acute, with frequent bloody diarrhea, fever and tenesmus. Crampy abdominal pain may be severe. Symptoms usually last from 2 to 7 days, but may be more protracted. Sigmoidoscopic

examination is not specific in appearance and biopsy may be indistinguishable from that found in ulcerative colitis. The treatment of choice is erythromycin by mouth 500 mg. q.i.d.

17. c) Viral diarrhea occurs regularly in adolescents and young adults. Epidemics occur in late fall and early winter. The clinical features include various combinations of diarrhea, nausea, vomiting, low-grade fever, abdominal cramps, headache and malaise lasting 24-48 hours. The agent most frequently implicated is the Norwalk agent. The treatment is symptomatic. Stool examination shows no leukocytes, thereby ruling out invasive bacterial processes.

18. e) Salmonella gastroenteritis is usually transmitted through a reservoir such as house pets (dogs, cats, and turtles) or through food products (particularly poultry and egg products). The incubation period is 8-48 hours and symptoms include abdominal cramps, vomiting and fever. Stools are foul smelling and bile coloured, and number 5-15/day. Bacteremia is more common in children than in adults.

Physical examination shows mild abdominal tenderness and hyperactive bowel sounds. Examination of the stool may reveal some white blood cells, and occasionally blood will be found.

Salmonella enteritis is self-limited except when bacteremia occurs. Oral antibiotics will not reduce either the symptoms or the fecal excretion of Salmonella. In fact, oral antibiotics prolong the carrier state and increase the risk of person-to-person transmission because of prolonged fecal carriage.

19. d) Shigellosis is more common in children than in adults, although it certainly occurs in all age groups. It is more common in certain institutional settings. The incubation period is 3-4 days, followed by fever, diarrhea and dysentery (bloody stools of small volume). The abdominal findings in Shigellosis are typical of invasive disease. Tenderness, hyperactive bowel sounds, and even rebound tenderness are occasionally seen. Sigmoidoscopy shows intense hyperemia with mucus, pus and multiple ulcerations. Microscopic examination of the stool reveals a large number of polymorphonuclear leukocytes.

Children with shigellosis should be treated, but adults normally have a self-limited, less severe illness. The drug of choice at the present time is trimethoprim-sulfamethoxazole, although ampicillin and tetracycline may be of value if the isolate is shown to be susceptible. In recent years, antibiotic-resistant Shigella species have become common. Treatment of shigellosis substantially shortens the period of diarrhea and fever in children. Antiperistaltic agents such as diphenoxylate, atropine and opiates are contraindicated in this and other invasive and toxigenic diarrheal diseases because they decrease the clearance of bacteria and toxins.

Reference

Parry M, Neu H. Infectious Diseases. Textbook of Family Practice 3rd edition; Rakel R, editor. W.B. Saunders Co., Philadelphia: 1984; pages 491-495.

PROBLEM #4: A 50 YEAR OLD MALE WITH JAUNDICE

20. A 50 year old male presents with anorexia, nausea, emesis and abdominal pain. He admits to abusing alcohol for the last 20 years. On examination his sclera are icteric and his liver is felt 7 cm. below the right costal margin. You suspect alcoholic hepatitis. Which of the following statements about alcoholic hepatitis is FALSE?

    a) Laennec's cirrhosis develops in approximately 10% of patients with alcoholic hepatitis
    b) serum bilirubin may often be 10-20 times the normal level
    c) serum ALT is almost always lower than serum AST
    d) hepatomegaly is seen in 80-90% of patients with alcoholic hepatitis
    e) a mortality rate of 10-15% is seen in acute alcoholic hepatitis

21. The most common cause of cirrhosis is:

    a) hepatitis A
    b) hepatitis B
    c) non-A, non-B hepatitis
    d) alcoholic hepatitis
    e) cytomegalovirus

22. A 21 year old female presents with nausea, vomiting, anorexia, aversion to her usual 2 pack/day smoking habit and right upper quadrant pain. On examination her sclera are icteric and her liver edge is tender. You suspect hepatitis A virus infection. Which of the following tests is most sensitive in predicting acute infection with HAA?

    a) anti-HAV-IgG
    b) anti-HAV-IgM
    c) hepatitis A core antigen
    d) anti-HAV-IgA
    e) hepatitis A surface antigen

23. The preferred method of treating the ascites that accompanies cirrhosis is:

    a) sodium restriction
    b) repeated paracentesis
    c) spironolactone
    d) peritoneovenous shunting
    e) none of the above

CODE: (a:1, 2 and 3; b: 1 and 3; c: 2 and 4; d: 4 only; e: all of the above)

24. Clinical manifestations of cirrhosis include:

   1) fatigue
   2) jaundice
   3) hypoalbuminemia
   4) splenomegaly

25. Indications for the use of hepatitis B vaccine (Heptavax) include:

   1) health care personnel
   2) hemodialysis patients
   3) patients requiring frequent blood transfusions
   4) male homosexuals

26. Initial screening for hepatitis B should include which of the following antigen/ antibody tests?

   1) anti-HBs
   2) anti-HBc
   3) HBeAg
   4) HBsAg

ANSWERS

20. a) The natural history of alcoholic liver disease is a slow process spanning many years and only 10-20% of chronic alcoholics go on to develop liver disease. Of those that do, the key morphologic lesion is alcoholic hepatitis. In this illness gastrointestinal complaints including anorexia, nausea, emesis and abdominal pain occur in over 50% of patients. Pain may be vague and poorly defined, but a significant proportion have it localized to the right upper quadrant. Fever is also common and usually implies more severe disease.

   Physical examination identifies hepatomegaly in 80-90% of cases. Other physical findings include jaundice, ascites, splenomegaly and spider angiomas.

   Diagnosis of alcoholic hepatitis can be suspected clinically but it requires laboratory confirmation. Hyperbilirubinemia is most often seen and may be 10-20 times normal. Serum transaminases are also elevated. The ratio of ALT to AST is peculiar to alcoholic hepatitis. ALT is almost always lower than AST and in fact may be only one-half as great. In viral hepatitis, ALT and AST values are almost always the same. Other laboratory abnormalities seen include elevation of alkaline phosphatase, low serum albumin and prolonged prothrombin time.

   Alcoholic hepatitis may run a mild course with few signs or symptoms, or it may run a fulminant course resulting in death. Overall, mortality is 10-15% for the acute event.

Treatment is mainly supportive, and the illness typically requires weeks to months to resolve. The first and most important step in therapy is cessation of alcohol consumption. Since many alcoholics are malnourished, increasing the caloric intake and vitamin supplementation may be useful. No pharmacologic therapy has been proven to be of significant benefit.

Laennec's cirrhosis develops in approximately 50% of patients surviving alcoholic hepatitis, and in the other half varying degrees of hepatic fibrosis develops.

21. d) The most common cause of cirrhosis is alcoholic hepatitis. Fifty percent of patients with alcoholic hepatitis go on to develop cirrhosis.

    Hepatitis A does not progress to chronic active hepatitis and subsequent cirrhosis. Ten percent of patients with hepatitis B infection and 40% of patients with non-A, non-B hepatitis infection go on to chronic persistent and chronic active hepatitis and possible subsequent cirrhosis.

    Cytomegalovirus infection does not go on to produce cirrhosis.

22. b) Acute infection with hepatitis A is confirmed by the demonstration of IgM antibodies to hepatitis A virus. These antibodies persist for approximately 12 weeks. IgG antibodies to hepatitis A virus are only diagnostic of previous exposure.

    Hepatitis A does not possess a recognizable core of surface antigen; these tests apply to hepatitis B. IgA antibodies are not useful in the diagnosis of hepatitis A infection.

23. c) The preferred method of treating the ascites that accompanies cirrhosis is diuretic therapy. Diuretics can overcome an increased level of sodium so that severe dietary restrictions are not necessary. Fluid restriction is also unnecessary in the therapy of ascites unless hyponatremia from water intoxication or inappropriate water retension occurs.

    Ascites is maintained by increased levels of aldosterone, which causes intense sodium and water retention. Logical diuretic therapy employs the aldosterone antagonist spironolactone. Approximately 75% of patients respond to 400 mg. daily, and the remaining 25% require addition of a second diuretic.

    Peritoneovenous shunting (Laveen shunt, Denver shunt) is used for intractable ascites. This involves placing one end of a catheter in the abdomen while the other is tunneled subcutaneously and inserted in the jugular vein.

    Paracentesis is not recommended as a form of treatment because the fluid that is removed rapidly reaccumulates.

24. e) Clinical manifestations of cirrhosis can be described as follows:

    1) systemic: weakness, fatigue, anorexia, weight loss, malaise and muscle wasting

2) hepatic: jaundice, hypoalbuminemia, splenomegaly, portal hypertension and ascites
3) renal: edema, hepatorenal syndrome
4) dermatologic: spider angiomas, palmar erythema, loss of body hair and clubbing of fingers
5) endocrinologic: gynecomastia, testicular atrophy, diabetes mellitus and hypoglycemia
6) hematologic: blood clotting abnormalities, purpura, hypersplenism, leukopenia, anemia and thrombocytopenia

25. e) Hepatitis B vaccine is available to persons at high and continued risk of hepatitis B infection. It is a non-infectious, formalin-inactivated fragment of the hepatitis B surface antigen and will induce formation of anti-Hbs. It is effective in reducing clinical infection as well as in serologic conversion following exposure to hepatitis B. Persons at high risk include all health care personnel, hemodialysis patients, patients requiring frequent blood transfusions, employees and residents of institutions for the mentally handicapped, male homosexuals, intravenous drug users and sexual contacts of chronic HBsAg carriers.

26. c) Hepatitis B antigen and antibody tests are a continuing source of confusion because of the number of tests available. Initial screening for hepatitis B should include HBsAg and anti-HBc. These two tests will identify most cases of acute hepatitis B. There is a "window" period between the clearance of HBsAg and the appearance of anti-HBs. This period can last for 4-6 weeks, and during this time the only marker for hepatitis B is anti-HBc. If acute hepatitis B is suggested from the initial screening, then further tests including the following should be done:
1) HBeAg: The presence of this antigen indicates a highly contagious state or a chronic infection.
2) anti-HBe: The presence of this antibody indicates low infectivity and predicts later seroconversion or resolution of hepatitis B.
3) anti-HBs: The presence of this antibody indicates past hepatitis B infection and current immunity.

Reference

Boydstun J, Barker J and Lawhorne L. Gastrointestinal Disorders. Textbook of Family Medicine 3rd edition; Rakel R, editor. W.B. Saunders Co., Philadelphia: 1984; pages 1019-1026.

PROBLEM #5: A 24 YEAR OLD COLLEGE STUDENT WITH PNEUMONIA

27. A 24 year old college student presents with a 3 day history of dry, hacking cough which initially was non-productive but which has become productive of scant, white sputum. The patient also complains of malaise, headache, fever and arthralgias.

    Physical examination reveals a temperature of 39 degrees Celcius and a few scattered rales in both lung bases. Chest X-ray reveals patchy perihilar and bilateral lower lobe infiltrates. The most likely organism responsible for this young man's illness is:

    a) Streptococcus pneumoniae
    b) Klebsiella pneumoniae
    c) Mycoplasma pneumoniae
    d) influenza A
    e) Haemophilus influenzae

28. The treatment of choice for the patient discussed in question #27 is:

    a) penicillin
    b) amoxicillin
    c) erythromycin
    d) gentamicin
    e) carbenicillin

29. A 55 year old female, previously healthy, and recovering from an episode of bronchitis suddenly develops a shaking chill followed by a high fever, pleuritic chest pain, and cough productive of purulent rusty sputum. On examination, the patient appears acutely ill, with a respiratory rate of 30/minute and chest splinting. Bronchial breath sounds are heard in the left lower lobe. Chest X-ray reveals a consolidation present in the left lower lobe. The most likely organism responsible for this patient's illness is:

    a) Streptococcus pneumoniae
    b) Klebsiella pneumoniae
    c) Mycoplasma pneumoniae
    d) influenza A
    e) Haemophilus influenzae

30. The treatment of choice for the patient described in question #29 is:

    a) penicillin
    b) erythromycin
    c) tetracycline
    d) gentamicin
    e) chloramphenicol

31. A 75 year old alcoholic with a history of chronic obstructive lung disease is admitted to hospital suffering from fever, shortness of breath, chest pain, and cough productive of purulent sputum and blood. Physical examination reveals a temperature of 39 degrees Celcius, a respiratory rate of 28/minute, and bronchial breath sounds heard in the right upper lobe. Chest X-ray confirms a right upper lobe pneumonia. The most likely organism responsible for this patient's illness is:

   a) Streptococcus pneumoniae
   b) Klebsiella pneumoniae
   c) Mycoplasma pneumoniae
   d) influenza A
   e) Haemophilus influenzae

CODE: (a:1, 2 and 3; b: 1 and 3; c: 2 and 4; d: 4 only; e: all of the above)

32. The drug(s) of choice for the patient described in question #31 is/are:

   1) erythromycin
   2) cephalothin
   3) penicillin
   4) gentamicin

ANSWERS

27. c) The patient described in this question has mycoplasma pneumonia. Mycoplasma pneumonia occurs most frequently in the young adult, although recent reports suggest that it occurs regularly in middle aged and older adults as well. The onset is usually gradual, with a hacking cough, originally non-productive, but later becoming productive with scant white and then purulent sputum. Systemic symptoms are prominent and include malaise, headache, and fever between 100-103 degrees Celcius. Rash, serious otitis media and joint symptoms may occasionally accompany the pulmonary complaints.

   Physical findings are usually unremarkable. Auscultation of the chest usually reveals only scattered rhonchi or fine localized rales. The chest X-ray in contradistinction to the benign physical examination is often impressive, with fine or patchy lower lobe or perihilar infiltrates. Laboratory data reveal a white blood cell count of 10,000 to 15,000/mm^3 with polymorphonuclear leukocyte predominance. Cold agglutinins may be helpful early in the disease but are not specific and are negative in approximately one third of cases. The diagnosis is confirmed by acute and convalescent Mycoplasma complement fixation titers.

   Clinically and radiologically, pneumonia caused by adenovirus is very difficult to differentiate from mycoplasma. H. influenzae is a common cause of pneumonia in children and sometimes occurs in debilitated patients. It is uncommon in young, healthy adults.

The other options listed in the question are discussed in subsequent sections of this problem or in other sections of this book.

28. c) The treatment of choice for Mycoplasma pneumoniae is erythromycin or tetracycline. The usual dose is 500 mg. q.i.d. for 10 days. Symptomatic improvement occurs with administration of either of these agents, but cough and malaise may persist. The organism is not easily eradicated from the sputum and therefore secondary cases in the family may still occur. Even in the absence of treatment, resolution is spontaneous in the vast majority of cases.

29. a) The patient described in this question presents a history that is classical of pneumococcal pneumonia. Streptococcus pneumoniae (pneumococcus) is the most common cause of pneumonia in the adult population.

    The classical presentation of pneumococcal pneumonia is that of a shaking rigor, followed by fever, pleuritic chest pain and cough with purulent or rusty sputum. Antecedent viral upper or lower respiratory tract infection is present in many cases. However, atypical presentations are common particularly in the elderly and alcoholic population. In such patients fever may be low grade, behavior disturbances may seem more significant than respiratory symptoms and cough may not be prominent. Patients appear acutely ill, frequently with dyspnea and chest splinting. Signs of consolidation are frequently present.

    Laboratory findings include an elevated white blood cell count with a left shift. Chest X-ray usually shows disease confined to one lobe (frequently a lower lobe), but several lobes may be involved with either consolidation or bronchopneumonia. Gram stain of the sputum will show polymorphonuclear leukocytes and "lancet shaped" gram-positive diplococci. Sputum cultures should be obtained, but up to 40% of patients with bacteremic pneumococcal pneumonia will have negative sputum cultures. Therefore, blood cultures should be obtained in all patients.

30. a) The treatment of choice for this patient is penicillin G. With this patient's clinical picture including a respiratory rate of 30/minute and chest splinting IV penicillin in a dose of 4-8 million units/day is indicated. Humidified oxygen would also be very beneficial in treatment. Amoxicillin and erythromycin could be used in place of penicillin G but would not be first-line drugs. Gentamicin and carbenicillin are not indicated for the treatment of pneumococcal pneumonia.

31. b) The most likely cause of pneumonia in an elderly, debilitated alcoholic is a gram-negative organism; most commonly Klebsiella pneumoniae. It frequently occurs in nursing home and hospitalized patients. The presentation is similar to pneumococcal pneumonia although it more frequently involves the upper lobes than the lower lobes. The onset is usually sudden with severe

toxicity. Pleuritic chest pain and hemoptysis are common features. Sputum is thick, often with blood, but in only 25% is it the characteristic "current jelly" sputum. Other important causes of pneumonia in elderly patients include other gram-negative organisms such as E. coli, H. influenzae as well as gram-positive organisms such as Streptococcus pneumoniae and Staphylococcus.

32. c) The treatment of choice until culture results are available is a combination of antibiotics that covers Klebsiella, E. coli, H. influenzae, Streptococcus pneumoniae and Staphylococcus. The best combination is a beta-lactam antibiotic like cephalothin (500 mg.-1.0 grams IV every 4 to 6 hours) and an aminoglycoside like gentamicin (3 mg./kg./day IV) in 3 divided doses.

Reference

Parry M, Neu H. Infectious Diseases. Textbook of Family Practice 3rd edition; Rakel R, editor. W.B. Saunders Co., Philadelphia: 1984; pages 498-502.

PROBLEM #6: A 78 YEAR OLD MALE WITH SUDDEN ONSET HEMIPLEGIA

33. A 78 year old male presents with an acute onset of leftsided hemiplegia and hemianesthesia, and a homonymous hemianopsia. His head and eyes are also deviating to the left side. The most likely artery involved with the symptoms described above is the:

    a) anterior cerebral artery
    b) right middle cerebral artery
    c) vertebral artery
    d) posterior cerebral artery
    e) none of the above

34. The diagnostic procedure of choice for the patient described in question #33 is:

    a) digital subtraction angiography
    b) carotid arteriography
    c) computerized cranial tomography
    d) lumbar puncture
    e) nuclear magnetic resonance imaging

35. The diagnostic procedure of choice for the patient described in question #33 is performed. It reveals an ischemic infarction. The neurologic deficits appear to be worsening. The drug of choice for the treatment of this patient in the acute phase is:

    a) warfarin
    b) aspirin
    c) dipyridamole
    d) heparin
    e) mannitol

36. The single most important risk factor for stroke is:

    a) hypertension
    b) age
    c) diabetes mellitus
    d) coronary artery disease
    e) cigarette smoking

37. The single most common cause of stroke is:

    a) embolism from a cardiac source
    b) intracranial hemorrhage secondary to hypertension
    c) thrombosis secondary to atherosclerosis of the carotid system
    d) subarachnoid hemorrhage
    e) thrombosis secondary to atherosclerosis of the vertebral system

38. Which of the following statements about transient ischemic attacks (TIA's) is
FALSE?

    a) transient ischemic attacks refer to episodes of neurologic dysfunction that
       last less than 24 hours
    b) almost all patients that experience TIA's go on to develop completed
       strokes
    c) the peak age for the development of TIA's is in the seventh decade
    d) transient ischemic attacks result largely from thromboembolism
    e) transient ischemia of the retina results in amaurosis fugax

CODE: (a:1, 2 and 3; b: 1 and 3; c: 2 and 4; d: 4 only; e: all of the above)

39. The drug(s) of choice for the prevention of transient ischemic attacks is/are:

    1) warfarin
    2) dipyridamole
    3) vitamin E
    4) aspirin

ANSWERS

33. b) The patient described in question #33 has the classical presentation of a
middle cerebral artery embolism or thrombosis. Involvement of the anterior
cerebral artery would produce a more profound degree of impairment in the
legs than in the arms. In this case urinary incontinence and primitive reflexes
(sucking or gasping) are often present.

34. c) Computerized cranial tomography will differentiate an ischemic stroke
from a hemorrhagic stroke. This is of critical importance in deciding whether
or not to use anticoagulants in the acute phase.

    Digital subtraction angiography is useless for this purpose. Carotid arteriog-
raphy is contraindicated in the acute phase of stroke and lumbar puncture for
the detection of subarachnoid hemorrhage has been replaced by CT scanning.

    Nuclear magnetic resonance imaging, although valuable in the detection of
cerebellar and cerebral pathology has not yet replaced CT scanning as the
diagnostic procedure of choice.

35. d) There is general agreement that anticoagulation with heparin should be
employed when the neurologic deficits are found to worsen progressively
(stroke in evolution), unless there is CT evidence of cerebral hemorrhage.
Prophylactic anticoagulation is also indicated in patients who have suffered a
cerebral embolism as a result of rheumatic heart disease or atrial fibrillation.
Although some authorities recommend delaying anticoagulation therapy for
48 hours after a stroke, immediate full-dose heparin appears to be safe,

provided CT scanning does not disclose a hemorrhage and there are no other contraindications to the administration of heparin. Anticoagulation is not recommended in patients with subacute bacterial endocarditis. Other specific therapies including the use of vasodilators and antiedema agents such as mannitol have not gained widespread acceptance.

Aspirin is recommended in the chronic phase of stroke and for the prevention of TIA's. Aspirin and dipyridamole are recommended for the prevention of cerebral embolism following insertion of an artificial heart valve. Warfarin is sometimes used in the treatment of TIA's if they are relatively recent in onset (within months).

36. a) Stroke remains the third leading cause of death in North America. The single most important risk factor for stroke is hypertension. The incidence of stroke has declined nearly 50% during the past 30 years, particularly in elderly patients. It is reasonable to suppose that antihypertensive therapy has been at least partially responsible for this decline.

Other factors that are important are age, coronary artery disease, cigarette smoking, diabetes mellitus, complicated migraine headaches and the use of the oral contraceptive pill.

37. c) The single most common cause of stroke is thrombosis secondary to atherosclerosis. The thrombus originates from the carotid artery system twice as often as from the vertebral artery system.

Cerebral embolism accounts for 16%-19% of strokes. The embolism most commonly arises from a cardiac source. These patients usually have something intrinsically wrong with the heart that allows the formation of a thrombus which embolizes. Problems such as mitral stenosis, artificial valves, atrial fibrillation and subacute bacterial endocarditis are usually responsible.

Subarachnoid hemorrhage accounts for 10% of the total number of strokes. This usually occurs secondary to a rupture of a congenital berry aneurysm around the area of the circle of Willis.

Intracerebral hemorrhage accounts for 5% of strokes, with most of this total being due to hypertensive intracerebral hemorrhage.

38. b) Cerebral transient ischemic attacks (TIA's) refer to episodes of neurologic dysfunction that develop suddenly, last five minutes to several hours (never more than 24 hours), and clear completely. Symptoms that develop during an attack generally point to disturbance of circulation in either the carotid or vertebrobasilar systems. The peak age for the development of TIA's is in the seventh decade. The incidence of stroke in patients with TIA's is not precisely known, although the majority do not go on to develop completed strokes. In general, if untreated, about one-third of patients with TIA's will suffer a completed stroke, one-third will continue to have TIA's without infarction, and one-third will have a spontaneous remission.

It is believed that transient ischemic attacks result largely from thromboembolism. Aggregated platelets or debris from ulcerated atheromatous plaques in the extracranial carotid system are the most common type of emboli. The transient nature of the attack is due to the rapid fragmentation and dissolution of the microemboli.

Transient ischemia of the retina, from reduced flow or microembolization in the ophthalmic branch of the internal carotid artery, causes transient blackness of vision (amaurosis fugax). Patients often feel as though a shade has been pulled down over one eye.

Cerebral hemisphere ischemia produces the sudden onset of such symptoms as contralateral monoparesis or hemiparesis, localized tingling or numbness, hemianopic visual loss or aphasia. The characteristic symptomatology of vertebrobasilar ischemia is referred to the posterior portion of the brain: the occipital lobe and the brainstem. In this syndrome, bilateral disturbance of vision results from insufficiency of the posterior cerebral arteries that supply the visual cortex. Visual symptoms are described as dim, grey, blurred vision, or even total blindness. Another common visual complaint is diplopia due to transient disturbance of conjugate gaze. Attacks of vertigo, unsteadiness, nausea, and vomiting point to circulatory disturbance either in the labyrinth or in the vestibular nuclei of the medulla. Brainstem symptoms include dysarthria, dysphagia, perioral numbness, and weakness or paresthesias of all four limbs.

So called drop attacks, in which there is a sudden loss of postural tone in the legs, are also characteristic of basilar insufficiency.

39. d) The drug of choice for the prevention of TIA's is aspirin in a dose of 325-650 mg. b.i.d. Dipyridamole in a dose of 100 mg./day is indicated in combination with aspirin for the prevention of cerebral embolism following insertion of an artificial heart valve and in the prevention of re-infarction following an myocardial infarction. It has not, however, been shown to be efficacous in the prevention of TIA's. Warfarin may be indicated in the treatment of TIA's (see above).

Vitamin E has no place to play in the treatment of TIA's.

References

Cutler R. Cerebrovascular Diseases. Scientific American Medicine; Rubenstein E and Federman D, editors. Scientific American Inc., New York: 1985; pages 11(X) 1-9.

Clifford J. Managing disability from stroke. Canadian Family Physician 1986; 32: 605-615.

PROBLEM #7: A 35 YEAR OLD FEMALE WITH FATIGUE

40. A 35 year old female presents with a 4 month history of fatigue. Her past history is unremarkable apart from heavy menstrual periods during the last year. She is not taking any medications. Physical examination is normal apart from mild pallor. Her hemoglobin is measured at 10 g/dl. The most likely diagnosis is:

    a) iron-deficiency anemia
    b) pernicious anemia
    c) hemolytic anemia
    d) folate deficiency
    e) hypothyroidism

41. The treatment of choice for the patient described in question #40 is:

    a) multivitamin complex b.i.d.
    b) ferrous sulfate 300 mg o.d. to t.i.d.
    c) Vitamin B-12 100 micrograms every 2 days decreasing to 100 micrograms monthly
    d) folic acid 5 mg o.d.
    e) levo-thyroxine 100 micrograms o.d.

42. Iron deficiency anemia is seen in what percentage of preschool children?

    a) <1%
    b) 5%
    c) 10%
    d) 20%
    e) 50%

43. The 70 year old grandmother of the patient described in question #40 complains of "lack of energy". On examination, she has marked pallor. Her hemoglobin level is 7.5 g/dl. A peripheral blood smear shows hypochromasia and microcytosis. Her previous hemoglobin level 1 year ago was 13.0 g/dl. The most likely cause of the grandmother's anemia is:

    a) malnutrition
    b) pernicious anemia
    c) folic acid deficiency
    d) gastrointestinal bleeding
    e) hypothyroidism

44. The most sensitive test for iron deficiency anemia is the:

    a) serum iron
    b) serum iron binding capacity
    c) serum ferritin
    d) serum transferrin
    e) reticulocyte count

CODE: (a:1, 2 and 3; b: 1 and 3; c: 2 and 4; d: 4 only; e: all of the above)

45. Which of the following disorders is/are often associated with anemia?

    1) rheumatoid arthritis
    2) non-Hodgkin's lymphoma
    3) renal failure
    4) myocardial infarction

46. A 75 year old female presents to your office with a 4 month history of fatigue, paresthesias, weakness, unsteady gait and severe gastritis. On examination, her skin is pale with a hint of jaundice and she has a number of neurologic findings including patchy impairment of touch and temperature sensation, loss of vibration and position sense, a positive Romberg sign, hyperreflexia and a bilaterally positive Babinski sign. Her hemoglobin is 6.8 g/dl. Which of the following statements is/are TRUE about this patient's condition?

    1) this patient has a hemolytic anemia
    2) oval macrocytes will be seen on the peripheral smear
    3) a CT scan of the brain should be performed
    4) a Schilling test should be performed to confirm the diagnosis

ANSWERS

40. a) Deficiency of iron is one of the most common organic diseases of man and is, by far, the most frequently encountered cause of anemia. If affects about 20% of adult women, 3% of adult men, 50% of pregnant women and 20% of preschool children. Normal hemoglobin levels for adult males remain above 14 g/dl and for females above 12 g/dl. Children greater than 6 months of age should have a hemoglobin of greater than 10.5 g/dl. The high prevelance of iron deficiency in women is explained by a combination of iron loss associated with menstruation and a lower intake of food than men. On the average, women lose about 2 mg of iron per day, or twice as much as men. This loss must be replaced by iron in the diet, which usually amounts to about 6 mg/1000 Kcal. A woman consuming a 2500 Kcal diet will take in about 15 mg of iron, of which about 10% will be absorbed. Obviously, therefore, many women exist in a precarious state of iron balance. In contrast, men not only lose less iron (1 mg/day) but they also consume more food, providing an ample margin of safety.

Pernicious anemia, folate deficiency, hemolysis and hypothyroidism are all forms of or conditions associated with anemia; however they are not nearly as common as iron deficiency.

41. b) The treatment of choice for an iron deficiency anemia is ferrous sulfate 300 mg o.d. to t.i.d. A typical regime is to begin with 1 tablet a day after the largest meal. After several days, if there are no substantial gastrointestinal side effects, the dose may be increased to BID and subsequently TID (if necessary). With optimal treatment reticulocytes increase in the blood, reaching a maximum volume 5 to 10 days after the first dose. The magnitude of the reticulocytosis is related to the degree of anemia. The anemia will usually be corrected in about two months, regardless of severity. Generally, by 3 weeks, the hemoglobin level has increased by about 60% of the interval between the starting level and the normal level.

42. d) Iron deficiency anemia may occur in up to 20% of preschool children. It usually begins after 4-6 months of age when the maternal iron stores become exhausted. Its etiology is most often inadequate intake, although as many as one-third of infants with severe iron deficiency in the United States have chronic intestinal blood loss produced by exposure to a heat labile protein in whole cow's milk.

43. d) The grandmother's hypochromic-microcystic picture, coupled with a drop in hemoglobin from 13.0-7.5 g/dl in 1 year is almost certainly due to blood loss from a gastrointestinal malignancy or other bleeding source. Any woman past the menopause or male of any age who develops a hypochromic-microcytic picture characteristic of iron deficiency anemia is considered to have bleeding from a malignancy until proven otherwise. The other common cause of iron deficiency anemia in elderly patients is malnutrition. Often poor, they have little extra money to spend on nutritious, iron-rich foods.

Pernicious anemia would be the most common megaloblastic anemia in elderly individuals. Folic acid deficiency and anemia due to hypothyroidism are also seen in the elderly.

44. c) The diagnosis of iron deficiency anemia is based on a direct or indirect demonstration that the iron stores in the body are reduced. The simplest demonstration of this is the serum ferritin level which may be less than 10 μg/litre in iron-deficiency anemia. The serum iron and the transferrin saturation will be decreased, and the total iron-binding capacity increased in iron-deficiency anemia, but these are all indirect measurements of iron stores. The reticulocyte count is not useful in assessing the degree of iron deficiency.

45. e) Anemia is a common manifestation of infectious, inflammatory, neoplastic, cardiovascular and renal disorders. These anemias are generally known as the "anemias of chronic disease". They are second only to iron deficiency in frequency and may be more common than iron deficiency in hospitalized patients. There is a rough but inconsistent correlation between severity of the

underlying illness and the degree of anemia. The characteristic mild to moderate anemia is usually asymptomatic, and if there are complaints of exercise intolerance or fatigue, they are more likely to be related to the chronic disease itself rather than to the anemia.

The anemia develops rapidly over the first month or two of the illness, after which it does not progress and, instead is stabilized at a hematocrit level of 30-40 ml/dl. Usually, the erythrocytes are normocytic and normochromic, but hypochromasia and microcytosis may be found in about 25-50% of patients. The reticulocyte count is usually normal; plasma iron and transferrin saturation reduced; and total iron binding capacity normal or reduced. Iron stores are typically normal to increased and their status is confirmed by a normal or elevated serum ferritin level.

46. c) The patient described in this question has pernicious anemia. Pernicious anemia is a disease resulting from a deficiency of Vitamin B-12. The lack of intrinsic factor, a glycoprotein normally found in the gastric juice, is the fundamental abnormality in the disorder. The normal absorption of Vitamin B-12 in the diet requires intrinsic factor. In its absence, vitamin B-12 deficiency supervenes, even though the diet contains adequate amounts of the vitamin. The neurological symptoms described are a result of the involvement of the dorsal and lateral columns of the spinal cord and possibly, the peripheral nerves as well. Classical pernicious anemia is invariably accompanied by severe, atrophic gastritis.

Oval macrocytes are the characteristic abnormality in the blood and their presence results in a greatly increased value for the MCV. Typically, hypersegmented neutrophilic leukocytes are found on microscopic evaluation, and their presence may be a relatively early sign of the disease. The anemia is characterized kinetically by "ineffective erythropoiesis" i.e., the production of a population of red cells that is destroyed before or shortly after its release from the marrow. Serum lactate dehydrogenase (LDH) levels also tend to be greatly increased, often to 10 X normal.

In pernicious anemia, serum vitamin B-12 is greatly reduced whereas the serum folate is normal. Once the presence of vitamin B-12 deficiency is established, the first step in diagnosis is to establish that intrinsic factor is lacking. This can be accomplished by means of a Schilling urinary excretion test. The body's stores of Vitamin B-12 are replaced by intramuscular B-12, beginning at 100 micrograms/daily and decreasing to a lifelong treatment of 100 micrograms/month.

This form of anemia does not have a hemolytic component and the neurological symptoms will resolve without further investigation (such as CT scan) or treatment.

Reference

Lee G. Gardner H. Textbook of Family Practice 3rd edition; Rakel R, editor. W.B. Saunders Company, Philadelphia: 1984, pages 1082-1091.

PROBLEM #8: A 55 YEAR OLD MALE WITH ACUTE CHEST PAIN

47. A 55 year old male presents to the emergency department following the acute onset of retrosternal chest pain that he describes as a "severe heartburn". His chest pain came on after attending a gourmet feast. He is hypertensive and smokes 2 packs of cigarettes/day. On examination his blood pressure is 150/100. His ECG shows 1 mm of ST segment depression. Which of the following statements about this patient's chest pain is FALSE?

    a) the patient may have suffered a myocardial infarction
    b) the patient's chest pain may be due to angina pectoris
    c) the patient's chest pain may be due to esophageal spasm
    d) the administration of sublingual nitroglycerine is a very sensitive diagnostic test in distinguishing angina pectoris from esophageal spasm
    e) the patient should be admitted to the coronary care unit until the origin of the chest pain is established.

48. The main indication for percutaneous transluminal coronary angioplasty is:

    a) when medical management fails and a greater than 50% stenosis of the left main coronary artery is present
    b) when medical management fails and there is a greater than 50% stenosis of two coronary arteries
    c) as a surgical option in any angina syndrome
    d) when medical management fails and a 70% or greater stenosis is present in a single coronary artery
    e) none of the above

49. The patient described in question #47 is admitted for observation. His pain subsides with intravenous nitroglycerine. His cardiac enzymes come back normal. Which of the following investigations is NOT INDICATED at this time?

    a) a treadmill stress test
    b) coronary angiography
    c) an upper gastrointestinal series
    d) a plasma lipid profile
    e) a fasting blood sugar

50. A 65 year old man with angina pectoris undergoes coronary angiography. The result is a 65% stenosis of the left main coronary artery. Which of the following treatment modalities is NOT a reasonable treatment option in this patient?

   a) coronary artery bypass surgery
   b) isosorbide dinitrate
   c) percutaneous transluminal coronary angioplasty
   d) propranolol
   e) diltiazem

CODE: (a:1, 2 and 3; b: 1 and 3; c: 2 and 4; d: 4 only; e: all of the above)

51. The drug(s) of choice for patients with angina pectoris is (are):

   1) nifedipine
   2) propranolol
   3) isosorbide dinitrate
   4) prazosin

52. Which of the following is (are) indications for coronary artery bypass surgery?

   1) disabling stable angina pectoris
   2) unstable angina pectoris
   3) angina due to left main coronary artery occlusion
   4) angina following myocardial infarction

53. A 65 year old male presents with chronic chest pain and hypertension. His blood pressure is 170/110. An exercise tolerance test suggests angina pectoris as the cause of his chest pain. Which of the following medication(s) would you consider as the agent(s) of first choice for the treatment of this patient?

   1) hydrochlorothiazide
   2) verapamil
   3) clonidine
   4) propranolol

ANSWERS

47. d) The patient who presents with acute chest pain is often a diagnostic problem. Patients with risk factors for coronary artery disease must be assumed to have had a myocardial infarction until proven otherwise and admitted preferrably to a coronary care unit. This patient's 1 mm ST segment depression is not diagnostic of anything. It may or may not be due to myocardial ischemia. Pain from esophageal spasm is often confused with pain

from myocardial ischemia. Indeed, sublingual nitroglycerine will often relieve both pains, thus decreasing the sensitivity of its administration as a diagnostic test.

48. d) The main indication of PTCA is when medical management of angina fails and there is a 70% or greater stenosis of a single coronary artery. Although some cases of multivessel coronary artery disease have responded to PTCA, more experience with such cases is needed before the procedure can be widely recommended.

At present, stenosis of the left main coronary artery is a contraindication to PTCA because of the potential consequences of post-procedural thrombosis.

49. b) Normal cardiac enzymes essentially rule out a myocardial infarction. However, the origin of the patient's chest pain is still unclear. Myocardial ischemia, esophageal spasm and musculoskeletal chest wall pain are the main diagnostic considerations. Because he is a high risk candidate for coronary artery disease, his other potential risk factors, including plasma lipid profile and plasma glucose, should be checked. A treadmill stress test will further delineate his risk of coronary artery disease and an upper gastrointestinal series may determine any contribution from reflux esophagitis. An invasive test such as coronary angiography should not be done until all of the other results are in and a probability figure for coronary artery disease can be arrived at.

50. c) As the potential for post-procedure thrombosis is ever present and would be devastating if it occurred in the left main coronary artery, stenosis of this artery is a contraindication to percutaneous transluminal coronary angioplasty. As a general rule, all patients with angina require medical therapy. Some also require coronary artery bypass surgery or PTCA. All patients following surgery or PTCA continue to require ongoing medical management. Therefore, isosorbide dinitrate, propranolol and diltiazem are all reasonable options for the patient in question. Because the left main coronary artery is involved with a stenosis of greater than 50%, coronary artery bypass surgery is recommended.

51. a) Traditionally, angina pectoris has been managed by a step care approach with sublingual nitroglycerine being the drug of choice for acute episodes, and long acting nitrates such as isosorbide dinitrate being used as the agents of first choice for prophylaxis. Beta-adrenergic receptor blockers such as propranolol were considered as the agents of second choice.

With the advent of the calcium channel blockers such as nifedipine, diltiazem, and verapamil the pharmacologic therapy of angina pectoris has been expanded. Many experts now consider the use of any one of the three classes of drugs mentioned above as acceptable first line therapy. Caution should be used in combining these agents as the negative inotropic and chronotropic properties may produce clinically significant hypotension. Prazosin is an alpha-adrenergic blocker which acts peripherally and is used in the treatment of hypertension. It is not indicated in the treatment of angina pectoris.

52. e) The main indications for coronary artery bypass surgery are:
    1. disabling stable angina pectoris that causes the patient to be disabled in
    2. spite of a vigorous medical treatment regime
    3. unstable angina pectoris that has not responded to medical therapy angina following myocardial infarction (The presence of angina in post-infarction patients is quite worrisome because it means that additional myocardium is in jeopardy in individuals who have already lost significant amounts of myocardial tissue)
    4. angina due to left main coronary artery occlusion of greater than 50%

53. c) A patient who initially presents with angina pectoris and hypertension should be treated with either a calcium channel blocker or a beta-blocker as the agent of first choice. Thus, verapamil or propranolol are the drugs of choice in this patient. Extreme caution should be used when combining these agents because of their additive negative inotropic and chronotropic effects. Hydrochlorothiazide and clonidine will treat the hypertension but not the angina. Thus, an agent that treats both is probably preferable. If the blood pressure is not well controlled, hydrochlorothiazide, clonidine or a number of other agents could be added to the treatment regime.

Reference

Brest A. Management of Angina Pectoris. Primary Care 1985; 12(1): 91-100.

PROBLEM #9: A 17 YEAR OLD FEMALE WITH WEIGHT LOSS, POLYURIA, AND POLIDYPSIA

54. A 17 year old female comes into your office with a 6 month history of weight loss in spite of increased appetite, along with polyuria and polydipsia. A spot blood sugar done in the office is 13.2 mmol./litre (240 mg./dl). Which of the following statements about this young girl's problem is INCORRECT?

    a) the diagnosis of diabetes should be confirmed with a glucose tolerance test
    b) a diabetic diet will be an essential part of treatment
    c) this illness may have been precipitated by a viral infection
    d) insulin will be required to control her disease
    e) hospital inpatient stabilization is not necessary to begin treatment

55. The patient in question #54 begins treatment for diabetes mellitus. Long term control of her disease will probably best be accomplished by:

    a) a single daily injection of intermediate acting insulin
    b) twice daily injections of intermediate acting insulin
    c) twice daily injections of intermediate acting and regular insulin
    d) twice daily injections of short acting insulin
    e) oral glyburide 5-10 mg./day

56. The patient described in question #54 is started on insulin therapy. The initial daily dose of insulin that the patient should receive is approximately:

    a) 1-2 units
    b) 5-10 units
    c) 15-20 units
    d) 30-50 units
    e) 50-75 units

57. A 65 year old asymptomatic obese female has a routine fasting sugar drawn at the time of her annual physical examination. The level comes back at 180 mg./dl (10 mmol./litre). Her urine is negative for ketones. The test is repeated the following day and comes back at the same level. Which of the following statements about this patient is INCORRECT?

    a) the patient has Type II diabetes
    b) insulin is the agent of first choice in the management of this condition
    c) a diabetic diet forms the cornerstone of therapy
    d) the complications of this type of diabetes include retinopathy and nephropathy
    e) monitoring of this type of diabetes is best done by measuring blood glucose at home

CODE: (a:1, 2 and 3; b: 1 and 3; c: 2 and 4; d: 4 only; e: all of the above)

58. Which of the following is/are criteria for the diagnosis of diabetes mellitus?

    1) a fasting glucose greater than 7.7 mmol./litre (140 mg./dl) on more than one occasion
    2) a single serum glucose level of 11.1 mmol./litre (200 mg./dl) or greater in the presence of classic symptoms of diabetes
    3) a serum glucose level of 11.1 mmol./litre (200 mg./dl) or greater twice within a 2 hour period following a 75 gram glucose load
    4) a single serum glucose level of 12.2 mmol./1 (220 mg./dl)

59. Which of the following drugs may increase the blood glucose level and lead to diabetes mellitus?

    1) thiazide diuretics
    2) indomethacin
    3) propranolol
    4) diazepam

60. Gestational diabetes is diagnosed when:

    1) the fasting blood sugar exceeds 5.8 mmol./1 (105 mg./dl) on two occasions
    2) a single random glucose level exceeds 12.2 mmol./1 (220 mg./dl)
    3) two of three values following a 100 gram oral glucose load exceed 10.5 mmol./1 (190 mg./dl) at 1 hour, 9.2 mmol./1 (165 mg.dl) at 2 hours, and 8.1 mmol./1 (145 mg./dl) at 3 hours
    4) the hemoglobin A_{1C} value exceeds 7%

ANSWERS

54. a) The patient described in question #54 has Type I diabetes mellitus. Although Type I diabetes may originate at any age, the onset is usually before 35 years of age. The classic symptoms of hyperglycemia include polyuria, polydipsia and recent weight loss in spite of an increased intake of food. There may also be complaints of recent onset of headaches, blurred vision, fatigue and malaise.

    Type I diabetes is characterized by an absolute insulin deficiency and dependence on injected insulin to prevent ketoacidosis and to sustain life. The inability of the pancreas to produce insulin is believed to be due to direct damage of the islet cells or to autoimmune destruction of the beta cells in genetically susceptible individuals.

    Insulin and a diabetic diet form the cornerstones of therapy. In this diet, 50% of the total calories come from complex carbohydrates, 30% from protein and 20% from fats.

    A single glucose level in excess of 11 mmol./litre (200 mg./dl) in the presence of the classic symptoms of diabetes is diagnostic; and therefore the glucose tolerance test is unnecessary.

Most new cases of diabetes mellitus (in the absence of ketosis) can be initially managed in an outpatient setting.

55. c) Most patients with Type I diabetes can be controlled on two daily injections of a combination of intermediate acting insulin (Humulin-N or NPH) and regular insulin (Humulin-R or Toronto). Twice daily injections are usually required for optimum control because the peak activity of intermediate acting insulin occurs in 6-14 hours and declines thereafter.

Human insulin (Humulin), which is synthesized artificially from DNA recombinant techniques is the insulin of choice because of lack of antigenicity and antibody formation. For patients who are already on pork or beef insulin and who are not having any problems it is reasonable to continue them on the same regime.

Intensive insulin therapy which refers to multiple injections (at least 4) of short acting (Humulin-R, Toronto) insulin or a continuous insulin pump, is not necessary for good control in most cases.

A usual treatment regime involves 2/3 of the total insulin dose in the morning and 1/3 in the evening, with 2/3 of each dose being an intermediate acting insulin and 1/3 of the total dose being a short acting insulin. Although the regime discussed above will usually be required for excellent control some authorities still begin with a single daily injection of an intermediate acting insulin (15-20 units) and proceed from there.

Oral hypoglycemic agents like glyburide are not indicated for the treatment of Type I diabetes.

56. c) The usual starting dose of insulin is 15-20 units/day. The average maintenance dose is 1 unit/kg. in children, 30 units per day in women, and 42 units/day in men. However, the dose must be individualized; some persons require much more and some persons require much less.

57. b) Type II diabetes is frequently insidious in onset, lacking many of the classic symptoms usually associated with diabetes. Patients in this group may present initially with vague symptoms of fatigue, weakness, blurred vision, vaginal and perineal pruritis, impotence, or paresthesias. Weight loss is uncommon in the patients, many of whom are quite obese and have a strong family history of obesity and diabetes.

As in this case, the onset of Type II diabetes is often so subtle that it is discovered only in the course of routine examination or examination for other illnesses.

As in Type I diabetes, a diabetic diet forms the cornerstone of therapy. If dietary manipulation is not sufficient, an oral hypoglycemic agent should be tried first. It has recently been shown that there is no difference between insulin and oral hypoglycemic agents in either hepatic glucose production or peripheral utilization. A second generation agent such as glyburide (average maintenance dose 5-10 mg./day) is a good choice. If an oral hypoglycemic agent is effective, insulin therapy is indicated.

The complications of diabetes including retinopathy, nephropathy, atherosclerotic vascular disease and peripheral neuropathy are just as prevalent as they are in Type I diabetes.

Home glucose monitoring remains the monitoring method of choice. In all patients, but especially in elderly patients, the renal threshold for glucose increases, making urine sugars inaccurate in correlation with blood sugar levels and therefore not recommended for monitoring.

58. a) The National Diabetes Data Group have established the following diagnostic criteria for diabetes mellitus:

    1) a fasting glucose greater than 7.7 mmol./l (140 mg./dl) on more than one occasion
    2) a single glucose level of 11.1 mmol./l (200 mg./dl) in the presence of classic symptoms of diabetes
    3) a serum glucose level that twice within a two hour period equals or exceeds 11.1 mmol./l (200 mg./dl) following a 75 gram glucose load

    A single serum glucose level of 12.2 mmol./l (220 mg./dl) is NOT diagnostic of diabetes mellitus.

59. a) Many drugs are known to raise the blood glucose level and lead in some cases to diabetes mellitus. These include thiazide diuretics, furosemide, corticosteroids, propranolol (and some other beta-blockers), indomethacin (and some other non-steroidal anti-inflammatory drugs), isoniazid, lithium, oral contraceptives and other estrogens, clonidine, diphenylhydantoin, tricyclic antidepressants and nicotinic acid. Diazepam does not raise the plasma glucose level.

60. b) Gestational diabetes is diagnosed when:

    1) a fasting blood sugar exceeds 5.8 mmol/l (105 mg./dl) on two occasions
    2) two of three values following a 100 gram oral glucose load exceed 10.5 mmol./l (190 mg./dl) at 1 hour, 9.2 mmol./l (165 mg./dl) at 2 hours, or 8.1 mmol./l (145 mg./dl) at 3 hours.
    A single random glucose level of 12.2 mmol./l (220 mg./dl) does not make the diagnosis of gestational diabetes.
    The value of hemoglobin A_{1C} (glycosylated hemoglobin) is a measure of long term control and has no bearing on the diagnosis of gestational diabetes. In non-diabetics and well controlled diabetics, the value is 4-7% of total hemoglobin. The greater the value, the worse the control.

References

Martin D. Type II diabetes. Insulin vs oral agents. New England Journal of Medicine 1986; 314 (20): 1314-1315.

Baker C, McFarland K. Endocrinology. Textbook of Family Practice 3rd edition; Rakel R, editor. W.B. Saunders Co., Philadelphia: 1984; pages 949-961.

PROBLEM #10: A 42 YEAR OLD MALE WITH A HISTORY OF ELEVATED CHOLESTEROL

61. A 42 year old obese male, with a history of hypercholesterolemia, alcohol abuse and a workaholic personality presents for his routine physical examination. He was told by another physician 3 years ago that he had "high cholesterol". He has no family history of hyperlipidemia or coronary artery disease. Physical examination reveals a blood pressure of 180/110 mm Hg. There are no xanthomas or corneal arcus seen. The patient is taking hydro-chlorothiazide and propranolol for his hypertension. Routine lipid analysis reveals a cholesterol and triglyceride level that are 8.0 mmol./litre and 3.4 mmol./litre (309 mg./dl and 302 mg./dl respectively). Which of the following statements about this patient is TRUE?

    a) this patient has a primary hyperlipidemia
    b) alteration of diet in this patient probably will have no effect
    c) drug therapy should be instituted promptly to lower both cholesterol and triglycerides
    d) a more complete lipoprotein analysis is needed to advise therapy
    e) none of the above statements are true

62. Which of the following dietary recommendations is NOT part of the American Heart Association's diet for hyperlipidemia: (expressed as % total daily caloric intake)

    a) saturated fats—20%
    b) poly and monounsaturated fats—25-30%
    c) carbohydrates—55%
    d) proteins—20%
    e) cholesterol less than 300 mg./day

63. Which of the following statements about serum HDL cholesterol is FALSE?

    a) HDL cholesterol is increased by weight reduction
    b) HDL cholesterol is increased by regular aerobic exercise
    c) HDL cholesterol is increased by moderate alcohol intake
    d) HDL cholesterol is atherogenic
    e) HDL cholesterol is decreased by smoking

64. The drug of choice for hypertriglyceridemia not responsive to dietary manipulations is:

    a) gemfibrozil
    b) cholestyramine
    c) colestipol
    d) clofibrate
    e) probucol

CODE: (a:1, 2 and 3; b: 1 and 3; c: 2 and 4; d: 4 only; e: all of the above)

65. Which of the following altered metabolic states or disease states is/are causes of hyperlipidemia?

   1) high simple carbohydrate intake
   2) hypothyroidism
   3) diabetes mellitus
   4) beta-adrenergic blocking agents

66. The drug(s) of choice for lowering serum cholesterol is/are:

   1) probucol
   2) gemfibrozil
   3) colestipol
   4) nicotinic acid

ANSWERS

61. e) None of the above statements are true. In clinical practice, the initial step in dealing with hyperlipidemias is to differentiate them into primary and secondary types. In this patient there is no history of premature coronary heart disease in first degree family members and he has no physical signs of hyperlipidemia such as xanthomas or corneal arcus. Thus, his hyperlipidemia is most likely secondary to an altered metabolic state (induced by excessive alcohol intake, excessive food intake and perhaps medications). Alteration of his diet will most likely be of benefit to this patient and certainly should be tried before the institution of drug therapy. As well, his hypertension should be reviewed with thought given to taking him off agents such as hydrochlorothiazide and propranolol that can adversely affect blood lipid values. In most cases a complex lipo-protein analysis will not influence your therapy.

62. a) The modified American Heart Association recommended diet for hyperlipidemia control (expressed as % total daily caloric intake) is as follows:

   1) fats:
      a) saturated fats 5-10%
      b) polyunsaturated and monounsaturated fats—25-30%
   2) carbohydrates:
      a) increase to about 55%
      b) increase complex carbohydrates (starches), decrease simple carbohydrates (sugars)
   3) proteins: 20% (with high biologic value)
   4) cholesterol: less than 300 mg./day

63. d) Most hygenic measures, including weight reduction, non-smoking, regular aerobic exercise, as well as moderate alcohol intake (about 60 mls./day) are helpful in raising the HDL cholesterol level. This is more complex than it first appears, in that HDL in itself is made up of certain subtypes which may have differing effects. As a general rule, however, the higher the HDL cholesterol and the lower the LDL and VLDL cholesterol, the lower the risk of coronary artery disease.

64. a) The drug of choice for lowering the triglyceride level in patients who do not respond to dietary therapy is gemfibrozil. There are 3 drugs which are useful in lowering plasma triglyceride levels: nicotinic acid, clofibrate and gemfibrozil. Gemfibrozil is preferred because it has fewer side effects and lower toxicity. Gemfibrozil is prescribed in a dose of 600 mg. b.i.d.

65. e) Hyperlipidemia secondary to altered metabolism and disease states can be broken down into the following categories.

1) metabolic and physiologic:

    a) weight gain after middle age
    b) pregnancy, after second trimester
    c) sedentary life style

2) dietary habits:

    a) high saturated fat intake
    b) high simple sugar intake
    c) high alcohol consumption

3) drug induced:

    a) steroids and hormones, estrogen, oral contraceptives
    b) thiazide diuretics
    c) beta-adrenergic receptor blockers (some)

4) disease states:

    a) hypothyroidism
    b) diabetes mellitus
    c) renal diseases
    d) hepatic diseases (obstructive jaundice)
    e) dysgammaglobulinemia

66. b) Hypercholesterolemia that is not responsive to dietary manipulations is best treated by combining a drug that facilitates degradation of cholesterol (such as colestipol) with another drug that blocks the increased lipid biosynthetic rate (such as probucol). Colestipol is usually administered as 15 grams b.i.d. and probucol is usually given as 500 mg b.i.d. Gemfibrozil is used mainly for the treatment of hypertriglyceridemia. Although nicotinic acid lowers serum cholesterol it has been associated with significant toxic effects including hepatic dysfunction, cholestatic jaundice, hyperglycemia, hyperuricemia and gouty arthritis.

Reference

Kuo P. When and How to Treat Hyperlipidemia. Primary Care 1985; 12(1): 77-87.

PROBLEM #11: AN OBESE 47 YEAR OLD MALE WITH HYPERTENSION

67. A 47 year old male presents to your office for a routine health assessment. He weighs 300 lbs, smokes 2 packs of cigarettes/day, works 18 hours/day at the office and drinks 8 oz. of hard liquor/day. His blood pressure is 180/105 mm. Hg. Which of the following statements about this patient's blood pressure is FALSE?

    a) a single blood pressure reading of diastolic 105 is satisfactory for a diagnosis of hypertension
    b) this patient's alcohol intake may be a significant contributing factor to his elevated blood pressure
    c) the patient should have his blood pressure rechecked after a period of rest in the office
    d) the patient should return for reassessment of his blood pressure in 1 weeks time
    e) the patient should not be started on antihypertensive medication at this time

68. A diagnosis of essential hypertension is established in the patient described in question #67. Therapy should be aimed at decreasing his blood pressure to as close to what level as possible?

    a) 150/90 mm. Hg.
    b) 140/90 mm. Hg.
    c) 130/90 mm. Hg.
    d) 120/80 mm. Hg.
    e) 110/70 mm. Hg.

69. The ideal daily dose of hydrochlorothiazide (the dose at which the efficacy/side effect ratio is greatest) is:

    a) 150 mg.
    b) 75 mg.
    c) 50 mg.
    d) 25 mg.
    e) 12.5 mg.

70. The level of blood pressure that constitutes hypertension in the elderly has not been clearly established. Most authorities, however, would try to lower an elderly patient's blood pressure to a level of:

    a) 180/110 mm. Hg.
    b) 180/90 mm. Hg.
    c) 170/100 mm. Hg.
    d) 160/90 mm. Hg.
    e) 120/80 mm. Hg.

CODE: (a:1, 2 and 3; b: 1 and 3; c: 2 and 4; d: 4 only; e: all of the above)

71. The patient described in question #67 is started on antihypertensive therapy. The drug(s) of first choice for controlling blood pressure in this patient is/are:

    1) hydrochlorothiazide
    2) prazosin
    3) propranolol (or other beta-blocker)
    4) captopril

72. The initial diagnostic workup of a patient with hypertension should include:

    1) electrolytes/BUN and creatinine
    2) IVP
    3) ECG
    4) 24-hour urine for metanephrines

73. A 50 year old male is being treated for hypertension. He is currently on a low salt diet, hydrochlorothiazide 25 mg./day and propranolol 120 mg. b.i.d. His blood pressure is 180/105 mm. Hg. Which of the following would be reasonable choice(s) for a third line agent?

    1) atenolol
    2) prazosin
    3) furosemide
    4) hydralazine

74. The patient described in question #73 has his blood pressure lowered to 160/100 mm. Hg. with the addition of a third line agent. Which of the following would be reasonable choice(s) for a fourth line agent?

    1) metoprolol
    2) pindolol
    3) reserpine
    4) captopril

75. Which of the following antihypertensive drug(s) decrease high density lipoprotein cholesterol and increase low density lipoprotein cholesterol and very low density lipoprotein cholesterol (LDL and VLDL)?

    1) propranolol
    2) pindolol
    3) hydrochlorothiazide
    4) prazosin

76. Which of the following metabolic side effects may occur with diuretic therapy?

1) hyperuricemia
2) hyperglycemia
3) hypokalemia
4) hyperlipidemia

For questions 77-86 match the lettered description to the numbered drug item. Each description may be used once, more than once, or not at all.

77) prazosin

78) pindolol

79) captopril

80) metoprolol

81) clonidine

82) labetalol

83) furosemide

84) amiloride

85) propranolol

86) diltiazem

a) a loop diuretic

b) a beta-blocker often used in the treatment of migraine headaches

c) a peripheral alpha-2 inhibitor

d) an agent that possesses both alpha and beta blocking activity

e) a beta-blocker with intrinsic sympathomimetic activity

f) a potassium sparing agent

g) a cardioselective beta blocker

h) an angiotensin converting enzyme inhibitor

i) a calcium channel blocker

j) a centrally acting alpha-receptor agonist

ANSWERS

67. a) Hypertension should not be diagnosed until a sustained elevation of blood pressure has been documented. For diagnosis, at least 3 readings, averaging greater than 140 systolic or 90 diastolic, and at least 1 week apart, should be recorded. Most experts agree that if a single diastolic reading of 110 mm.Hg. is obtained, it is unlikely to return to normal on subsequent readings.

   Alcohol abuse is a significant cause of hypertension. Any patient that presents with hypertension should be questioned about alcohol intake. Studies have shown that blood pressure increases in anyone who intakes more than an average of 2 drinks/day.

   The patient described in this question should have his blood pressure taken again after 5 minutes of rest. This will give you a better idea of the baseline reading for this visit. A patient whose blood pressure goes down after a period of rest has "labile hypertension". Roughly 1/2 of these patients will go on to develop sustained hypertension.

   Some experts believe that baseline blood pressure readings obtained at home are much more representative of true blood pressure, and recommend routine monitoring and reporting by the patient. This regime has the added advantage of involving the patient in the evaluation and treatment of his problem.

   The patient should not be started on antihypertensive medication until it is established that his blood pressure elevation is sustained.

68. d) Epidemiologic studies have shown that risk for atherosclerotic cardiovascular disease increases with sustained blood pressure above 150 mm.Hg. systolic and 82 mm.Hg. diastolic. It is generally agreed that the goal of antihypertensive therapy in patients under age 60 is to reduce the blood pressure to a level of as close to 120/80 mm.Hg. as possible.

69. d) The ideal dose of hydrochlorothiazide appears to be approximately 25 mg./day. The efficacy of 25 mg./day appears to be equal to that of any higher dose, but the side effects including hypokalemia, hyperglycemia, hyperlipidemia and hyperuricemia are considerably less than with a higher dose.

70. d) The level of blood pressure needed to establish the diagnosis of hypertension in elderly patients (>65 years) has not been established with certainty. However, it is known that both systolic and diastolic hypertension contribute to cardiovascular and cerebrovascular mortality. Many hypertension experts recommend that the blood pressure of patients over the age of 65 years be reduced to 160/90 or less. Even if the diastolic pressure is 90 mm.Hg. or less, an attempt should be made to lower the systolic pressure to less than 170 mm.Hg.

71. b) The drugs of first choice for controlling blood pressure are the thiazide diuretics and the beta-blockers. One of these agents should be selected for treatment if non-drug methods including dietary modification (decreased sodium, decreased calories, and increased potassium), and increased activity are not effective. At this time many physicians are leaning towards the beta-blockers as the drugs of first choice except in black patients and elderly patients (where they do not appear to be as effective as thiazide diuretics). The usual starting dose of propranolol is 20 mg. b.i.d. increasing to a maximum of 360 mg./day. The initial dose of hydrochlorothiazide is 25 mg. o.d.

72. b) The hypertensive workup is aimed at uncovering secondary causes of hypertension in a cost-effective manner, and uncovering signs of end-organ damage. The basic workup should include a complete urinalysis, electrolytes, BUN and creatinine, CXR and ECG. An IVP and a 24-hour urine for metanephrines (for the detection of pheochromocytoma) are only indicated in specific clinical circumstances. For example, a patient over the age of 55 who has been previously normotensive and who suddenly develops hypertension should be suspected of having renal artery stenosis. This would necessitate an IVP and renal angiograms. A young person with hypertension accompanied by palpitations and sweating should be suspected of having a pheochromocytoma or hyperthyroidism. In this case a 24-hour urine for metanephrines would be indicated.

73. c) After beta-blockers and thiazide diuretics have been introduced as step 1 and 2 agents, a vasodilator such as prazosin or hydralazine should be added as a step 3 agent. Prazosin is given in a dose of 4-20 mg./day (after a test dose of 0.5 mg. is administered and slowly increased) and hydralazine as 100-200 mg./day in divided doses.

Atenolol is a beta-blocker and thus would not be indicated as propranolol has already been given in high dose.

Furosemide is a loop diuretic and is usually only indicated in the treatment of hypertension if concomitant renal insufficiency exists.

Other appropriate third line agents include clonidine and guanabenz.

74. d) The fourth line agent of choice is the angiotensin enzyme converting inhibitor captopril. It is usually begun as 12.5 mg. b.i.d. and gradually increased up to 100 mg. t.i.d. Because of the risk of a hypotensive reaction it is better to discontinue other antihypertensive medications (especially beta-blockers and vasodilators) before beginning therapy with captopril. A new angiotensin-converting inhibitor, enalapril, has recently been introduced. Metoprolol and pindolol are beta-blockers and thus are not indicated when propranolol is being used.

Reserpine is a centrally acting agent which has many side effects and which now is rarely used in hypertension management.

75. b) The influence of antihypertensive agents on plasma lipid values has become an area of increasing concern. In some studies antihypertensive treatment has not lowered mortality. This may be explained by the fact that a decrease in mortality because of lowered blood pressure is balanced by a concomitant increase in mortality due to altered metabolic parameters including blood lipids.

Some beta-blockers including propranolol may have an adverse effect on the ratio of HDL cholesterol to LDL and VLDL cholesterol. Other beta-blockers like pindolol do not appear to affect this ratio. Hydrochlorothiazide likewise can adversely affect this ratio. Prazosin actually increases the ratio of HDL to LDL and VLDL cholesterol.

76. e) Diuretic therapy (both thiazide diuretics and loop diuretics) may produce a number of metabolic side effects. These include hyperuricemia, hyperglycemia, hypokalemia, and hyperlipidemia. These side effects may be significant in increasing the tendency to atherosclerosis or ventricular ectopy, thus negating the beneficial effects of blood pressure reduction. Therefore, the dose of diuretic should be kept to a minimum.

77. c) Prazosin is a peripheral alpha-adrenergic inhibitor which acts as a vasodilator and which is generally used after beta-blockers and thiazide diuretics have failed to control the blood pressure.

78. e) Pindolol is a beta-adrenergic receptor blocker agent with intrinsic sympathomimetic activity. Of all the beta-blockers, this is the agent least likely to produce symptoms in a patient with a history of bronchial hyperreactivity. Because of its intrinsic sympathomimetic activity it is less likely to produce Raynaud's phenomenon.

79. h) Captopril is an angiotensin converting enzyme inhibitor. It is generally indicated for the treatment of hypertension that does not respond to a beta-blocker, a thiazide diuretic, and a vasodilator.

80. g) Metoprolol is a cardioselective beta-blocker which inhibits the B_1 receptors to a greater degree than the B_2 receptors. At high doses, however, this cardioselectivity is lost.

81. j) Clonidine is a centrally acting alpha-2 receptor agonist. It is used in patients who do not respond to beta-blockers or thiazide diuretics and also in elderly patients with isolated systolic hypertension.

82. d) Labetalol is an agent that possesses both alpha-1 (post synaptic) and beta-blocking activity.

83. a) Furosemide is a potent loop diuretic that blocks sodium reabsorption in the ascending loop of Henle and in the proximal and distal convoluted tubule. It is useful in treating hypertension in patients with renal insufficiency.

84. f) Amiloride is an antikaluretic agent with mild natriuretic and antihypertensive properties. It is sometimes combined with hydrochlorothiazide to produce a diuretic that will spare potassium and produce a significant antihypertensive effect.

85. b) Propranolol is the original beta-blocker. It has many indications including hypertension, angina and most recently, prophylactic treatment of migraine headaches.

86. i) Diltiazem is a calcium channel blocking agent that is used both in the treatment of angina and hypertension. Most experts predict that the use of calcium channel blockers in the treatment of hypertension will increase over the next few years. Even at present, diltiazem and the other calcium channel blockers (verapamil and nifedipine) are considered as good first line agents in the treatment of hypertensive patients that also have angina pectoris.

References

Drayer et al. Where to start in hypertension therapy. Patient Care 1985; 19(20): 18-54.
Moore M. Current Management of Hypertension. American Family Physician 1985; 32(6): 129-136.

PROBLEM #12: A 31 YEAR OLD FEMALE WITH HEAT INTOLERANCE AND PALPITATIONS

87. A 31 year old female presents with a 3 month history of anxiety, heat intolerance, palpitations and fatigue. On examination, her thyroid gland feels slightly enlarged. Which of the following tests will provide the most useful information in diagnosing or excluding hyperthyroidism?

   a) serum T-3
   b) serum T-4
   c) free thyroxine index
   d) thyroid binding globulin
   e) serum TSH

88. A diagnosis of hyperthyroidism is confirmed in the patient described above. The most common cause of hyperthyroidism in this patient would be:

   a) thyrotoxicosis (Grave's disease)
   b) toxic multinodular goiter
   c) toxic adenoma
   d) subacute thyroiditis
   e) autoimmune thyroiditis

89. The treatment of choice for the patient described above would be:

   a) propylthiouracil
   b) propranolol
   c) radioactive iodine
   d) surgery
   e) none of the above

90. A 25 year old female is seen for a complete physical assessment. Her past history is unremarkable, she is feeling well at present and is currently taking the oral contraceptive pill. A routine T-4 level done is elevated at 13 micrograms/dl. (169 nmol./litre). The most likely explanation for the elevated T-4 level is:

   a) thyrotoxicosis
   b) toxic nodular goiter
   c) an elevated TBG level
   d) laboratory error
   e) none of the above

91. The differentiation of hyperthyroidism due to thyrotoxicosis from hyperthyroidism due to thyroiditis is best made by:

    a) thyroid antibody level
    b) radioactive iodine uptake (I-131 uptake)
    c) thyroid scan
    d) level of elevation of serum T-4
    e) level of thyroglobulin level

92. The major complication of I-131 therapy for the treatment of hyperthyroidism is:

    a) carcinoma of the thyroid
    b) allergic reaction to the iodine
    c) leukemia
    d) hypothyroidism
    e) genetic damage to women in the childbearing years

93. A 65 year old male presents with a 6 month history of lethargy, weakness, psychomotor retardation, cold intolerance, constipation, hair loss and weight gain. You suspect hypothyroidism. Which of the following tests will provide the most useful information for diagnosing or excluding hypothyroidism?

    a) serum T-3
    b) serum T-4
    c) free thyroxine index
    d) thyroid binding globulin
    e) serum TSH

94. The most common cause of hypothyroidism is:

    a) autoimmune thyroiditis
    b) post I-131 hypothyroidism
    c) iodine deficiency
    d) idiopathic hypothyroidism
    e) post-thyroidectomy hypothyroidism

CODE: (a:1, 2 and 3; b: 1 and 3; c: 2 and 4; d: 4 only; e: all of the above)

95. Which of the following is/are signs or symptoms of hypothyroidism?

    1) menstrual disturbance
    2) slow reflex relaxation
    3) edema
    4) bradycardia

ANSWERS

87. c)The free thyroxine index (FTI) is the most widely used test for excluding and diagnosing both hyperthyroidism and hypothyroidism. The index is calculated from the T-4, a measure of circulating thyroxine, and the T-3 resin uptake, a test that indirectly measures the amount of thyroid binding globulin in the serum. Unless there is some disagreement with the clinical impression, these are the only tests needed to assess thyroid function, although additional tests may be needed to determine the etiology of the thyroid abnormality. In hyperthyroidism, the FTI will be elevated. Occasionally, the serum T-3 will be elevated when the serum T-4 is normal. This is known as T-3 thyrotoxicosis. The serum TSH will be elevated when the functional thyroxine index is low and a state of primary hypothyroidism exists.

88. a) Thyrotoxicosis is a relatively common disorder with a prevalence rate of 19 per 1000 women and 1.6 per 1000 men. The most common cause of hyperthyroidism is thyrotoxicosis (Grave's disease). Subjective findings in Grave's disease include nervousness, heat intolerance, palpitations, dyspnea, fatigue, weakness, weight loss and eye symptoms. Objective findings include goiter; tachycardia; tremor; hypertension; warm, moist hands; a thyroid bruit and lid lag. Other causes of hyperthyroidism including toxic multinodular goiter, toxic adenoma, subacute thyroiditis, and autoimmune thyroiditis are not nearly as common as thyrotoxicosis.

89. a) The treatment of choice for thyrotoxicosis is antithyroid drug therapy. The chief advantage of antithyroid drug therapy is that it does not cause permanent thyroid damage, and a significant number of patients experience permanent remission of hyperthyroidism following several months of therapy with propythiouracil or methimazole. Clinical improvement of the hyperthyroidism may be evident in one or two weeks, and usually the patient becomes euthyroid between two and three months after the initiation of therapy. Once the patient is euthyroid, the dose of antithyroid medication may be reduced by one-third every couple of months as long as the patient remains euthyroid. There is no clear indication of how long the drug should be continued after the patient has been rendered completely euthyroid, but commonly the drugs are continued for 6 months to a year. The basic regime is to start with propythiouracil 300 mg./day or methimazole 30 mg./day in divided doses.

90. c) The most likely explanation for the elevated T-4 level in this patient is an elevated TBG level secondary to the estrogen component of the oral contraceptive pill. The amount of serum thyroxine bound to TBG depends on two factors: the amount of thyroxine produced and the level of protein available for binding. As the level of TBG rises, the amount of bound thyroxine also increases. TBG increases in patients who are on estrogen supplementation, as well as in pregnant patients. On the other hand, if there is a decrease in the

amount of TBG, the amount of bound thyroxine will decrease. This occurs in patients with chronic liver disease and those on androgens or other anabolic steroids. There are also a number of drugs that compete with T-4 for binding to the serum proteins; among the most common are phenytoin, heparin, salicylate and clofibrate.

91. b) The differentiation of hyperthyroidism due to thyrotoxicosis (Grave's disease) from hyperthyroidism due to thyroiditis is best made by radioactive iodine uptake (I-131 uptake). In most cases, the normal radioiodine uptake is below 25%. The I-131 uptake is usually greatly increased in patients with Grave's disease and moderately elevated in those with toxic nodular goiter. Patients with hyperthyroidism due to subacute thyroiditis, autoimmune thyroiditis or factitious hyperthyroidism have a low I-131 uptake.

92. d) The major complication of I-131 therapy for the treatment of hyperthyroidism is permanent hypothyroidism. Eventually, most patients treated with I-131 will become hypothyroid. Therefore, every patient who receives I-131 must understand that hypothyroidism is the expected consequence of therapy, and that replacement therapy with thyroxine will probably be necessary for life. A period of anti-thyroid drug therapy should precede and follow treatment with I-131 in severely symptomatic patients because several months may elapse before the patient becomes euthyroid after treatment with the radioisotope alone.

    Past concerns regarding a high risk of carcinoma of the thyroid, leukemia, or genetic damage to the offspring of women in childbearing years have not been substantiated by follow-up of treated patients (as long as 30 years). Radioiodine is however ABSOLUTELY CONTRAINDICATED in pregnancy. An allergic reaction to iodine is not a contraindication to the use of I-131 because the amount of iodine used in so small.

93. c) The most useful test for diagnosing or excluding hypothyroidism is the free thyroxine index. In hypothyroidism, the free thyroxine index will be depressed (see critique of question #87). The serum TSH will differentiate primary from secondary hypothyroidism. Primary hypothyroidism is hypothyroidism that is due to thyroid disease. Secondary hypothyroidism is hypothyroidism that is due to pituitary or hypothalamic disease.

94. b) The most common cause of hypothyroidism is post I-131 treatment of hyperthyroidism. Other causes of hypothyroidism without goiter include 1) post-thyroidectomy hypothyroidism, 2) idiopathic hypothyroidism, 3) hypothyroidism that is due to pituitary or hypothalamic defects and 4) developmental defects.

    Causes of hypothyroidism with goiter include 1) autoimmune thyroiditis, 2) drug-induced hypothyroidism, 3) iodine deficiency or 4) an inherited defect in the synthesis of thyroid hormone.

95. e) The signs and symptoms of hypothyroidism include lethargy/weakness, slow movement and speech, cold intolerance, constipation, hair loss, menstrual disturbance, paresthesias, slow reflex relaxation, dry skin, edema, impaired memory, weight gain, deafness and bradycardia. The treatment of hypothyroidism is simple and effective. Levo-thyroxine in a dose of 0.10-0.20 mg./ day will restore the T-4 and TSH levels to the normal range within a few weeks.

Reference

Baker C, McFarland K. Endocrinology. Textbook of Family Practice 3rd edition; Rakel R, editor. W.B. Saunders Co., Philadelphia: 1984; pages 963-974.

PROBLEM #13: A 32 YEAR OLD FEMALE WITH FEVER, WEIGHT LOSS AND CHRONIC DIARRHEA

A 32 year old female presents to the office with a 6 month history of loose bowel movements. She has lost 20 pounds in that period of time. For the last 3 weeks she has had an intermittent fever.

For each of the following lettered options, select "a" if the numbered option is associated with "a" only; select "b" if the numbered option is associated with "b" only; select "c" if the numbered option is associated with both "a" and "b"; and select "d" if the numbered option is associated with neither "a" nor "b".

a) ulcerative colitis
b) Crohn's disease
c) both ulcerative colitis and Crohn's disease
d) neither ulcerative colitis nor Crohn's disease

96) most common chronic inflammatory disease of the colon

97) disease confined to the mucosa

98) transmural involvement of all layers of the bowel

99) predominant clinical symptom is bloody diarrhea

100) more commonly associated with toxic megacolon

101) commonly associated with fistulas, perianal abscesses and fissures

102) carcinoma of the colon is a major complication

103) X-ray appearance commonly shows "skip lesions"

104) sulfasalazine is effective in maintaining remissions

105) prednisone is effective in inducing remissions

106) steroid-containing enemas are the treatment of choice for localized disease

107) bowel obstruction is a common complication

108) clindamycin is frequently implicated as a cause

109) malabsorption is a common problem

110) Clostridium difficile is frequently implicated as a cause

ANSWERS

96. a) The most common chronic inflammatory disease of the colon is ulcerative colitis. The cause of the disease is unknown. Symptomatic ulcerative colitis usually develops between age 25 and 45. Females are more often affected than males.

97. a) The hallmark of ulcerative colitis is continuous involvement of the colonic mucosa, with no intervening normal areas. The inflammation can be mild, so that the examiner sees only loss of the normal vascular pattern, or it can be marked with the mucosa appearing congested, highly vascular and friable.

98. b) Pathologically, Crohn's disease presents as a chronic inflammatory process involving the entire bowel wall and the surrounding mesentery and lymph nodes. The bowel wall is thickened and edematous, which narrows the lumen, causing stricture formation. The mucosa has a cobblestone appearance because of deep transverse and longitudinal fissures and ulcers.

99. a) The predominant clinical symptom of ulcerative colitis is bloody diarrhea, followed by crampy abdominal pain often relieved by defecation. As a general rule, the more colon that is involved, the more severe are the symptoms. With ulcerative pancolitis (entire colon inflamed) systemic symptoms of fever, anemia, and prostration may be of primary importance. With these symptoms the diagnosis of ulcerative colitis can be suspected clinically. The sigmoidoscopic examination is diagnostic if bacterial and amoebic infection can be ruled out. A barium enema examination can also be diagnostic, but it may be normal in early or mild disease.

Because Crohn's disease can involve any part of the alimentary tract from the mouth to the anus, the presenting symptoms are more variable than ulcerative colitis. Diarrhea is usually of secondary importance to abdominal pain and cramping. Patients may also present with fever, weight loss, arthritis, perirectal abscesses and fistulas, and generalized fatigue.

100. a) Toxic megacolon is a major complication of ulcerative colitis. Toxic megacolon can be severe in ulcerative pancolitis and is the result of transmural colonic inflammation. This more extensive inflammation causes systemic toxicity and loss of colonic muscular tone. The colon is dilated to greater than 6 cm. in diameter and the chance of colonic perforation makes this a medical emergency. Mortality following colonic perforation in this setting still approaches 50%. Megacolon usually occurs in the setting of known ulcerative colitis, but 20% or more of the cases appear as the initial episode of colitis.

Treatment of toxic megacolon consists of correction of fluid and electrolyte disturbance, nasogastric suction to prevent swallowed air from adding to the colonic dilatation, and corticosteroids in doses equivalent to 100-200 mg. of prednisone. Toxic megacolon can occur with Crohn's colitis but is distinctly less common.

101. b) Crohn's disease is commonly associated with fistulas, perianal abscesses and fissures. These complications may actually be the first sign of the disease.

102. a) The risk of colon cancer is dramatically higher in patients with ulcerative colitis than in the general population. This is related to duration of the disease, so that 25 years after the diagnosis, the incidence approaches 25%. Currently, 10 years is an accepted duration of the disease in which the risk of cancer is minimal. In the past, prophylactic proctocolectomy was advised after 10 years. Since the advent of the widespread use of colonoscopy in the past decade, some experts have begun surveillance programs on their population at risk. The patients undergo yearly colonoscopy and multiple biopsies are taken. If dysplastic or "precancerous" changes are seen, surgery is advised.

103. b) The small bowel series and the barium enema in a patient with Crohn's disease demonstrate a variety of changes. The thickened loops of bowel are separated from adjacent loops; the lumen is narrowed and the bowel proximal to the narrowed segment is dilated; the mucosal folds are blunted, irregular and ulcerated; and ulcers extend deep into the wall of the bowel. Skip areas of disease interposed with normal bowel are characteristic. The most common areas of the bowel involved with Crohn's disease are the terminal ileum, the cecum and the ascending colon.

104. c) Sulfasalazine is effective in maintaining remissions initially induced by corticosteroids in ulcerative colitis and in Crohn's disease confined to the colon. It is not, however, effective in Crohn's disease that is present in the small intestine. Sulfasalazine is usually begun in a dose of 1-2 grams four times daily, and gradually reduced after 3 weeks to 1.5-2.0 grams daily. A new agent, 5-aminosalicylic acid, which lacks the sulfa part of the molecule is now regarded by many authorities as the agent of choice for maintaining remissions.

105. c) Prednisone in doses of 30-60 mg./day is effective inducing remissions in inducing both ulcerative colitis and Crohn's disease. The dose of prednisone should be gradually tapered over several weeks.

106. a) Steroid containing enemas are the treatment of choice for localized ulcerative colitis confined to the rectum and lower part of the sigmoid. This condition is known as ulcerative proctitis. Rectal steroids reduce inflammation, are usually adequate therapy, and do not have the systemic side effects of

prednisone. Until recently it was felt that patients with ulcerative proctitis do not have an increased risk of colon cancer. Unfortunately, colonoscopy has blurred the once clear distinction between ulcerative colitis and proctitis. Biopsies taken at intervals above the apparent demarcation between normal and abnormal mucosa have shown histologic inflammation involving the entire colon with more severe involvement distally. Whether most patients with proctitis have pancolonic inflammation is unknown. Ulcerative proctitis still appears to have a low potential for malignant degeneration.

107. b) Crohn's disease is a transmural disease, and this can cause stricture formation with resulting obstruction. Small bowel obstruction occurs in a third of patients hospitalized with Crohn's disease, but this is from the edema associated with active disease as well as strictures.

108. d) Clindamycin is the antibiotic most closely associated with pseudomembranous colitis and has nothing to do with either ulcerative colitis or Crohn's disease. It seems to trigger the propagation of Colstridium difficile, which elaborates a toxin that is responsible for the onset of the disease.

109. b) Because of the common location of Crohn's disease in the small bowel, malabsorption is common. This occurs because of surgical resection of the bowel or because of inflamed areas that cannot perform their appropriate function. Compounding this problem is the fact that many patients with narrowed segments are afraid to eat because abdominal pain is worsened after meals. Consequently, the patient loses weight. Dietary instruction in low-residue and high protein/high calorie diets may be beneficial. Supplementation with elemental diets, and vitamins and minerals is often necessary. Vitamin B_{12} should be adminstered monthly after resection or when more than 100 cm. of distal ileum is diseased.

110. d) Clostridium difficile is the organism most closely associated with the production of toxin that results in pseudomembranous colitis. It has nothing to do with ulcerative colitis or Crohn's disease. It is most often associated with clindamycin. Considering all antibiotics, however, ampicillin is the most common cause of antibiotic-induced diarrhea.

Reference

Boydstun J, Barker J and Lawhorne L. Gastrointestinal disorders. Textbook of Family Practice 3rd edition; Rakel R, editor. W.B. Saunders Co., Philadelphia: 1984; pages 1002-1004.

PROBLEM #14: AN 80 YEAR OLD FEMALE WITH PAINFUL FINGER JOINTS

111. An 80 year old female presents with stiffness in her hands bilaterally and bony swellings at the margins of the distal interphalangeal joints. Which of the following statements about this patient is TRUE?

    a) these swellings may represent Heberden's nodes
    b) these swellings may represent Bouchard's nodes
    c) this patient will most likely demonstrate an elevated ESR and positive rheumatoid factor
    d) synovial fluid analysis will probably demonstrate low viscosity and normal mucin clotting
    e) the total leukocyte count in the synovial fluid will probably be less than 1000 cells/mm.

112. Which of the following statements regarding the pathogenesis and symptomatology of osteoarthritis is FALSE?

    a) pain is the chief symptom of osteoarthritis and is usually deep and aching in character
    b) stiffness of the involved joint is common but of relatively brief duration
    c) the pain of osteoarthritis does not originate from the degenerating cartilage
    d) the major physical finding in osteoarthritis is bony crepitus
    e) the presence of osteophytes is sufficient for the diagnosis of osteoarthritis

113. A 65 year old female with moderately severe osteoarthritis of her hip comes into your office requesting an exercise prescription. She wishes to "get into shape". You should advise her that:

    a) exercise is not good for osteoarthritis; rest is much more appropriate
    b) a graded exercise program that consists of brisk walking gradually increasing the distance to 3-4 miles/day will probably not cause pain and will be good for her
    c) a passive isotonic exercise program is preferable to an active exercise isometric one
    d) any exercise program will probably hasten her need for total hip replacements
    e) swimming is the best exercise prescription you can give her as it promotes cardiovascular fitness and at the same time keeps pressure off the weight-bearing joints

CODE: (a:1, 2 and 3; b: 1 and 3; c: 2 and 4; d: 4 only; e: all of the above)

1) narrrowing of the joint space
2) bony sclerosis
3) osteophyte formation
4) subchondral cysts

115. Which of the following is/are useful treatment modalities in osteoarthritis?

1) weight loss in obese patients
2) canes, crutches, and walkers
3) the application of heat to involved joints
4) nonsteroidal anti-inflammatory agents

ANSWERS

111. a) The patient described in this question has osteoarthritis. The pathogno-monic finding in osteoarthritis is Heberden's nodes, which are bony swel-lings of the margins of the distal interphalangeal joints. Bourchard's nodes represent similar swellings at the margins of the proximal interphalangeal joints. Osteoarthritis is most commonly associated with a normal age-adjusted ESR and a negative rheumatoid factor. Synovial fluid analysis will probably demonstrate high viscosity and normal mucin clotting. The total leukocyte count in the synovial fluid will probably be less than 1000 cells/mm.

112. e) Pain is the chief symptom of osteoarthritis and is usually deep and aching in character. The pain is increased by usage of the involved joint and improves with rest. Stiffness of the involved joints is common but is of relatively brief duration, generally subsiding within 30 minutes. It is often characterized as a gelling sensation, which develops following a period of inactivity. It is espe-cially common in weight-bearing joints and often subsides completely after the patient has taken a few steps. The pain of osteoarthritis does not arise from the degenerating cartilage. Synovial inflammation, which is usually of rel-atively low intensity may be a significant source of the pain. In addition, microfractures in the subchondral bone, irritation of the periosteal nerve endings, stress on ligaments due to bone deformity or synovial effusion, venous congestion due to remodeling of the subchondral bone, muscle strain, and associated soft tissue bursitis or tendinitis may be responsible for the pain.

The major physical finding in osteoarthritis is bony crepitus, that is, the palpable or audible sensation of grating caused by bone rubbing on bone during joint motion. Soft tissue swelling and ultimately bony swelling due to osteophytes may be detected on physical examination. The sole presence of osteophytes is insufficient for the diagnosis of osteoarthritis and appears to be related to age. Less than 1% of patients who had osteophytes as the only radiologic abnormality in the hip developed joint space narrowing and further changes of osteoarthritis when reevaluated a decade later.

113. e) A graduated exercise program helps to decrease muscle spasm and prevent muscle atrophy. Active rather than passive exercises and isometric rather than isotonic exercises are preferred. With no involvement of weight-bearing joints, swimming is an ideal exercise and in this patient it is the best recommendation. A graded exercise program that includes walking 3-4 miles/day will result in trauma to the joints and should not be advised. It may very well hasten the need for total hip replacement. When walking it is best to advise the patient to keep pressure off the involved joint; patients should be encouraged to use canes and other devices to accomplish that goal.

114. e) The radiologic changes in osteoarthritis reflect the pathology of the affected joint. Narrowing of the joint space results from loss of articular cartilage. In the hip and knee, this narrowing may be seen in x-ray films obtained during weight bearing, even when no changes are present on standard films of non-weight bearing. Bony sclerosis (due to thickening of subchondral bone) is often prominent radiologically. Subchondral cysts may result from the transmission of pressure through the disrupted cartilage surface into the underlying bone. Osteophytes (bony spurs) occur at the margins of the joint and are representative of newly formed bone and cartilage. With progression of the disease obvious deformity and malalignment occur.

115. e) The treatment aims of osteoarthritis are to:
    1) decrease the pressure loading on the involved joint and retard progression of the disease. This is best accomplished by encouraging weight loss in obese patients and by the use of canes, crutches and other devices.
    2) decrease the muscle spasm and prevent muscle atrophy. This can be accomplished by the application of heat for muscle spasm and a graduated exercise program that does not involve weight bearing.
    3) to relieve pain. This can be accomplished by the use of acetominophen, aspirin or any of the other non-steroidal anti-inflammatory agents.

Reference

Eyanson S, Brandt K. Osteoarthritis. Primary Care 1984; 11(2): 259-269.

PROBLEM #15: A 75 YEAR OLD MALE WITH TREMOR AND A SLOW SHUFFLING GAIT

116. A 75 year old male presents with generalized slowness and poverty of spontaneous movement, a shuffling gait, rigidity of the limbs, facial immobility, a stooped over posture and a rhythmic tremor. Where is the lesion associated with this disease located?

a) the caudate nucleus
b) the hypothalamus
c) the substantia nigra
d) the putamen
e) the globus pallidus

117. The patient described in question #116 has a deficit of which of the following neurotransmitters?

a) acetylcholine
b) serotonin
c) gamma-aminobutyric acid
d) dopamine
e) norephinephrine

118. Which of the following statements regarding the tremor associated with the disease described in question #117 is FALSE?

a) the tremor is usually first noted as a rhythmic alternating flexion and extension of the thumb and digits
b) the frequency of the tremor is four to five cycles/second and is known as a pill-rolling tremor
c) the treatment of choice for the tremor described is propranolol
d) the tremor is prominent in the resting limb
e) the tremor disappears briefly during the course of movement

119. Which of the following medications IS NOT a cause of drug-induced Parkinsonism?

a) diazepam
b) haloperidol
c) largactil
d) perphenazine
e) reserpine

120. The drug of choice for treatment of severe symptoms of Parkinson's disease is:

    a) amantadine hydrochloride
    b) trihexyphenidyl
    c) hydroxyzine
    d) levodopa
    e) bromocriptine

CODE: (a:1, 2 and 3; b: 1 and 3; c: 2 and 4; d: 4 only; e: all of the above)

121. Which of the following statements about benign essential tremor is/are CORRECT?

    1. it is commonly familial
    2. a nodding head tremor and tremulousness of speech are often observed
    3. it predominantly affects the hands
    4. it is a resting tremor

122. Treatment of benign essential tremor may include which of the following agents?

    1. propranolol
    2. diazepam
    3. alcohol
    4. levodopa-carbidopa

ANSWERS

116. c) The patient described in this question has Parkinson's disease. Parkinson's disease (paralysis agitans) is a degenerative disorder of the basal ganglia of unknown etiology. The principal pathologic feature is degeneration of the substantia nigra, particularly the zona compacta. Neurons of the substantia nigra project to the corpus striatum (caudate nucleus and putamen), where they release the neurotransmitter dopamine. Loss of the striatal dopamine is the principal biochemical defect in Parkinson's disease.

    The principal clinical features of Parkinson's disease are generalized slowness and poverty of spontaneous movement, rigidity of the limbs, facial immobility, disorders of posture and gait, and a rhythmic resting tremor. Most disabling to the patient are muscle rigidity and bradykinesia. The patient often describes these symptoms as tiredness and weakness, but it is usually not the power of muscles but rather their speed of movement that is primarly affected. The gait is usually slow and shuffling. A loss of associated arm swinging may develop as well.

117. d) Parkinson's disease is characterized by a deficit of the striatal dopamine (See critique of question #116 for a detailed explanation).

118. c) The tremor of Parkinson's disease is usually first noted as a rhythmic, alternating flexion and extension of the thumb and digits at a frequency of four to five cycles/second. This is known as the so-called "pill-rolling tremor". The tremor is prominent in the resting limb, disappears briefly during the course of the movement, and reappears when the limb is held in a static, unsupported posture. Tremor of the head, lips, tongue and feet may also occur.

   Propranolol is the treatment of choice for essential tremor, not the tremor of Parkinson's disease.

119. a) Several environmental agents induce symptoms of Parkinsonism, and it has been suggested that most cases of the disease result from the combination of neuronal loss from aging and exposure to other agents. Drugs probably represent the number one environmental agent. The most common classes of drugs producing Parkinsonism are the antipsychotics including both the phenothiazines and butyrophenones. Examples of these drugs include haloperidol, largactil and perphenazine. The antihypertensive agent reserpine which was formerly extensively used is also a potential cause. Diazepam is not associated with the production of Parkinsonism symptoms.

120. d) The principal pharmacologic agent for treating Parkinson's disease is levodopa (L-Dopa). The rationale for its use is to provide a precursor for dopamine synthesis in the basal ganglia. Dopamine itself does not cross the blood-brain barrier. The drug is usually administered in combination with carbidopa, an aromatic amino acid decarboxylase inhibitor. Because of the nearly inevitable complications of long term levodopa therapy including sleep disorders, confusion, agitation, depression, hallucinations, involuntary movements (dyskinesias and akinesia), many neurologists continue to treat mild cases of Parkinson's disease or drug-induced Parkinsonism with anticholinergic and antihistaminic agents. An anticholinergic agent such as trihexyphenidyl (2 mg. t.i.d.) may be used. When the symptoms become more pronounced, amantadine, which stimulates the release of dopamine from nerve terminals, may be tried. This agent is usually begun as a single morning dose of 100 mg. If adverse reactions do not occur this may be increased to 100 mg. b.i.d. In more advanced cases of Parkinson's disease in which symptoms interfere with the quality of life, the treatment of choice is levodopa combined with carbidopa. Three combinations of levodopa plus carbidopa (Sinemet) are available: 100 mg./10 mg., 100 mg./25 mg. and 250 mg./125 mg. Treatment must be individualized but commonly starts with 100 mg. levodopa and 10-25 mg. carbidopa orally two to four times/day. Severe cases may require a dose of 250 mg. levodopa and 25 mg. carbidopa orally six times/day.

   Bromocriptine, which acts as a dopamine receptor agonist, is currently under study for the treatment of Parkinson's disease. Unfortunately, it has as many side effects as levo-dopa and therefore its usefulness is limited.

121. a) Benign essential tremor is one of the most commonly encountered disorders of movement. It commonly has a hereditary pattern and is then known as familial tremor. In a sense, essential tremor represents an exaggeration of the "physiologic tremor" that occurs at times of stress, such as after drinking too much coffee. It predominantly affects the hands; the trunk and legs are infrequently involved. A nodding head tremor and tremulousness of speech are often observed. The tremor is characteristically an action tremor, prominent during the maintenance of a static posture or during fine manipulative activity such as handwriting.

122. a) The treatment of choice for benign essential tremor is propranolol. A dose of 40 to 60 mg. by mouth four times/day is generally required. In some patients propranolol is contraindicated or produces significant side effects; these patients may benefit from modest doses of alcohol or diazepam (5 mg tid). Levodopa-carbidopa is not indicated for the treatment of benign essential tremor.

Reference

Cutler R. Neurology: Degenerative and Hereditary Diseases. Scientific American Medicine: Rubenstein E and Federman D, editors. Scientific American Inorporated, New York: 1984; pages 11: IV, 4-7.

PROBLEM #16: A 35 YEAR OLD FEMALE WITH BILATERAL PAINFUL JOINTS IN HER WRISTS AND HANDS

123. A 35 year old female presents with a 3 month history of morning stiffness, pain on motion of both wrists and swelling in the metacarpal-phalangeal joints of both hands. The most likely diagnosis is:

   a) non-articular rheumatism
   b) synovitis
   c) gonococcal arthritis
   d) rheumatoid arthritis
   e) systemic lupus erythematosus

124. The single most common cause of arthritis in females aged 15-35 is:

   a) rheumatoid arthritis
   b) systemic lupus erythematosus
   c) gonococcal arthritis
   d) rubella
   e) traumatic arthritis

125. The drug of first choice for suppressing inflammation in patients with rheumatoid arthritis is:

   a) aspirin
   b) gold
   c) D-penicillamine
   d) naproxen
   e) indomethacin

126. The drug of first choice for the induction of remission in rheumatoid arthritis is:

   a) aspirin
   b) gold
   c) D-penicillamine
   d) naproxen
   e) indomethacin

127. The treatment of choice for the prevention of joint deformity in a single joint or multiple small joints in a patient with rheumatoid arthritis who is already on remission-inducing therapy is:

    a) systemic corticosteroids
    b) intra-articular corticosteroids
    c) D-penicillamine
    d) gold
    e) aspirin

128. Instability of the cervical spine is a major problem in patients with rheumatoid arthritis. This instability usually develops between:

    a) C5 and C6
    b) C4 and C5
    c) C3 and C4
    d) C2 and C3
    e) C1 and C2

ANSWERS

123. d) The patient presented in this question has definite rheumatoid arthritis by criteria laid down by the American Rheumatologic Society. The criteria (based on a duration of at least 6 weeks) are:

    1) morning stiffness
    2) pain on motion or tenderness in at least one joint
    3) swelling (soft-tissue thickening of fluid, not bony overgrowth alone) in at least one joint
    4) swelling of at least one other joint
    5) symmetrical joint swelling with simultaneous involvement of the same joint on both sides of the body; terminal phalangeal joint involvement will not satisfy this criteria
    6) subcutaneous nodules over bony prominences, on extensor surfaces, or in juxta-articular regions
    7) roentgenographic changes typical of rheumatoid arthritis (which must include at least bony decalcification localized to or greatest around the involved joints and not just degenerative changes
    8) positive agglutination (anti-gammaglobulin) test
    9) poor mucin precipitate from synovial fluid
    10) characteristic histologic changes in synovial membrane
    11) characteristic histologic changes in nodules

    If a patient has 7 of 11 categories positive he (she) has classic rheumatoid arithritis; 5 of 11 positive are definite rheumatoid arthritis; and 3 of 11 positive are probable rheumatoid arthritis. The patient described in question #123 has at least 5 criteria positive and therefore has definite rheumatoid arthritis.

With the joint involvement described non-articular rheumatism is by definition not a consideration. Synovitis is a pathological diagnosis and not a disease. Gonococcal arthritis is the single most common cause of arthritis in young sexually active females but usually has an acute onset affecting only one joint. None of the other organ manifestations that would make systemic lupus erythematosus a consideration are present.

124. c) The single most common cause of arthritis in females ages 15-35 years is gonococcal arthritis. This is much more common than any of the other entities listed in the question. Gonococcal arthritis is secondary to gonococcal septicemia from an acute episode of pelvic inflammatory disease. With gonococcemia characteristic skin lesions also develop. These are small hemorrhage-like spots 5 to 6 mm. in diameter with 1-2 mm. of central necrosis. Inflammation around tendon sheaths is characteristic of the condition. Single joints, especially those of the wrist, hand, ankle and foot are most often affected. Before beginning therapy with high dose intravenous penicillin, cultures of blood, skin and joint fluid should be performed to document sensitivity to penicillin.

125. a) The drug of first choice for suppressing inflammation in patients with rheumatoid arthritis is aspirin. Aspirin must be given in sufficient dose to reach a serum concentration of 20-30 mg./dl. of serum. Usually the dose is increased to maximum tolerated serum level (the level at which tinnitus occurs) and then cut back slightly. This is often in the range of 12-20 tablets/day. A much easier to take and more tolerable regime with fewer gastrointestinal side effects is enteric-coated aspirin which provides 650-975 mg. of aspirin in each tablet. Salicylate levels in the range of 20-30 mg./dl. are therapeutic.

   Gold and D-penicillamine are agents used to induce remission if spontaneous natural remission does not occur. Naproxen and indomethacin are non-steroidal anti-inflammatory agents that can be used in place of aspirin if intolerance, side effects, or other reasons preclude its use. Consideration should be given to the addition of antacids or stomach-coating agents such as sulcralfate to the treatment regime, as the anti-inflammatory agents will be used for indefinite period of time and are a major cause of gastric irritation and ulceration.

126. b) The drug of first choice for the induction of remission in rheumatoid arthritis is gold. Until recently, this was always given as an intramuscular injection of 50 mg. each week. Auranofin, a new conjugated oral gold compound will probably eliminate the need for intramuscular injections of gold. The usual starting dose for oral gold is 6 mg./day. D-penicillamine is the second-line agent but has considerably more toxicity than gold. Aspirin, naproxen, and indomethacin are non-steroidal anti-inflammatory agents and have no effect on inducing remission of the disease.

127. b) The prevention of deformities is a major aim of the treatment regime of patients with rheumatoid arthritis. Often, even after inflammation has been suppressed with aspirin or other non-steroidal anti-inflammatory agents and remission has been induced with oral gold one or more joints will flare up. By removing the accumulation of synovial fluid and injecting a long-acting steroid intraarticularly dramatic relief is often obtained. Oral corticosteroids can also be used but have many more side effects (especially a tendency to osteoporosis).

128. e) Cervical spine instability in patients with rheumatoid arthritis is often of life-threatening significance. Because of the synovitis attacking ligaments in the first and second cervical vertebral region a large proportion of patients with chronic rheumatoid arthritis (30-40%) develop significant instability of the cervical spine. About 5 % of these rheumatoid patients eventually go on to cord injury and myelopathy as a result of the cervical spine instability. The usual instability is anterior displacement of C-1 on C-2. The risk of cord injury during anaesthesia is particularly significant.

References

Connolly J, Jardon D. Orthopedics in Family Practice. Textbook of Family Practice 3rd edition; Rakel R, editor. W.B. Saunders Co., Philadelphia: 1984; pages 743-746.
Dorward B. Rheumatoid Arthritis. Primary Care 1984; 11(2): 233-241.

PROBLEM #17: A 51 YEAR OLD MALE WITH EPIGASTRIC PAIN

129. A 51 year old male presents with epigastric pain that begins several hours after meals and is relieved by foods or antacids. The pain often wakes him up in the middle of the night. Which of the following statements about this man's pain is FALSE?

    a) an upper gastrointestinal series is the diagnostic procedure of choice
    b) cigarette smoking may aggravate the condition
    c) alcohol may aggravate the condition
    d) the patient should be placed on a bland diet
    e) this condition may be aggravated by the ingestion of certain medications

130. The patient discussed in question #129 is diagnosed as having a duodenal ulcer. He is placed on antacid therapy. Which of the following statements regarding antacid therapy in the treatment of peptic ulcer disease is FALSE?

    a) antacids should be given 1 hour and 3 hours after meals and before bedtime
    b) antacids in tablet form are just as effective as antacids in liquid form
    c) magnesium hydroxide may produce diarrhea and hypokalemia
    d) aluminum hydroxide may produce constipation
    e) antacid treatment should continue for 4-6 weeks

131. The patient described in question #129 is placed on antacid therapy for the appropriate time interval. His symptoms recur 2 months after stopping therapy. Which of the following is the most appropriate course of action at this time?

    a) repeat the upper gastrointestinal series
    b) perform fiberoptic gastroscopy
    c) begin antacid therapy again
    d) select another anti-ulcer agent for therapy
    e) c or d

132. With which of the following conditions are non-steroidal anti-inflammatory drugs MOST CLOSELY associated?

    a) duodenal ulcer
    b) gastric ulcer
    c) reflux esophagitis
    d) duodenitis
    e) gastritis

CODE: (a: 1, 2 and 3; b: 1 and 3; c: 2 and 4; d: 4 only; e: all of the above)

133. Which of the following statements regarding cimetidine is/are TRUE?

    1) cimetidine is an H-1 histamine receptor antagonist
    2) cimetidine may be combined with antacids to increase the efficacy of treatment
    3) recurrence of peptic ulcer after 6 weeks of cimetidine therapy is unusual
    4) cemetidine is usually given in a dose of 1200 mg./day in two to four divided doses

134. With which of the following drugs does cimetidine interact?

    1) warfarin
    2) doxepin
    3) diazepam
    4) theophyllines

135. Which of the following statements regarding sucralfate is/are TRUE?

    1) sucralfate is usually given in a dose of 1 gram q.i.d. 1 hour before meals
    2) peptic ulcer recurrence rate with sulcralfate is similar to cimetidine
    3) peptic ulcer healing rate with sulcralfate is similar to cimetidine
    4) constipation is a significant side effect of sucralfate

ANSWERS

129. d) The patient presented in this question has a history typical of peptic ulcer disease. The diagnosis of peptic ulcer disease can often be suspected from the history. The classic pattern is described as a burning epigastric pain that begins several hours after meals and is relieved by food, antacids, or vomiting. The patient is often awakened at night by pain. As is true with many "classics" in medicine, this pattern is not seen in the majority of peptic ulcer patients and the diagnosis must be suspected in anyone complaining of upper abdominal pain.

An upper gastrointestinal series is the diagnostic procedure of choice. It will identify a duodenal ulcer in 80-90% of cases. If a gastric ulcer is seen endoscopy should be carried out as it is difficult to differentiate a benign from a malignant ulcer on the basis of an X-ray.

Both cigarette smoking and alcohol have been shown to aggravate peptic ulcer. The ingestion of certain medications, especially aspirin and the other non-steroidal anti-inflammatory drugs can aggravate or produce a peptic ulcer. There are absolutely no good studies that show that a bland diet or other special diets help heal ulcers. Frequent feedings and bedtime snacks will actually increase acid production.

130. b) Antacid therapy is still the cornerstone of ulcer management. It has been well documented that 30 mls of liquid antacid 1 hour and 3 hours after meals and at bedtime will give a buffering capacity of greater than 1000 meq. This will essentially eliminate gastric acidity for about 4 hours after each meal.

    Most antacids are combinations of aluminum hydroxide and magnesium hydroxide. Magnesium hydroxide tends to produce diarrhea with possible subsequent hypokalemia. Aluminum hydroxide tends to be constipating. When these two compounds are combined the side effects cancel each other. Calcium carbonate, which is the active component in a number of antacids may lead to hypercalcemia and the milk-alkali syndrome.

    Antacid therapy given in the liquid form has a much greater acid binding capacity than when given in the tablet form. The liquid form is therefore the preferred formulation. Antacid therapy should be continued for 4-6 weeks to allow adequate healing time for the ulcer.

131. e) Peptic ulcer disease should be thought of as a recurrent disease. Relapses are the rule, with 60-90% of patients relapsing within 12 months. The recurrence rate appears to be the same, regardless of therapy. If recurrent symptoms are identical to previous episodes, no diagnostic tests need to be run, and treatment can be restarted immediately. You have the option of restarting the same treatment regime used previously or using another agent. In the case of the patient discussed in this case either restarting antacids or beginning therapy with cimetidine or sulcralfate would be appropriate.

132. e) Non-steroidal anti-inflammatory drugs are notorious for causing gastrointestinal side effects. All of the drugs in this class, including aspirin, have been implicated in the development of gastritis, duodenitis, and peptic ulceration. Gastritis is the most common condition produced by these agents. For this reason, non-steroidal anti-inflammatory drugs should be prescribed to be taken with meals or milk. Another option is to use sucralfate 1 gram along with each dose of anti-inflammatory drug.

133. c) Cimetidine is an H-2 histamine receptor antagonist that is now the most commonly prescribed treatment for peptic ulcer disease. The total daily dose of cimetidine for peptic ulcer disease is 1200 mg./day, divided into 2-4 doses, and given for 4-6 weeks. This will produce healing in 90% of patients. Cimetidine should not be combined with antacids; there is no increase in efficacy of treatment with this regime. Recurrence of peptic ulcer occurs at the same rate regardless of the treatment provided. Some experts are recommending prophylaxis with cimetidine 400 mg. hs on a long-term basis.

134. e) Cimetidine delays hepatic microsomal metabolism of any drug that is primarily excreted by the liver. Examples of these drugs include the anticoagulant warfarin, all drugs in the tricyclic antidepressant group (including doxepin), diazepam and all of its derivatives and all drugs in the theophylline class. Because of the delay of excretion induced by cimetidine, the dose of the other agents has to be adjusted accordingly.

135. e) Sucralfate is a complex of sulfated sucrose and aluminum hydroxide which acts locally on the gastrointestinal tract. Upon contact with gastric acid it is transformed into a viscous adhesive with a high affinity for defective mucosa. It forms a protective shield which prevents acid pepsin and bile salts from reaching the ulcer. It also complexes with plasma proteins contained in the ulcer, protecting them from the action of pepsin. Peptic ulcer patients treated with sucralfate have the same heading rates and recurrence rates as patients treated with cimetidine or antacids. Constipation is a significant side effect, occuring in up to 10% of patients. Sucralfate is usually given in a dose of 1 gram q.i.d. before meals.

Reference

Boydstein J, Barker J and Lawhorne L. Gastrointestinal Disorders. Textbook of Family Practice 3rd edition; Rakel R, editor. W.B. Saunders Co., Philadelphia: 1984; pages 1008-1011.

PROBLEM #18: A 50 YEAR OLD MALE ADMITTED TO THE EMERGENCY DEPARTMENT WITH RETROSTERNAL CHEST PAIN

136. A 50 year old male is admitted to the emergency department with acute retrosternal chest pain. As he is being assessed he suddenly lapses into unconsciousness. Quick-look paddles reveal ventricular fibrillation. Initial treatment of the patient described above should be:

a) synchronized cardioversion at 100 joules
b) defibrillation at 200-360 joules
c) defibrillation at 100-200 joules
d) lidocaine 1 mg./kg. bolus followed by an infusion of 2 mg./min
e) bretylium 5 mg./kg bolus

137. The patient described in question #136 is treated appropriately and sinus rhythm is restored. An acute myocardial infarction is documented on the ECG. You are concerned about dysrhythmias developing in the next 24 hours. The drug of choice for the prevention of ventricular dsyrhythmias is:

a) bretylium
b) procainamide
c) lidocaine
d) dopamine
e) isoproterenol

138. The patient described in question #136 is doing well until 18 hours post-admission. At that time his blood pressure drops from 110/70 to 70/50 and his ECG shows sinus bradycardia at a rate of 40 beats/minute. Your next course of action should be:

a) observation only
b) isoproterenol infusion at 2-20 micrograms/minute
c) atropine 0.5 mg. IV
d) instillation of a temporary transvenous pacemaker
e) dopamine infusion at 1-2 μg./kg./min

139. A 65 year old male is admitted to the emergency room with an acute onset of a "fluttering heart". His blood pressure is 100/70 and a rhythm strip shows ventricular tachycardia. The treatment of choice at this time is:

a) synchronized cardioversion at 50 joules
b) synchronized cardioversion at 20 joules
c) lidocaine 1 mg./kg. bolus and a lidocaine infusion of 2 mg./min
d) a precordial thump followed by synchronized cardioversion at 50 joules
e) procainamide 100 mg. bolus (20 mg./min) followed by a procainamide infusion of 2 mg./min

140. CPR is in progress on a 60 year old male who collapsed in the emergency department. A blood gas sample is drawn and the following results are obtained.

    pH- 7.10
    pCO_2- 60 mm.Hg
    pO_2- 75 mm.Hg
    pCO_3- 15 mmol./litre

    This represents:

    a) metabolic acidosis with respiratory alkalosis
    b) respiratory acidosis with metabolic alkalosis
    c) pure metabolic acidosis
    d) pure respiratory acidosis
    e) mixed respiratory and metabolic acidosis

141. Which of the following factors is the MOST important predictor of late mortality following myocardial infarction?

    a) age of the patient
    b) history of angina pectoris
    c) reduced left ventricular ejection fraction
    d) presence of systolic hypertension on admission
    e) presence of premature ventricular contractions in the late in-hospital phase

CODE: (a:1, 2 and 3; b: 1 and 3; c: 2 and 4; d: 4 only; e: all of the above)

142. Which of the following is/are important prognostic factors in the actue phase for patients who have suffered a myocardial infarction?

    1) age of the patient
    2) history of previous angina or myocardial infarction
    3) evidence on the CXR of cardiac enlargement and pulmonary congestion
    4) systolic arterial pressure at the time of admission

143. Regarding the rehabilitation of patients who have suffered a myocardial infarction, which of the following statements is/are TRUE?

    1) psychologically induced invalidism is extremely common following myocardial infarction
    2) marital sexual relations can usually be resumed at 3-4 weeks after infarction
    3) exercise treadmill tests in the second or third week after myocardial infarction has been demonstrated to be safe in selected uncomplicated cases
    4) a progressive increase in physical activities aimed at a return to normal function in about six months should be a prime objective in convalescence after acute myocardial infarction

144. The use of which of the following medications has been shown to reduce mortality in the first three years following a myocardial infarction?

    1) aspirin
    2) sulfinpyrazone
    3) dipyridamole
    4) timolol

ANSWERS

136. b) Witnessed cardiac arrest caused by ventricular fibrillation should be treated immediately by defibrillation at 200-360 joules. If the first shock is unsuccessful it should be repeated at maximal energy level (360 joules). If the second shock is unsuccessful drug therapy including epinephrine and lidocaine should be administered. Synchronized cardioversion is not used for ventricular fibrillation but rather for ventricular tachycardia, acute atrial fibrillation and acute atrial flutter. Defibrillation at lower than 200 joules will result in a lower conversion rate than defibrillation at 200 joules or greater. Lidocaine and bretylium are useful anti-arrhythmic drugs but should be given only after the dysrhythmia has been converted (unless 2 unsuccessful attempts have already been made).

137. c) Lidocaine is still the number one agent for the treatment of ventricular dysrhythmias. It is usually given as a bolus dose of 1 mg./kg. to be repeated to a total dose of 225 mg; and an infusion rate of 2-4 mg./min is begun at the time the first bolus dose is given. Bretylium and procainamide are both second line agents that may be used if lidocaine fails. Bretylium is usually given as a bolus dose of 5 mg./kg. and repeated every 10-15 minutes at a dose of 10 mg./kg. to a maximum dose of 30 mg./kg. Alternatively, after the first bolus dose an infusion of 2-4 mg./min is then established. Dopamine is used to correct hypotension and increase perfusion of vital organs. Isoproterenol is not useful in the treatment of dysrhythmias; it produces dysrhythmias by its beta-receptor stimulating action.

138. c) Hemodynamically significant sinus bradycardia should first be treated with a parasympatholytic agent such as atropine 0.5 mg. IV. The increase in heart rate produced by atropine should raise the cardiac output and correct the hemodynamic compromise. If atropine is unsuccessful isoproterenol by infusion at 2-20 μg./minute should be given. Sinus bradycardia rarely has to be treated by pacemaker insertion, which is the next step. Dopamine could be used in this situation to raise the blood pressure but is not the drug of choice.

139. c) The treatment of choice for ventricular tachycardia depends on whether or not there is hemodynamic compromise. In a patient with a blood pressure of 100/70 conservative treatment with lidocaine 1 mg./kg. bolus and a lidocaine infusion of 2 mg./min should be initiated. If, on the other hand, the patient is hemodynamically compromised synchronized cardioversion at 50-200 joules should be initiated. If ventricular tachycardia develops under supervision a precordial thump can be tried prior to electrical conversion. The patient should be sedated with diazepam or similar medication prior to electrical conversion.

140. e) Most patients who are undergoing cardiopulmonary resuscitation have a mixed respiratory and metabolic acidosis. Normal pCO_2 is 40 mm.Hg. The patient in this case has a markedly elevated pCO_2 of 60 mm.Hg. and thus is being hypoventilated. The patient's bicarbonate level of 15 mmol./litre is below the normal range of 21-28 mmol./litre and thus the patient has a metabolic acidosis as well. It is quite likely that bicarbonate therapy would not be needed in this case; checking the airway and increasing the alveolar ventilation will probably correct the problem.

141. c) Reduced left ventricular ejection fraction is the single most important predictor of late mortality following myocardial infarction. Left ventricular ejection fractions of less than 50% are associated with much higher mortality rates than ejection fractions greater than 50%. Older age, a history of angina pectoris, and the presence of systolic hypertension on admission are important risk factors in the early in-hospital phase. The other significant predictor of late mortality is a history of multiple myocardial infarctions.

142. e) A prognostic index based on six clinical features that can be determined soon after admission including age, history of previous angina or infarction, systolic arterial pressure at the time of admission, type of ECG pattern, and evidence on the CXR of cardiac enlargement and pulmonary congestion identifies patients at high risk for mortality during the acute phase.

143. a) Psychologically induced invalidism is extremely common following myocardial infarction. Preventing this invalidism is often the greatest contribution the family physician can make.

    Marital sexual activity can usually be resumed by 3-4 weeks post-infarction. Marital sexual activity in middle-aged men typically increases the heart rate to only 120-130 beats/minute and is comparable to walking up one flight of stairs.

Treadmill exercise testing in the second or third week after acute myocardial infarction has been demonstrated to be safe in selected uncomplicated cases. Such testing often shows arrhythmias or ischemic ST segment changes that might not have been recognized otherwise. These findings may have prognostic value and affect the advice given to the patient regarding activity and return to work. Perhaps the greatest value of early exercise tests is that many patients show good exercise performance without ischemia or arrhythmia; in these patients rehabilitation can be rapid and complete and the psychologic support from the test performance is great. The prime objective in cardiac rehabilitation after acute myocardial infarction should be a progressive increase in physical activities aimed at a return to normal function about two months after acute infarction, not six months as suggested in the question.

144. d) Only the beta-blocking agents including timolol, propranolol, metoprolol, atenolol and nadolol have been shown to be associated with decreased mortality in the first 3 years after myocardial infarction. Aspirin, sulfinpyrazone and dipyridamole have not been shown to be of significant benefit, although large studies are now under way.

References

McIntyre K, Lewis A; editors. Textbook of Advanced Cardiac Life Support. American Heart Association, 1983.

Wenger N. Rehabilitation of the Patient with Myocardial Infarction. Primary Care 1981; 8(3): 491-507

PROBLEM #19: A 40 YEAR OLD OBESE MALE WITH AN ACUTELY INFLAMED LEFT GREAT TOE

145. A 40 year old obese male presents to the office after waking up with an acutely swollen left great toe. On examination, an erythematous, tender, swollen left great toe is seen. He has hypertension which is currently being treated with hydrochlorothiazide 100 mg./day. He is also an alcohol abuser. The most likely diagnosis is:

   a) acute rheumatoid arthritis
   b) acute gouty arthritis
   c) acute gonococcal arthritis
   d) acute septic arthritis
   e) acute osteomyelitis

146. For the disease described in the patient in question #145, the diagnostic test of choice is:

   a) a plasma level
   b) a random urine determination
   c) a 24 hour urine determination
   d) a synovial fluid analysis
   e) a Gram stain plus culture and sensitivity

147. The drug of choice for the initial management of the patient described in question #145 is:

   a) indomethacin
   b) colchicine
   c) naproxen
   d) aspirin
   e) phenylbutazone

148. The patient described in question #145 has a 24 hour urine collected. His 24 hour urine output of uric acid is 400 mg. His serum uric acid level is 550 mmol./litre (9.1 mg./dl). The first step that should be undertaken in this patient's treatment to reduce the chance of subsequent attacks is:

   a) begin treatment with probenecid
   b) begin treatment with sulfinpyrazone
   c) begin treatment with allopurinol
   d) begin treatment with indomethacin
   e) decrease the dose of hydrochlorothiazide

149. The treatment of choice for asymptomatic hyperuricemia is:

   a) probenecid
   b) sulfinpyrazone
   c) allopurinol
   d) a or b
   e) none of the above

CODE: (a:1, 2 and 3; b: 1 and 3; c: 2 and 4; d: 4 only; e: all of the above)

150. The drug(s) of choice for the prophylaxis of gouty arthritis in patients that are underexcretors of uric acid is/are:

   1) indomethacin
   2) probenecid
   3) allopurinol
   4) sulfinpyrazone

151. The drug(s) of choice for the prophylaxis of gouty arthritis in patients that are overproducers of uric acid is/are:

   1) indomethacin
   2) probenecid
   3) sulfinpyrazone
   4) allopurinol

152. Which of the following statements is/are TRUE regarding pseudogout?

   1) pseudogout is caused by the deposition of calcium carbonate crystals within the joint
   2) the crystals associated with pseudogout are rhomboidal or rectangular in shape
   3) pseudogout is most often detected in the small joints of the hand
   4) the crystals associated with pseudogout are positively birefringent

ANSWERS

145. b) The most likely diagnosis is acute gouty arthritis. The presentation given in this question is typical for acute gouty arthritis. Aggravating factors in this patient's case include a high purine diet associated with obesity, hydrochloro-thiazide treatment for hypertension and alcohol abuse. None of the other options listed are reasonable choices. Acute rheumatoid arthritis usually affects larger joints such as knees, wrists and ankles. Acute gonococcal arthritis is the most common cause of acute arthritis in young sexually active females (often secondary to pelvic inflammatory disease). Acute septic arthritis and acute osteomyelitis do not usually present in the great toe.

146. d) The first important step in the management of gout is to establish the correct diagnosis. The precise method of diagnosis is the demonstration of crystals in synovial fluid. The aspiration of fluid from a joint or tendon sheath is safe, and identification of crystals provides a solid diagnostic platform upon which to base years of potential treatment. In addition, the critical diagnosis of septic arthritis can be ruled out by appropriate stains and cultures of the same specimen of synovial fluid. The appearance of needle-shaped crystals which are negatively birefringent under a polarizing microscope is a diagnosis of urate crystals, and therefore gout.

147. a) Until recently, the drug of choice for the treatment of acute gout was colchicine. However, this agent has many gastrointestinal side effects which limit its usefulness. Many authorities now recommend indomethacin 50 mg. t.i.d. as the agent of choice. If given 1/2 hour before meals and taken with an antacid, the gastrointestinal side effects of indomethacin will be minimized. I have found the use of sucralfate 1 gram t.i.d. with indomethacin a useful adjuvant. The indomethacin should ideally be given for 1-2 weeks until treatment aimed at decreasing the uric acid pool is begun.

Aspirin in small doses (>2.0 grams) per day can actually aggravate the problem. Naproxen and other non-steroidal anti-inflammatories may be just as effective as indomethacin but experts seem to favor indomethacin because of its superior anti-inflammatory activity. Phenylbutazone is an excellent anti-inflammatory agent but has now been associated with bone marrow suppression and aplastic anemia.

148. e) The first step in the treatment of this patient should be to decrease his dose of hydrochlorothiazide. Prior to his attack of acute gouty arthritis he was taking 100 mg./day. Recent studies have shown that there is little increase in efficacy of treatment of hypertension past 25-50 mg./day; while side effects including hyperuricemia, hyperglycemia, hyperlipidemia and hypokalemia increase. His dose of hydrochlorothiazide should probably be decreased to 25 mg./day and his blood pressure watched carefully. If his serum uric acid decreases to less than 440 mmol./litre probably no treatment other than life style changes including decreasing his intake of red meat and alcohol should be advised. If these measures do not reduce the serum uric acid, then either probenecid (250-500 mg./day) or sulfinpyrazone (100-400 mg./day) should be begun once the acute attack has subsided. These agents are used when the patient is an "underexcretor" (<700 mg. uric acid/24 hour urine) rather than an "overproducer" (>700 mg. uric acid/24 hour urine). This patient's 24 hour urine uric acid of 400 mg. indicates that he is an "underexcretor". Allopurinol is used only when the patient is an "overproducer" of uric acid; has gouty tophi; has a history of renal calculi or has uric acid nephropathy. The daily dose is 100-300 mg./day. Indomethacin is useful only in the treatment, not the prevention, of acute gout.

149. e) It is currently felt that asymptomatic hyperuricemia should not be treated because only 10% of hyperuricemic patients eventually develop gout. Rather, efforts should concentrate on dietary modification to decrease the meat (purine) intake, decrease alcohol intake, and decrease or discontinue medications such as diuretics or ASA.

150. c) See critique of question #148.

151. d) See critique of question #148.

152. c) Although pseudogout does not usually produce the intense inflammation that gout does, synovial fluid analysis may lead to confusion. The crystals of pseudogout, which are composed of calcium pyrophosphate, are rectangular or rhomboidal in shape and are positively birefringent. They are most often found in synovial fluid aspirated from large joints such as the knee.

Reference

Wisner P, Simkin P. Management of Gout and Hyperuricemia. Primary Care 1984; 11(2): 283-294.

PROBLEM #20: A 45 YEAR OLD MALE WEIGHING 320 POUNDS AND COMPLAINING OF FATIGUE

153. A 320 pound, 45 year old male presents to your office complaining of fatigue. You decide that his fatigue is mainly due to his morbid obesity and send him for dietary counselling. The dietician puts him on a 1300 Kcal/day diet and calculates his ideal weight at 170 lbs. Assuming that his activity level does not change, that his total energy expenditure is 2300 Kcal/day, and that he sticks to his diet, how long will it take him to reach his ideal weight?

   a) 125 days
   b) 225 days
   c) 325 days
   d) 425 days
   e) 525 days

154. Obesity is generally defined as:

   a) an increase in the ponderal index of 20% above normal
   b) a decrease in the ponderal index of 30% below normal
   c) an increase in the body mass index of 20% above normal
   d) an increase in the body mass index of 30% above normal
   e) none of the above

155. The overall incidence of obesity in North Americans is:

   a) 1%
   b) 5%
   c) 10%
   d) 20%
   e) 50%

156. Which of the following conditions is MOST CONSISTENTLY associated with obesity?

   a) alveolar hypoventilation syndrome
   b) hypertension
   c) hyperlipidemia
   d) diabetes mellitus
   e) angina pectoris

157. The use of severe calorie restricted diets (<800 Kcal/day) has been responsible for many deaths. The most common cause of death in these cases has been:

   a) sudden cardiac death
   b) congestive cardiac failure secondary to anemia
   c) hepatic failure
   d) renal failure
   e) septicemia

CODE: (a:1, 2 and 3; b: 1 and 3; c: 2 and 4; d: 4 only; e: all of the above)

158. Many therapeutic options have been tried in an effort to help patients lose weight. Which of the following options have been shown to be efficacious and safe?

    1) the prescription of amphetamines and other anoretic drugs
    2) the prescription of a diet sheet with first follow-up in one months time
    3) the jejunoileal bypass procedure
    4) behavior modication programs

ANSWERS

153. e) Each additional pound of fat represents an accumulation of 3500 extra Kcal. Therefore, if his total energy expenditure per day is 2300 Kcal and he is only taking in 1300 Kcal, his energy deficit is 1000 Kcal/day. His excess weight above ideal weight of 150 lbs corresponds to 525,000 Kcal. Therefore, it will take him 525 days to lose the 150 extra pounds IF he sticks to his diet.

154. c) The definition of obesity has been the subject of much controversy. It is generally accepted that an increase in relative weight for height (body mass index) greater than 20% above normal is considered as obesity and less than 20% is simply designated as being overweight. Ponderal index is a measure of height/weight.

155. d) The overall incidence of obesity in North Americans is approximately 20% of the population. In certain groups the incidence is as high as 40-50%. The highest incidence appears in those individuals in the lowest socioeconomic groups with improvement with change to higher levels.

156. b) Obesity is associated with many chronic diseases. These include cardiomyopathy, alveolar hypoventilation syndrome, angina pectoris and sudden cardiac death, hyperlipidemia, diabetes mellitus, degenerative joint disease, cholelithiasis, gout, varicose viens, thromboembolic disease and endometrial carcinoma. However, the disease most consistently correlated with obesity is hypertension. In the Framingham study hypertension was 10X more common among obese individuals than among non-obese ones.

157. a) The most common cause of death recorded in patients on severe calorie restricted diets has been sudden cardiac death. This in many cases appears to have been secondary to hypokalemia-induced dysrhythmias (particularly ventricular fibrillation). The other causes listed have not been frequently documented as causes of death.

158. d) The therapy of obesity has a relatively low success rate. Amphetamines and anorectic drugs should not be given. They have cardiovascular and central nervous system side effects and are not recommended. The handing out of a diet sheet to a patient, with instructions to follow it and report back, has resulted in a greater than 90% failure rate. The jejunoileal bypass operation has a greater than 50% morbidity (including hepatic dysfunction) and a mortality rate of 8-10%. Behavior modification programs which encourage sensible eating habits and educate the patient about the causes of overeating still offer the best hope for long-term success.

Reference

Steffie W. The Medical Syndrome of Obesity. Primary Care 1982; 9(3): 581-593.

PROBLEM #21: A 45 YEAR OLD MALE WITH CHRONIC RENAL FAILURE

159. A 45 year old male with chronic renal failure presents with a 1 month history of constipation. Which of the following laxatives are CONTRAIN-DICATED in this patient?

    a) mineral oil
    b) docusate sodium
    c) psyllium (Metamucil)
    d) senekot
    e) magnesium hydroxide

160. The most common cause of chronic renal failure is:

    a) glomerulonephritis
    b) chronic pyelonephritis
    c) hypertensive renal disease
    d) diabetes mellitus
    e) congenital anomalies

161. The least common cause of chronic renal failure among thoses causes listed below is:

    a) glomerulonephritis
    b) chronic pyelonephritis
    c) hypertensive renal disease
    d) diabetes mellitus
    e) congenital anomalies

162. Which of the following antihypertensive agents are CONTRAINDICATED in patients with chronic renal disease?

    a) hydrochlorothiazide-triamterene
    b) furosemide
    c) prazosin
    d) captopril
    e) alpha-methyldopa

163. The major cause of death in patients with chronic renal failure is:

    a) uremia
    b) malignant hypertension
    c) hyperkalemia-induced arrhythmias
    d) myocardial infarction
    e) subarachnoid hemorrhage

164. The anemia associated with chronic renal failure usually is:

    a) hypochromic
    b) macrocytic
    ʼc) normochromic-normocytic
    d) microcytic
    e) hypochromic-microcytic

CODE: (a:1, 2 and 3; b: 1 and 3; c: 2 and 4; d: 4 only; e: all of the above)

165. Which of the following metabolic abnormalities is/are commonly seen in patients with chronic renal failure?

    1) hypernatremia
    2) hypertriglyceridemia
    3) hyperparathyroidism
    4) hypokalemia

ANSWERS

159. e) Most patients with chronic renal failure have hypermagnesemia. Therefore, laxatives containing magnesium or antacids containing magnesium should be avoided or severe hypermagnesemia and related muscle weakness may result.

160. a) The most common cause of chronic renal failure is glomerulonephritis. Glomerulonephritis is the cause of renal failure in about 40% of patients. Another 33% result from congenital anomalies, hypertensive renal disease, diabetes mellitus or infections. Slightly more than 25% of patients have chronic renal failure as a result of a number of rarer causes.

161. b) Chronic pyelonephritis was once thought to be a common cause of chronic renal failure, but it is now known to be very rare. Because many patients on dialysis have small kidneys they are assumed to have pyelonephritis; however, most of them do not. Pyelonephritis in relation to chronic renal failure is seen only when something is wrong with the collecting system as well; that is, when obstruction is present.

162. a) Potassium-sparing diuretics such as hydrochlorothiazide-triamterene should not be administered to patients with chronic renal failure. The decreased urine output seen with chronic renal failure subsequently causes the concentration of potassium in the extracellular fluid to increase. This hyperkalemia will be aggravated by potassium-sparing diuretics. All of the other agents including hydrochlorothiazide (alone), furosemide, prazosin, captopril and alpha-methyldopa are safe in chronic renal failure.

163. d) The major causes of death in patients with chronic renal failure are myocardial infarction and cerebrovascular accidents, secondary to atherosclerosis and arteriolosclerosis. Uremia itself can usually be controlled by dialysis or renal transplantation. Hypertension is usually controllable by step-care therapy. Arrhythmias, although they do occur in these patients, are not the major cause of death. Subarachnoid hemorrhage, as a subset of cerebrovascular accident, does occur, but is less common as a cause of death than myocardial infarction.

164. c) Anemia is a common finding in chronic renal failure and is usually normochromic-normocytic. Hematocrit often starts to decrease when the serum creatinine reaches 200-300 micromoles/litre (2-3 mg./dl.), or when the glomerular filtration rate has decreased to about 20-30 mls/minute. Uremic patients usually do not make enough red blood cells. It is not clear why erythropoiesis is decreased but it has been suggested that uremic patients also suffer a decrease in kidney-produced erythropoietin.

165. a) A wide range of metabolic abnormalities including hypernatremia, water retention, hyperkalemia, hypermagnesemia, hypertriglyceridemia, hyperuricemia, hyperglycemia, hyperprolactinemia and elevation of serum growth hormone occur in chronic renal failure. Hypokalemia does not occur in chronic renal failure.

Reference

Lazarus J. When Chronic Renal Failure accelerates. Patient Care 1981; 15(11): 119-140.

PROBLEM #22: A 65 YEAR OLD MALE WITH NEW ONSET SEIZURE

166. A 65 year old male is brought to the emergency department after suffering a seizure while eating a meal in a restaurant. His wife states that this is his first seizure. The most common cause of a new onset seizure in a patient over the age of 40 years is:

   a) idiopathic
   b) a metabolic problem
   c) head trauma
   d) an old stroke
   e) a brain tumor

167. Characteristics of temporal lobe epilepsy (psychomotor seizures) include all of the following except:

   a) a visceral aura
   b) déjà vu symptoms
   c) behavioral abnormalities
   d) lip smacking
   e) 3/second spike and wave complexes on the EEG

CODE: (a:1, 2 and 3; b: 1 and 3; c: 2 and 4; d: 4 only; e: all of the above)

168. In contrast to generalized seizures, partial seizures:

   1) are bilaterally symmetric without local onset
   2) may exhibit Todd's paralysis
   3) rarely become generalized
   4) are usually accompanied by an aura

169. The drug(s) of choice for the treatment of alcohol withdrawal seizures is/are:

   1) phenytoin
   2) phenobarbitol
   3) carbamazepine
   4) diazepam

170. The drug(s) of first choice for typical absence epilepsy is/are:

   1) ethosuximide
   2) phenytoin
   3) valproic acid
   4) phenobarbitol

171. Regarding anticonvulsant therapy, which of the following statements is/are TRUE?

    1) plasma concentration of anticonvulsants are of little practical value in treating patients with epilepsy
    2) polytherapy is generally preferred to monotherapy
    3) most anticonvulsants do not interact with one another
    4) fever, fatigue, exhaustion and alcohol use may provoke seizures and require an adjustment of anticonvulsant dose

ANSWERS

166. e) The common causes of new onset seizures by age are:

    a) less than 10 years: i) idiopathic
                            ii) congenital
                            iii) birth injury
                            iv) metabolic
    b) 10-40 years of age: i) idiopathic
                            ii) head trauma
                            iii) preexisting focal brain disease
                            iv) drug withdrawal
    c) greater than 40 years: i) brain tumor
                               ii) old stroke
                               iii) trauma

167. e) Temporal lobe (psychmotor) epilepsy refers to seizures with complex symptomatology that originate in the temporal lobe. The initial complex is often of visceral origin, such as abdominal pain, "butterflies", and "funny feelings". Lip-smacking, repetitive motion of the extremities, behavioral abnormalities, lack of responsiveness, and other automatisms are characteristic features during which the patient is usually unresponsive to the environment. There is usually a period of post-ictal confusion and some drowsiness or amnesia for the event. The treatment of choice is carbamazepine, phenytoin, or phenobarbitol. A spike or sharp wave discharge on the electroencephalogram helps confirm the diagnosis. The 3/second spike and wave discharge is characteristic of petit mal rather than temporal lobe epilepsy.

    Carbamazepine is usually given in a dose of 600 mg./day, although 800-1200 mg./day may be required. Phenytoin is usually given in a dose of 300-400 mg./day and phenobarbitol in a dose of 90-180 mg./day.

168. c) Partial seizures may originate from the frontal, parietal or temporal lobes. They are usually accompanied by an aura, often visceral in origin. This can be a vague sensation of "butterflies" or "funny feelings". Partial seizures may exhibit Todd's paralysis (a persistence of the focal deficit for up to 24 hours

after the seizure). Partial seizures may become secondarily generalized and bilaterally symmetric but not without focal onset. Generalized seizures are bilaterally symmetric from the outset, usually not accompanied by an aura and they do not exhibit Todd's paralysis.

169. d) The drugs of choice for alcohol withdrawal seizures are diazepam and chlordiazepoxide. None of the usual anticonvulsants including phenytoin, phenobarbitol or carbamazepine are effective. Chlordiazepoxide is usually begun as 50-100 mg. IV, then 50 mg. in 2-4 hours if necessary. Diazepam is usually begun as 10 mg. IV and repeated in 2-4 hours in necessary.

170. b) Absence seizures (petit mal epilepsy) constitute an idiopathic primary generalized seizure disorder that is not associated with underlying structural pathology. The age of onset is between 5 months and 12 years of age, and over 75% of patients are in remission before they reach adulthood. Petit mal epilepsy has a characteristic pattern of ongoing activity, altered level of consciousness, staring spells with no gross body movements, but associated symptoms of eye-flickering and mild twitching. The child snaps out of the seizure as abruptly as he went into it, and there is no post-ictal confusion or altered consciousness. Usually, the episode lasts from 5-20 seconds. These seizures are usually augmented by hyperventilation or reproduced by it and this serves as a useful clinical test. The drugs of choice are ethosuximide or valproic acid. The classical electroencephalogram pattern is one of synchronous bursts of generalized, three/second spike and wave complexes that are usually reproducible and/or augmented with hyperventilation.

171. d) Plasma concentrations are essential to gauge therapy in patients with epilepsy. Keeping the drug(s) in the therapeutic range will ensure optimal control. As well, significant drug-drug interactions (between different classes of anticonvulsants) raise or lower serum levels of the first drug when the second one is added. For this and other reasons, monotherapy is preferable to polytherapy. Fever, fatigue, exhaustion and alcohol may decrease the seizure threshold and make alteration in medication dose essential.

Reference

Pohowalla P, Hogen V, McIntyre H. Evaluation of the Patient with New Onset Seizures. Primary Care 1984; 11(4): 625-642.

PROBLEM #23: A 26 YEAR OLD MALE WITH ACNE

172. A 26 year old male presents to your office with multiple facial acne scars. He is depressed and wishes to have the scars removed. You should tell him that:

    a) there is no hope for removing existing acne scars
    b) the treatment of choice is collagen implant
    ·c) the treatment of choice is dermabrasion
    d) a prolonged course of isotretinoin should significantly improve his complexion
    e) cryotherapy is the treatment of choice

CODE: (a:1, 2 and 3; b: 1 and 3; c: 2 and 4; d: 4 only; e: all of the above)

173. Which of the following foods and/or drugs has been implicated in the pathogenesis of acne?

    1) halogens, especially iodide in seafood, salt and health foods
    2) lithium carbonate
    3) phenytoin
    4) chocolate

174. Which of the following statements is/are TRUE regarding the use of benzoyl peroxide in the treatment of acne?

    1) it normalizes keratinization
    2) it is often used as a drying and desquamating agent
    3) it is generally applied three times/day
    4) the gel form is usually more effective than the lotion

175. Which of the following antibiotic(s) is/are effective when used in topical form for the treatment of acne vulgaris?

    1) erythromycin
    2) tetracycline
    3) clindamycin
    4) gentamicin

176. The antibiotic(s) of choice for the systemic therapy of acne vulgaris is/are:

    1) clindamycin
    2) tetracycline
    3) chloramphenicol
    4) erythromycin

177. Which of the following statements about the use of oral isotretinoin (Accutane) is/are TRUE?

    1) it is the only drug that works against all components of acne genesis
    2) isotretinoin is used in a dose of 0.5-1.0 mg./kg./day for 16-24 weeks
    3) isotretinoin prevents scarring and improves existing scars
    4) isotretinoin often causes significant elevation of serum cholesterol

ANSWERS

172. c) The treatment of choice for the removal of sharp-bordered, deep acne scars is dermabrasion. Collagen implant can be used to treat isolated shallow depressions but it is not useful for sharp-bordered "ice-pick" scars.

173. a) Ingestion of certain foods and drugs can cause acne eruptions. Halogens, especially an excess of iodide in seafood, salt and health foods can worsen acne. In controlled studies, chocolate has not been found to have a significant effect. High dose corticosteroids can cause a pustular form of acne, especially on the trunk. Stubborn acne is also seen in depressed patients on lithium therapy, as well as in epileptics who are taking phenytoin or phenobarbitol.

174. c) The topical agent chosen most often for initial treatment of acne vulgaris is benzoyl peroxide. The agent acts primarily as an antibiotic against Propionibacterium acnes, but also is often used for drying and desquamation to counteract excess sebum. It also causes superficial peeling and loosens comedones. Because of its drying and desquamating properties, benzoyl peroxide is often irritating to sensitive or relatively dry skin.

    Benzoyl peroxide products are available in acetone or water-based lotions, creams, or gels and washes in 2.5%, 5%, and 10% concentrations. As a rule of thumb, gels are most effective. Acetone bases should be used only on excessively oily skin. Water-based products are ideal for delicate or even dry skin. The usual protocol is to apply the medication in the morning after facial washing.

    Another first-line topical agent is tretinoin (Vitamin A acid gel). This is a retinoic acid that fights acne at its genesis; the microcomedo. It normalizes follicular keratinization and loosens horn cells. This product is available as a gel or a cream. Although the gel is more effective, it can cause excessive peeling or drying. The manufacturers emphasize the importance of using only mild soap and water 20 minutes before applying tretinoin. Tretinoin is usually applied at night and is begun at a concentration of 0.01%.

175. a) Antibiotics are often as effective when applied topically as when given in low dose oral form. Erythromycin, tetracycline and clindamycin are all available in topical lotion form. These products, when applied to a clean skin surface with a sponge applicator twice daily are effective in decreasing the level

of P. acnes. The destructive hydrolytic enzymes and chemotactic factors of P. acnes are decreased; lessening inflammation. Gentamicin is not available in a topical lotion and is not effective in treating acne vulgaris.

176. c) Oral antibiotics are still the foundation of many acne treatment protocols, with tetracycline and erythromycin being the most widely used. These agents act against P. acnes, reducing their number and consequently lessening inflammation. Tetracycline is usually begun as 250 mg. q.i.d. and tapered to 250-500 mg. daily for prolonged maintenance therapy. Erythromycin is given in divided doses of 750-1000 mg./day. Clindamycin is a major cause of pseudomembranous colitis and is not used systemically for acne treatment. Chloramphenicol is associated with aplastic anemia and is not appropriate for acne treatment.

177. a) Oral isotretinoin (Accutane) is now the treatment of choice for severe, recalcitrant nodulocystic acne. It is the only drug that works against all components of acne genesis. It is not only active against P. acnes, but it impedes comedogenesis and significantly inhibits sebum production. Remarkably, this drug is able to prevent scarring and also improve existing scars. It produces lasting remissions. Isotretinoin is initiated at 0.5 mg./kg. daily for 2-4 weeks as a single daily dose or in 2 divided doses. Maintenance therapy should be adjusted between 0.1 and 1 mg./kg./day. Therapy should be continued for 16-24 weeks.

Isotretinoin is a well-established teratogen. Pregnancy must be excluded before initiation of treatment. All women of childbearing potential who use the drug must use an adequate birth control method (preferrably the oral contraceptive pill). Because of the severe CNS defects seen in offspring of women who have taken the drug during pregnancy, abortion should be strongly considered should pregnancy occur during treatment.

Elevated serum triglycerides and liver enzymes are often seen in patients taking isotretinoin. Therefore, baseline levels should be drawn before therapy is commenced. Although serum cholesterol may be minimally elevated, the major change in cholesterol metabolism on isotretinoin is a decrease in the level of high density lipoprotein cholesterol.

Reference

Puissegur L. Acne vulgaris. Postgraduate Medicine 1985; 78(7): 76-84.

PROBLEM #24: A 25 YEAR OLD FEMALE WITH DYSURIA

178. A 25 year old female presents for her first prenatal assessment. A routine urine culture is performed and reveals a mixed growth of E.coli and Staph. epidermitis each at 10^4 organisms/ml. At this point you should:

   a) ignore the result as it is probably insignificant
   b) begin therapy with ampicillin to prevent pyelonephritis
   c) repeat the culture as two organisms grown probably indicate contamination
   d) consult a urologist
   e) begin therapy with trimethoprim-sulfamethoxazole to prevent pyelonephritis

179. The patient who is described in question #178 has a urine culture done at 20 weeks gestation because of a one week history of dysuria. The culture result shows E.coli growing at a concentration greater than 105 organisms/ml. While awaiting sensitivity results, which of the following antibiotics should NOT be used?

   a) ampicillin
   b) amoxicillin
   c) trimethoprim-sulfamethoxazole
   d) tetracycline
   e) a cephalosporin

180. The most common organism involved in urinary tract infections is:

   a) E.coli
   b) Klebsiella
   c) group D Streptococcus
   d) Streptococcus pneumoniae
   e) Staphylococcus aureus

181. A 24 year old female presents with a 1 week history of dysuria and frequency. Microscopic examination of the urine shows pyuria but not bacteriuria. The most likely organism causing this syndrome is:

   a) E.coli
   b) Chlamydia trachomatis
   c) T-strain mycoplasma
   d) Proteus mirabilis
   e) Serratia

CODE: (a:1, 2 and 3; b: 1 and 3; c: 2 and 4; d: 4 only; e: all of the above)

182. The treatment(s) of choice for uncomplicated urinary tract infection is/are:

    1) a single dose of amoxicillin 3.0 grams and 1.0 gram of probenecid
    2) a single dose of two double strength tablets of trimethoprim-sulfamethoxazole
    3) a single dose of 2.0 grams of sulfamethoxazole
    4) ampicillin 500 mg. q.i.d. for fourteen days

183. Which of the following statements concerning pyelonephritis is/are correct:

    1) acute episodes of pyelonephritis in adults often lead to chronic pyelonephritis
    2) any child with a urinary tract infection should be investigated to rule out structural abnormalities
    3) chronic pyelonephritis rarely presents focal areas of involvement
    4) acute pyelonephritis is manifested by loin pain, fever, chills, and symptoms of cystitis.

ANSWERS

178. c) In more than 95% of urinary tract infections, a single bacterial species is responsible for the infection. Therefore, whenever mixed bacterial species are grown out of culture, the likelihood of contamination is quite high and the culture should be repeated. Treatment with antibiotics is not appropriate until the second culture result comes back. Instruction in the proper collection of a mid-stream urine should be undertaken. A consultation with a urologist is not necessary at this time. Asymptomatic bacteriuria of pregnancy that is true bacteriuria should be treated, as 25% of untreated patients develop acute pyelonephritis.

179. d) Urinary tract infections in pregnancy can be safely treated with a 1 week course of ampicillin, amoxicillin, trimethoprim-sulfamethoxazole (except in the last month of pregnancy), or cephalosporins. Trimethoprim-sulfamethoxazole should not be used in the last month as it may displace bilirubin from binding sites during the neonatal period and lead to kernicterus. Tetracycline should not be used in pregnancy because it produces yellow discoloration in the teeth of the newborn.

180. a) E.coli is the most common organism involved in urinary tract infection-occurring in 89% of cases. Other organisms include Proteus mirabilis, Klebsiella pneumoniae, Pseudomonas aeruginosa, Serratia marcescens, and Staphylococcus aureus.

181. b) Dysuria and frequency with microscopic evidence of pyuria but no bacteriuria is best explained by the anterior urethral syndrome. In women presenting
with dysuria and frequency 1/3 of them have the anterior urethral syndrome
and 2/3 have bacterial cystitis. Chlamydia trachomatis is the most common
cause of the anterior urethral syndrome, followed by Mycoplasma species.
The treatment of choice is tetracycline or erythromycin 500 mg. t.i.d. for 1
week.

182. a) In uncomplicated urinary tract infections single dose therapy with either
ampicillin 3.5 grams plus 1.0 gram probenecid, amoxicillin 3.0 grams plus 1.0
gram probenecid, 2.0 grams of sulfamethoxazole or two double strength
tablets of trimethoprim-sulfamethoxazole is appropriate therapy that will
produce a cure in 85% of acute bacterial urinary tract infections. Compliance
is much greater with single dose therapy and thus the cure rate is theoretically
greater. Ampicillin in a dose of 500 mg. q.i.d. for 14 days does not result in an
increased cure rate and is much more difficult to comply with; it is therefore
not recommended for initial therapy.

183. c) Acute pyelonephritis usually presents with flank pain, fever, rigors, dysuria,
frequency and other systemic symptoms. Episodes of acute pyelonephritis in
adults rarely lead to chronic pyelonephritis and pathologically often appear as
focal areas of renal infection with intervening normal non-infected areas.

In children, the anatomy of the urinary tract makes the possibility of
vesicoureteral reflux secondary to structural abnormalites and subsequent
chronic pyelonephritis much more likely, especially in males. Therefore, even
one episode of urinary tract infection in a boy should be investigated with
intravenous pyelography and voiding cystourethrography. A girl should be
investigated after the second episode.

Reference

Rubin R. Infections of the urinary tract. Scientific American Medicine. Rubenstein E. and
Federman D., editors. New York: 1984; 7(8) XXIII; 1-12.

PROBLEM #25: A 75 YEAR OLD MALE WITH INFLUENZA

184. A 75 year old male presents with headache, non-specific myalgias, cough, fever and chills. You suspect influenza. The most common initial symptoms in influenza is:

    a) cough
    b) headache
    c) myalgia
    d) fever
    e) chills

185. Influenza vaccination is extremely effective in the prevention of influenza. For which of the following groups is routine immunization NOT recommended?

    a) diabetics
    b) immunocompromised individuals
    c) patients over the age of 65
    d) children under the age of 1 year
    e) patients with chronic renal disease

186. The major cause of death from influenza is due to:

    a) viral meningitis
    b) staphylococcal pneumonia
    c) pneumococcal pneumonia
    d) acute viral encephalopathy
    e) dehydration

CODE: (a:1, 2 and 3; b: 1 and 3; c: 2 and 4; d: 4 only; e: all of the above)

187. Which of the following statements regarding influenza viral infections is/are CORRECT?

    1) infections with Type A influenza are more common than infections with Type B
    2) influenza B most commonly affects children
    3) the two major antigens of the influenza virus are hemagglutinin (H) and neurominidase (N)
    4) influenza viral vaccine offers excellent protection against both influenza A and influenza B

188. Which of the following statements regarding amantadine prophylaxis of influenza is/are CORRECT?

    1) amantadine (Symmetrel) is as effective as vaccination in preventing influenza
    2) the adult daily dose of amantadine is 200 mg.
    3) amantadine is effective not only in preventing influenza A but also in treating the disease after symptoms appear
    4) amantadine has significant side effects which limit its usefulness.

189. In which of the following situations is/are amantadine prophylaxis recommended for the prevention of influenza?

    1) in outbreaks of new Type A influenza strain when a vaccine is usally not available
    2) in unvaccinated high risk individuals at the start of an influenza outbreak
    3) in patients with an allergy to eggs
    4) in hospitalized patients, including the elderly in nursing homes who are not immunized and who may have been exposed to Type A virus during an outbreak

ANSWERS

184. b) Influenza can easily be recognized clinically during a major epidemic. The incubation period is 48-72 hours. The most common initial symptom is severe generalized or frontal headache, often accompanied by retro-orbital pain. Diffuse myalgia often occurs in the legs and over the lumbosacral area. Fever and chills may appear initially, but are more often preceeded by headache and myalgia. Fever and myalgia usually subside within two or three days. Some degree of prostration is common; the face is flushed and the skin is hot and dry. Respiratory symptoms are prominent-particularly cough, which is productive in about 30% of patients. Approximately half of the patients experience substernal chest pain, which is accentuated by coughing.

185. d) Immunization with influenza vaccine is 70-90% effective in preventing influenza A. The United States Public Health Service Committee on immunization practices recommends immunization for the following high risk groups:

    1) the elderly, especially in nursing homes and hospitals
    2) patients with chronic respiratory conditions
    3) congenital or chronic cardiovascular disorders
    4) chronic renal disease

5) diabetes mellitus or other chronic metabolic disorders
6) immunocompromised patients

In children with chronic disease, only subunit vaccine should be used, since whole virus vaccine is too reactogenic. Although healthy infants show excess morbidity during influenza outbreaks, the risks associated with vaccinating this group outweigh the benefits.

186. c) The most common cause of death from influenza is secondary pneumococcal pneumonia. This also demonstrates the importance of administering pneumococcal vaccine to patients with chronic disease, immunocompromised patients and the elderly. Other causes of death include Staphylococcal pneumonia and a direct effect of the virus itself. Viral meningitis and acute viral encephalopathy are very uncommon complications of influenza. Dehydration can be a contributing factor in death from any infection.

187. e) Infections with influenza type A are much more common than type B infections in all age groups. Influenza B, when it occurs, most often affects children, predominantly those of school age.

The virus surface carries spikes containing the two glycoproteins of influenza-hemagglutinin (H) and neuraminidase (N). Antibodies produced against these antigens are responsible for protection against infection and disease.

Influenza viral vaccine offers a protection rate of 70-90% against both influenza A and influenza B.

188. a) When early immunization is not feasible, or when the vaccine is contraindicated amantadine can be used to prevent influenza A. It should be used as long as an epidemic situation exists in the community. Tests of the drug's efficacy in preventing influenza A clearly demonstrate that amantadine is as effective as the vaccine. All type A strains are sensitive to the drug; type B strains are not. The adult daily dose of amantadine is 200 mg.; this can be given as a single dose of two 2(100 mg.) capsules. Amantadine is effective not only in preventing influenza A but also in treating the disease after symptoms appear. When given in the same dose as that used for prophylaxis the drug specifically inhibits the replication of influenza A virus. Amantadine shortens the duration of fever by at least 24 hours and reduces upper and lower airway respiratory symptoms. Recently, amantadine therapy was found to accelerate the resolution of peripheral airway abnormalities in patients with uncomplicated influenza. Although it is not yet known whether amantadine can prevent the complications of influenza A this observation may have significant implications for more severe lower respiratory problems.

Side effects have occasionally been noted during amantidine prophylaxis in healthy individuals; however, the side effects are usually mild, short lived and totally reversible and occur mainly during the first week of drug administration. Insomnia, light-headedness, difficulty in concentrating and drowsiness, alone or in combination, have been observed in 6-7% of patients receiving amantadine.

189.   e) The National Institute of Health recommends amantadine prophylaxis in the following situations:

1) in outbreaks of new Type A strain when a vaccine is generally not available
2) in unvaccinated high-risk individuals at the start of an influenza A outbreak: these individuals should be vaccinated promptly and placed on amantadine prophylaxis for at least 2 to 3 weeks.
3) in patients with an allergy to eggs — such individuals should be placed on amantadine and should not be vaccinated
4) in hospitalized patients, including the elderly in nursing homes, who are not immunized and who may have been exposed to Type A virus during an outbreak

References

Monto A. Prevention and Drug Treatment of Influenza. American Family Physician 1985; 28(6): 33-37 (quiz), 165-169.

Acres S et al. Statement of influenza vaccination for the 1986-1987 season. Canadian Medical Association Journal 1986; 135; 337-339.

PROBLEM #26: A 45 YEAR OLD HYPERTENSIVE MALE NOT TAKING HIS MEDICATION

A 45 year old male with a blood pressure of 210/120 presents to your office for a blood pressure assessment. He was started on medication one year ago and was asked to return in one month. This is his first visit since that time.

Questions 190-199 are TRUE or FALSE questions. If the answer is TRUE, mark a; if it is FALSE mark b.

190. Estimates for non-compliance in short-term therapies is as high as 90%.

191. Estimates for non-compliance in long-term therapies rarely exceed 25%.

192. Biological assays are generally the most accurate method for measuring patient compliance.

193. Previous iatrogenic side-effects have a marked influence on patient compliance.

194. Acceptance of the diagnosis is a particularly important factor in determining patient compliance.

195. Satisfaction with the doctor-patient relationship markedly influences patient compliance.

196. Patient complicance is reduced when the drug regime is complex.

197. Physician-patient contracts including instructions and rewards do not seem to increase patient compliance.

198. Patient knowledge about disease and treatments always increases patient compliance.

199. A social support network increases patient compliance in long-term treatment regimes.

ANSWERS

190. a) True. Studies have shown that non-compliance in short-term therapies such as treatment of otitis media and pharyngitis may be as high as 92%.

191. b) False. Non-compliance rates for long-term therapy such as hypertension, congestive cardiac failure and diabetes are usually 60% or greater.

192. a) True. Biological assays are generally the most accurate method of determining patient compliance. Pill-counts are intermediate in accuracy and interviews are generally the least accurate.

193. a) True. Previous iatrogenic side-effects from other medications decreases patient compliance for the current treatment regime. Studies have shown that 41% of the population have had adverse effects to prescription drugs. This large segment of the population will, generally speaking, be less compliant and more wary of potential side-effects.

194. a) True. Modifying general and specific health beliefs is important in increasing patient compliance. Physicians need to monitor their patient's health beliefs by asking if the patient cares about his health, agrees with and accepts the diagnosis, preceives the condition as serious, feels the recommended treatment will work, fears regimen side effects, or believes the regimen will be difficult to follow.

195. a) True. Satisfaction with the patient-physician relationship and other aspects of medical encounters can alter patient compliance. Studies have shown positive correlations between compliance and patient satisfaction with the visit, including perceptions of convenience and waiting time. Conversely, impersonality and brevity of the encounter have been shown to negatively affect patient compliance. Satisfaction and resulting compliance are greater when patients feel their expectations have been fulfilled, the physician elicits and respects patients' concerns, responsive information about condition and progress are provided, and sincere concern and sympathy are shown.

196. a) True. Compliance is reduced when the regimen is complex, of long duration, dependent on an alteration of the patient's lifestyle, inconvenient, or expensive. For example, for patients with diabetes or congestive heart failure, medication errors were less than 15% when only one drug was prescribed, increased to 25% when two or three drugs were taken; and exceeded 35% when five or more drugs were taken.

197. b) False. One way to modify compliance is via the contingency contract, wherein both parties set forth a treatment goal, the specific obligation of each party in attempting to accomplish that goal, and a time limit set for its achievement. Beyond increasing the likelihood of adherence to therapy, contracts also offer: a written outline of expected behavior; the involvement of the patient in the decision making process concerning the regimen, and the opportunity to discuss potential problems and solutions with the physician; a formal commitment to the program from the patient; and rewards, which are especially important in contracts with children.

198. b) False. Knowledge about disease and treatments influences patient decisions, but its effect on patient compliance is unclear. Patients must have both knowledge and an understanding of recommendations in order to comply. A considerable amount of non-compliance may be involuntary, due to disparity in patient and provider understanding.

A good start towards enhancing compliance can be made by basing physician instructions on these points: patients remember best the first instructions presented; instructions that are emphasized are better recalled; and the fewer the instructions given, the greater will be the proportion remembered.

199. a) True. Modification of social interaction factors such as social networks and supervision of the patient improve compliance. The family can also enhance supervision of the patient, as well as assist and encourage patient compliance. Social support is crucial to long-term treatment plans that require continuous action on the part of the patient.

Reference

Eraker S, Kirscht J, Becker M. Understanding and Improving Patient Compliance. Annals of Internal Medicine 1984; 100(2): 258-268.

PROBLEM #27: A 25 YEAR OLD FEMALE WITH DIFFUSE MUSCULOSKELETAL PAIN

200. A 25-year old female patient presents with a chronic aching pain in her cervical, shoulder, pectoral and proximal lumbosacral areas. On examining these areas you discover rather marked tenderness. On the basis of these findings your provisional diagnosis is:

    a) fibromyalgia
    b) polymyalgia rheumatica
    c) hysterical conversion reaction
    d) diffuse musculoskeletal pain NYD
    e) myasthenia gravis

201. A 75 year old female presents with the acute onset of a diffuse, proximal musculoskeletal aching and stiffness. In the morning she is unable to reach up and comb her hair. In addition, she complains of fatigue, a 4 kg. weight loss and intermittant fever since the illness began. Her erythrocyte sedimentation rate is 75 mm./hr. On the basis of these findings your provisional diagnosis is:

    a) fibromyalgia
    b) polymyalgia rheumatica
    c) acute onset rheumatoid arthritis
    d) myasthenia gravis
    e) late onset hyperthyroidism

202. The upper limit of normal for erythrocyte sedimentation rate in female patients over the age of 65 years is:

    a) 20 mm./hr
    b) 30 mm./hr
    c) 45 mm./hr
    d) 60 mm./hr
    e) 80 mm./hr

CODE: (a:1, 2 and 3; b: 1 and 3; c: 2 and 4; d: 4 only; e: all of the above)

203. The treatment(s) of choice for the patient who is described in question #200 is/are:

    1) reassurance about the benign nature of the condition
    2) non-steroidal anti-inflammatory agents
    3) muscle relaxants
    4) intralesional injections of corticosteroids

204. The treatment(s) of choice for the patient who is described in question #201 is/are:

    1) reassurance about the benign nature of the condition
    2) non-steroidal anti-inflammatory agents
    3) muscle relaxants
    4) systemic corticosteroids

ANSWERS

200. a) This patient describes a classical case of "fibromyalgia". This syndrome can best be defined as diffuse aching, stiffness, tenderness, and pain around the joints, in muscles, and in fibrous and subcutaneous tissues. Fibromyalgia probably accounts for the majority of patients who complain of generalized musculoskeletal pain. The condition is often referred to as "fibrositis", but biopsies of tissue from these painful areas have yielded no evidence of inflammation.

The typical patient with fibromyalgia is a woman between 25 and 50 years old who complains of an aching pain in the cervical, shoulder, pectoral, and proximal lumbosacral regions. The pain is not severe and is never associated with any mechanical or functional abnormality. Neither is it acute in onset; patients almost always report long-standing symptoms. Fibromyalgia frequently occurs in chronically tense people or in those experiencing physical or emotional stress.

Physical examination is normal apart from the characteristic and reproducible abnormality of tenderness at certain "trigger points" present in the areas previously described. In many patients, as in the patient described, multiple sites are tender. Laboratory evaluation, including erythyrocyte sedimentation rate is entirely normal.

Polymyalgia rheumatica usually occurs in older individuals and is associated with an elevated erythrocyte sedimentation rate.

There are no symptoms such as altered sensation, ataxia, paralysis or involuntary movements that may be associated with an hysterical conversion reaction.

Diffuse musculoskeletal pain NYD, although sufficient in description is not a diagnosis.

Myasthenia gravis is usually found in older individuals and is associated with progressive weakening and tiring of muscular groups.

201. b) The provisional diagnosis in this case is polymyalgia rheumatica. Polymyalgia rheumatica is almost exclusively a disease of women over the age of 60. Characteristically, the patient complains of diffuse, primarily proximal, musculoskeletal aching and stiffness. Patients usually complain of a worsening of symptoms after a period of rest. In the morning, for example, the patient, as in this case, may be unable to reach up to comb her hair or get a dish out of the cabinet.

This illness may be difficult at times to differentiate from rheumatoid arthritis. Rheumatoid arthritis usually presents with more joint symptoms than polymyalgia, but this too can be misleading. Physical examination usually reveals a generalized stiffness and soreness in the proximal muscles. Passive range-of-motion movements are usually normal.

The characteristic laboratory abnormality of polymyalgia rheumatica is an elevated erythrocyte sedimentation rate. This can be grossly elevated to greater than 100 mm./hr. The sensitivity of this test in patients with polymyalgia rheumatica is extremely high.

The patient described has no symptoms of hyperthyroidism. Some of the symptoms described, may however, be associated with hypothyroidism, and thus the checking of the T-4 is worthwhile. The other choices are discussed in question #200.

202. c) The normal values for erythrocyte sedimentation rate quoted for young patients (less than 10 mm./hr for males and 20 mm./hr for females) do not apply to elderly patients. Over the age of 65 years normal values may be as high as 30 mm./hr for males and 45 mm./hr for females.

203. e) The treatment of fibromyalgia should begin with reassurance and explanation to the patient. The patient should be told that they have a benign condition. Often the form of an analogy (such as to headaches) will help them understand the condition. Specific therapy includes nonnarcotic analgesics, non-steroidal anti-inflammatory drugs, mild sedatives, or muscle relaxants. Occasionally, local injections of lidocaine or long-acting corticosteroids into particularly painful trigger areas are indicated. Heat, massage and exercise programs often help. Occasionally, if a psychiatric condition is causing or contributing to the fibromyalgia, referral to a psychiatrist or the use of psychoactive drugs may be required.

204. d) The treatment of choice for patients with polymyalgia rheumatica is systemic corticosteroid therapy. The condition is extremely responsive to low doses of prednisone; 10-20 mg./day. Symptoms often improve in 24-48 hours, and the ESR generally returns to normal in seven to ten days. Fatigue, weight loss, fever and other symptoms respond more gradually.

Although non-steroidal anti-inflammatory agents may be of some benefit, they are certainly not the treatment of choice. Muscle relaxants are usually not beneficial.

Polymyalgia rheumatica is not a benign condition, and unless treated aggressively, may be associated with blindness secondary to temporal arteritis. Therefore, patients should be questioned about headaches, visual symptoms, jaw claudication and scalp tenderness; and the temporal arteries should be palpated. Reassurance about the benign nature of the condition is not appropriate.

Reference

Pasten R. Diffuse Musculoskeletal Pain. Diagnosis 1985; 2(4): 42-48

PROBLEM #28: A 30 YEAR OLD FEMALE WITH LOWER ABDOMINAL PAIN

205. A 30 year old female presents to the office with a 6-month history of lower abdominal pain associated with bloating, increased flatulence, and alternating diarrhea and constipation. With respect to the classical irritable bowel syndrome, which of the following statements is FALSE?

    a) the typical location is in the lower abdomen
    b) defecation frequently relieves the pain
    c) there is often a feeling of incomplete emptying of the rectum
    d) the abdomen is usually not tender
    e) bowel action is often irregular

206. Which of the following investigations are indicated in a patient you suspect of having the irritable bowel syndrome?

    a) complete blood count and erythrocyte sedimentation rate
    b) sigmoidoscopy
    c) barium enema
    d) a and b
    e) all of the above

207. Which of the following diseases is the irritable bowel syndrome often associated with?

    a) diverticulosis
    b) chronic appendicitis
    c) chronic cholecystitis
    d) chronic pancreatitis
    e) none of the above

208. Which of the following treatments have been found to be beneficial in the treatment of the irritable bowel syndrome?

    a) phenobarbitol
    b) antispasmodics
    c) high fibre diet
    d) antihistamines
    e) none of the above

CODE: (a:1, 2 and 3; b: 1 and 3; c: 2 and 4; d: 4 only; e: all of the above)

209. Which of the following locations may be associated with the pain of the irritable bowel syndrome?

    1) the right iliac fossa
    2) the right upper quadrant
    3) the epigastrium
    4) the splenic flexure

ANSWERS

205. d) The classical irritable bowel syndrome presents with lower abdominal pain, often left sided, which is usually eased, sometimes very transiently, by bowel action or the passing of flatus. Bowel action is often irregular, with constipation or diarrhea of small volume. The stools may be thin and ribbon-like, or rather like rabbit droppings. There is often a feeling of incomplete emptying of the rectum.

   On examination, the patient does not usually look ill, unless tense and depressed. However, the sigmoid colon may be palpable and tender, and pressure may reproduce the pain. Sigmoidoscopy is normal, but air sufflation of the sigmoid may reproduce the pain.

206. e) The classical irritable bowel syndrome is usually a diagnosis of exclusion. A complete evaluation is indicated before coming to the conclusion that the patient has an irritable bowel. Investigations should include a complete blood count and erythrocyte sedimentation rate, electrolytes, BUN and creatinine, serum proteins, sigmoidoscopy and a barium enema. Depending on the location of the pain an upper GI series and follow-through may or may not be indicated.

207. a) Diverticulosis is often associated with the irritable bowel syndrome. Left sided diverticular disease is associated with muscle hypertrophy which is assumed to be the cause of the pain. There appears to be no consistent clinical feature that distinguishes the symptoms of patients with an irritable bowel from uncomplicated diverticular disease, and psychogenic factors may play a part in both groups.

   Appendicitis, cholecystitis, pancreatitis and other abdominal conditions have no known association with the irritable bowel syndrome. Sometimes, however, a patient presents with atypical irritable bowel syndrome manifested by right upper quadrant pain. This may be attributed to the poorly defined entity of "biliary dyskinesia". In a recent survey of 22 such patients, 16 of whom had undergone 38 fruitless operations, 21 had their pain reproduced by distension of segments of the small bowel or right colon. Thus, it seems that this syndrome is a variant of the irritable bowel syndrome.

208. e) The most important facet in managing patients with the irritable bowel syndrome is to explain to the patient the nature of the disorder and the probable mechanisms behind the symptoms. The benign nature should be emphasized and the patient warned that symptoms could recur at any time. Patients should be told that their condition does not shorten life, and that a bowel which causes symptoms for a long period of time is not more vulnerable to the development of cancer and other complications.

The initial enthusiasm for a high fibre diet has not withstood the test of time. Double blind studies have not shown a significant difference between a high fibre and a regular diet. Obviously, if constipation is a major problem, an increase in the fibre content of the diet makes good sense.

Medications including phenobarbitol, antispasmodics, antihistamines and others have not been demonstrated to be effective in the treatment of this syndrome. An exception to this is the depressed patient who presents with abdominal pain as a component of an endogenous depressive illness. Obviously, treatment of the primary depression with a tricyclic antidepressant will relieve the somatic symptoms of depression.

209. e) Often, the pain associated with the irritable bowel syndrome is not confined to the typical lower abdominal location. Pain in the right iliac fossa may mimic appendicitis or an twisted ovarian cyst. Pain in the right upper quadrant may mimic acute or chronic cholecystitis. Pain in the epigastrium may mimic appendicitis or a twisted ovarian cyst. Pain in the right upper quadrenal problem. It is important to bear these atypical locations in mind, and consider an irritable bowel as a cause when investigations for other conditions are negative.

Reference

Dawson A. The irritable bowel. The Practitioner 1984; 228: 797-800.

PROBLEM #29: A 51 YEAR OLD FEMALE WITH SEVERE NAUSEA, VOMITING, AND ADVANCED OVARIAN CARCINOMA

210. A 51 year old female with advanced ovarian carcinoma presents with severe anorexia, nausea and vomiting. In addition, she describes a sore mouth, diarrhea and difficulty breathing. With respect to her anorexia, which of the following treatments may be indicated:

    a) prednisone 5 mg. t.i.d.
    b) alcohol 1 oz. prior to meals
    c) cyproheptadine 4 mg. t.i.d.
    d) maltevol 12 multivitamin preparation
    e) all of the above may be of benefit

211. The patient described in question #210 has a 3 day history of severe nausea and vomiting. Which one of the following treatments is NOT recommended for this patient?

    a) prochlorperazine 5-10 mg. q4h
    b) haloperidol 0.5-1.0 mg. b.i.d.
    c) chlorpromazine 10-25 mg. q4h
    d) metoclopramide 10 mg. t.i.d.
    e) intravenous fluids

212. The patient described in question #210 has had a sore mouth for the past 3 days. Which of the following may be helpful in the treatment of this problem?

    a) nystatin oral suspension 100,000 units q4h
    b) anetholtrithion (Sialor) 25 mg. t.i.d.
    c) lemon-glycerine swabs
    d) a and c
    e) all of the above

213. The patient described in question #210 undergoes palliative radiotherapy for severe bone pain that develops one month after the problems described above. Following this, she develops bloody diarrhea. Which of the following treatments may be helpful in the treatment of this problem?

    a) diphenoxylate HCl 2.5 mg. t.i.d. to a maximum of 20 mg./day
    b) loperamide HCl 2 mg. after each unformed stool to a maximum of 16 mg./day
    c) pentazocine 50 mg. q4h prn
    d) a and b
    e) all of the above

CODE: (a:1, 2 and 3; b: 1 and 3; c: 2 and 4; d: 4 only; e: all of the above)

214. The patient described in question #210 becomes increasingly short of breath. Which of the following treatments may be useful in alleviating this symptom?

   1) palliative radiotherapy
   2) prednisone 10-15 mg. t.i.d.
   3) morphine sulfate 5-10 mg. q4h
   4) dexamethasone 8-12 mg. daily

215. The patient described in question #210 becomes severely depressed with the deterioration of her condition. Which of the following may be indicated in the treatment of this problem?

   1) amitriptyline 25-50 mg. at HS
   2) trazodone 50-150 mg. at HS
   3) supportive psychotherapy
   4) diazepam 5 mg. t.i.d. and at HS

ANSWERS

210. e) Anorexia is a very common and distressing symptom occurring in all types of cancer. Mouth discomfort, changes in sense of taste, dehydration, malnutrition, some drugs, and chemotherapy may all contribute to it.

   Small food helpings on small plates with patients' preferred foods attractively prepared will make meals more appealing. Prednisone 5 mg. t.i.d. may improve appetite. Maltevol 12 may be used or cyproheptadine 4 mg. t.i.d. before meals. Alcohol, such as 1 oz of brandy may also be beneficial. It is important to reassure the patient and compulsive family members that large feeds are unnecessary.

211. e) Nausea and vomiting may result from stimulation of the emetic centre in the brain stem by impulses from the gut, vestibular apparatus, cerebral cortex, or the chemoreceptor trigger zone. There are multiple causes including the following:

   a) drugs — digoxin, morphine, and estrogens
   b) biochemical changes — uremia, hypercalcemia, liver failure and ketosis
   c) bowel obstruction
   d) psychological causes

   If nausea and vomiting are caused by an oral narcotic, a phenothiazine should be given concurrently. These work on the chemoreceptor trigger zone in the medulla and have a tranquillizing action. The most widely used are:

a) metoclopramide 10 mg. q.i.d.
b) chlorpromazine 10-25 mg. q4h
c) haloperidol 0.5-1.0 mg. b.i.d.
d) prochlorperazine 5-10 mg. q4h

In addition to working on the central chemoreceptor zone, metoclopramide also works on the upper gut to increase gastric peristalsis and to relax the pyloric antrum.

Intravenous fluids have no part to play in the management of terminal malignancy unless the dehydration is a major factor to the patient's comfort level, and oral fluids cannot be tolerated.

212. e) Sore mouth can be caused by monilial infection, ill-fitting dentures, aphthous ulcerations, vitamin deficiency, and blood dyscrasias. Monilial infection is treated with nystatin oral suspension 100,000 units (1 ml.) q4h until 48 hours after clinical cure. Dentures must be treated with the same solution.

If dry mouth is the problem, the main complaint will be thirst. This can be treated by good mouth care including ice chips, lemon candies, or lemon-glycerine swabs. Vaseline to the lips is helpful. If the mouth is painful, use viscous Xylocaine mouth rinse before eating. A useful drug is Sialor 25 mg. t.i.d. to increase salivation.

213. d) The diarrhea in this case is most likely due to the effect of the radiotherapy on the bowel. In this case, both diphenoxylate and loperamide are good treatment choices. Pentazocine is a narcotic agonist-antagonist and has no place in the management of symptoms in the terminally ill patient.

214. e) The dyspnea described in this patient may be the result of metastatic lung disease, lymphatic carcinomatosis or a malignant pleural effusion.

Palliative radiotherapy may have an important role to play in some patients. Steroids such as Prednisone 10-15 mg. t.i.d. or dexamethasone 8-12 mg. daily can be useful to provide quick relief of dyspnea in some patients by causing shrinkage of nodes and relief of bronchospasm. Steroids can also be helpful with superior vena cava obstruction either alone or combined with radiotherapy. Pleural effusions that are symptomatic should be tapped and the cause treated.

Small doses of oral morphine such as 5-10 mg. every 4 hours is effective during the terminal event to relieve the sensation of dyspnea and relax the patient by reducing the respiratory drive. With severe terminal dyspenea an injection of morphine 5-10 mg. IV or s.c. may give compassionate relief.

215. a) If symptom control is adequate and the patient is free from pain there is less incidence of depression. The dying patient has many vegetative symptoms including anorexia, weight loss, and malaise. This makes the clinical diagnosis of a true unipolar depression difficult. The tricyclic anti-depressants are known to be effective as co-analgesics in several chronic pain syndromes

including post-herpetic neuralgia and superficial dysesthetic pain. The tricyclic antidepressants are also indicated if the patient presents with full clinical depression in spite of attention to the patient's physical, mental and spiritual distress. Amitriptyline 25-50 mg. at H.S. has been standard therapy for some time. Imipramine 25-50 mg. H.S. or any other tricyclic antidepressant will probably work equally well.

Diazepam has no place in the treatment of depression. Its strictly sedative properties may actually increase the patient's and relative's distress, as it may result in confusion.

Supportive psychotherapy is a cornerstone of treatment, and should be the first therapy attempted. In this case, involvement of all staff and family members is essential.

Reference

Saunders C. Principles of Symptom Control in Terminal Care. Medical Clinics of North America 1982; 66(2): 1169-1183.

PROBLEM #30: A 75 YEAR OLD MALE WITH TERMINAL CANCER PAIN

216. A 75-year old male was discovered to have Stage IV cancer of the prostate. As he was not sympomatic at the time of diagnosis, therapy was postponed. Six months after diagnosis he develops mild pain in the lumbar region. A bone scan reveals increased uptake of radionuclide in the L2-L5 area compatible with metastatic disease. No other abnormal areas are seen on the bone scan. The treatment of choice for *mild* bone pain due to secondary deposits of cancer is:

    a) morphine sulfate
    b) palliative radiotherapy
    c) non-steroidal anti-inflammatory drugs
    d) Brompton's cocktail
    e) acetaminophen

217. The most common type of pain in patients with terminal cancer is:

    a) visceral pain
    b) bone pain
    c) nerve root compression pain
    d) soft-tissue inflammatory pain
    e) pain due to secondary infection

218. A patient with terminal cancer of the colon is suffering from abdominal pain that is not responsive to acetaminophen or codeine. It is decided to begin therapy with morphine sulfate. The patient weighs 70 kg. The initial treatment with morphine sulfate should begin as:

    a) 20 mg.IM every 4 hours
    b) 10 mg.IV every 6 hours
    c) 10 mg.orally every 6 hours
    d) 5 mg.orally every 4 hours
    e) 50 mg.orally every 8 hours

CODE: (a:1, 2 and 3; b: 1 and 3; c: 2 and 4; d: 4 only; e: all of the above)

219. Which of the following medications may be indicated as adjuvant therapy along with morphine sulfate?

    1) colace (docusate sodium)
    2) metoclopramide
    3) senekot
    4) chlorpromazine

220. Which of the following medications SHOULD NOT be used in the treatment of patients with terminal cancer pain?

    1) pentazocine
    2) aspirin
    3) meperidine
    4) codeine phosphate

221. Which of the following statements regarding the use of analgesics in patients with terminal cancer pain is/are TRUE?

    1) cancer pain is continuous pain requiring regular preventive treatment
    2) the dose of the analgesic used should be the lowest compatible with pain control
    3) the next dose is given before the effect of the previous one has worn off and therefore before the patient may think it is necessary
    4) psychological dependence (addiction) does occur in terminal cancer patients on narcotic analgesics

ANSWERS

216. c) The treatment of first choice for mild bone pain due to secondary cancer is a non-steroidal anti-inflammatory drug. Tumors in bone, and possibly elsewhere, liberate prostaglandins which sensitize nerve endings to painful stimuli. Anti-inflammatory drugs such as aspirin, ketoprofen and naproxen inhibit prostaglandin synthesis and are therefore effective at the site of the pain, whereas narcotic analgesics act centrally.

   If this was not effective, the next step in analgesia would be a weak narcotic such as codeine. This could be added to aspirin or another nonsteroidal anti-inflammatory drug, as these two classes of drugs act by different mechanisms. Thereafter, morphine sulfate should be considered.

   Palliative radiotherapy could be used as a treatment option following the failure of a non-steroidal agent. However, it may be better to try a narcotic analgesic first and keep palliative radiotherapy as a future consideration.

   Acetaminophen has little role to play in the treatment of bone pain.

   Brompton's cocktail is a mixture of medications in a morphine base and as such, probably has no place to play in the 'step-care' management of terminal pain.

217. a) The most common type of cancer pain encountered is visceral pain (29%). Following this, in order, are bone pain (17%), soft-tissue infiltration pain (10%), nerve root compression pain (9%), and pain due to secondary infection (6%).

   It should be mentioned that patients with terminal pain often have more than one kind of pain, with each one requiring somewhat different therapy.

218. d) Morphine sulfate should be given as 5 mg. orally every 4 hours as a starting dose. It is important to give the medication on a 4-hourly basis to prevent pain from recurring. The aim is to titrate the dose of the morphine against the patient's pain, gradually increasing the dose until the patient is pain free. The next dose is given before the effect of the previous one has fully worn off-and therefore before the patient may think it is necessary. In this way it is possible to erase the memory and fear of pain.

Intramuscular and intravenous morphine are not needed to control terminal cancer pain. If the patient cannot tolerate oral medication, morphine by rectal suppository is the preferred route of administration.

219. e) Colace and Senekot are usually needed to control the constipating effect of narcotic analgesics. Docusate sodium (a stool softener) is usually given on a b.i.d. basis and Senekot (a peristaltic stimulant) is usually given at bedtime.

Metoclopramide (a GI tract motility modifier and anti-nauseant) is the treatment of choice for nausea associated with narcotic analgesia. Alternatively, chlorpromazine may be used both for its anti-nauseant and sedative properties.

220. b) Pentazocine, which is a narcotic agonist-antagonist has no place in the treatment of chronic pain. If combined with narcotic analgesics, it will actually increase the pain, due to its antagonist properties. As well, it has a very short half-life (2-3 hours) and thus is also inappropriate for that reason.

Meperidine also has a very short half-life, and thus should not be used in the treatment of terminal cancer pain.

Aspirin and codeine are the first two of the three basic analgesics in the treatment of cancer pain. The third basic agent is morphine sulfate.

221. a) The following priniciples in the treatment of cancer pain with analgesics apply:
1) cancer pain is continuous pain requiring regular preventive treatment.
2) the dose of analgesic should be the lowest compatible with pain control.
3) the exact dose is found by titrating the analgesic against the patient's pain, increasing the dose until the patient is pain free.
4) the next dose is given before the effect of the previous one has worn off and therefore before the patient may think it necessary.
5) oral medication is preferable to injection.
6) psychological dependence (addiction) does not occur in cancer patients.
7) tolerance is a minor problem and is usually self-limiting after a few weeks.
8) continued reassessment is needed as old pains worsen and new pains may occur.
9) adjuvant therapy will be necessary. Laxatives are almost always needed for constipation, and antiemetics are sometimes needed for nausea and vomiting.

References

Twycross R. Analgesics. Postgraduate Medical Journal 1984; 60: 876-880.
Baines M. Cancer pain. Postgraduate Medical Journal 1984; 60: 852-857.

PROBLEM #31: A 45 YEAR OLD MALE WITH A HEADACHE

222. A 45 year old male awakes in the middle of the night with a deep burning headache centered behind the left orbit. It is excruciating and associated with lacrimation, facial flushing, nasal discharge, conjuctivitis, ptosis and pupillary constriction. The most likely cause of the headache in this case is:

   a) subarachnoid hemorrhage
   b) tension-migraine syndrome
   c) atypical migraine
 ₵ d) cluster headache
   e) left-sided cerebrovascular accident

223. With respect to migraine headache, which of the following statements is INCORRECT?

 ⌐ a) during a migraine attack extracranial vasodilation is followed by intra-cranial vasoconstriction
   b) the neurological symptoms preceeding the headache are caused by intra-cranial arterial constriction and cerebral ischemia
   c) alteration of arterial tone is associated with liberation of vasoactive substances including catecholamines, histamines, serotonin, kinins, neuro-peptides, and prostaglandins
   d) the pounding headache is presumed to be related to neurogenic vasodilata-tion and a sterile inflammatory response generated by the interaction of these substances with blood vessels and nerves

224. The treatment of choice for acute migraine headache is:

   a) meperidine
   b) acetylsalicylic acid
 ⌐ c) an ergot alkaloid
   d) haloperidol
   e) morphine sulfate

CODE: (a:1, 2 and 3; b: 1 and 3; c: 2 and 4; d: 4 only; e: all of the above)

225. Which of the following medications is/are useful for the prophylaxis of migraine headache?

   1) amitriptyline
   2) cyproheptadine
   3) propranolol
   4) nifedipine

226. Which of the following treatments is/are useful in chronic benign tension headache?

    1) relaxation techniques
    2) methysergide
    3) tricyclic antidepressants
    4) meperidine

ANSWERS

222. d) The patient described in this question has a classical "cluster" headache. Cluster headaches often awaken a patient from sleep and may recur with a clock-like regularity during a 24-hour period. Cluster headache is occasionally chronic but most often occurs in bouts lasting from weeks to months during which time the patient has one or several headaches per 24 hours.

     Cluster headache, which usually occurs in males, is described as a deep, burning or stabbing pain. It is often excruciating; the patient may even be suicidal. The associated symptoms of cluster headaches are most often ipsilateral to the pain and include lacrimation, facial flushing and nasal discharge. The eye is often red; conjunctival vessels are dilated, and ptosis and pupillary constriction often occur.

     The treatment of cluster headache is essentially the same as migraine, with ergotamine being the mainstay of treatment in the acute situation. Ergotamine tartrate may be given sublingually in a dose of 2 mg. This dose may be repeated to a maximum of 6 mg. Oxygen by mask at 7-10 litres/minute is also very effective. Methysergide and pizotyline are both moderately effective in prophylaxis.

223. a) During a migraine attack, intracranial vasoconstriction is followed by extracranial vasodilation. The neurological symptoms preceding the painful phase are caused by intracranial arterial constriction and cerebral ischemia, and pain is related to dilatation of the extracranial and some intracranial arteries. Alteration of arteriolar tone is associated with liberation of vasoactive substances including catecholamines, histamines, serotonin, kinins, neuropeptides, and prostaglandins. The pounding headache is presumed to be related to neurogenic vasodilatation and a sterile inflammatory response generated by the interaction of these substances with blood vessels and nerves.

224. c) The treatment of choice in acute migraine headache is an ergot alkaloid (ergotamine). Ergotamine can be given orally, sublingually, by oral inhalation, parenterally or by rectal suppository. Ergotamine abolishes the headache by causing extracranial vasoconstriction. Nausea, vomiting, and epigastric discomfort are signs of toxicity.

     The combination of ergotamine with an anti-emetic such as metoclopramide 10-20 mg. will often increase the efficacy of the treatment of the acute attack.

Some authorities are now recommending intravenous chlorpromazine as the treatment of choice.

225. e) The drugs useful in the prophylactic treatment of migraine headaches include the following agents:
1) amitriptyline — this agent can be given in doses of 10-150 mg./day. It is best introduced gradually to avoid excessive sedation. It presumably works by an action independant of its antidepressant action.
2) cyproheptadine — this agent is a central serotonin-agonist with platelet anti-aggregating properties. The dose varies from 8-24 mg./day.
3) propranolol — this beta blocker is often given in doses of 40-320 mg./day. Its mechanism of action is uncertain but it may be related to its central effects rather than peripheral beta-blockade.
4) calcium-channel receptor blockers (nifedpine, and verapamil). These agents have recently come into use in the prophylaxis of migraine and cluster headaches. The usual doses are nifedipine 60 mg./day, and verapamil 240 mg./day.

226. b) muscle contraction headaches are most effectively treated by muscle relaxation techniques and elimination of a stressful environment. In addition, simple analgesics such as acetaminophen and aspirin are useful in treatment. Tricyclic antidepressants have also been found to be effective. Methysergide (Sansert) and meperidine (Demerol) have no part to play in the treatment of chronic recurrent tension headache.

Reference

Atkinson R, Appenzeller O. Headache. Postgraduate Medical Journal 1984; 60: 841-846.

PROBLEM #32: A 25 YEAR OLD COLLEGE STUDENT WITH A FEVER

227. A 25 year old college student presents with a 3 week history of fatigue, malaise, fever, chills and sore throat. You suspect infectious mononucleosis. Of the following clinical features of acute infectious mononucleosis, the least common is:

   a) splenomegaly
   b) hepatomegaly
   c) fever
   d) exudative tonsillitis
   e) generalized lymphadenopathy

228. Which one of the following findings is so specific for infectious mononucleosis that serologic testing becomes unnecessary?

   a) combination of fever, tonsillitis, and generalized lymphadenopathy
   b) splenomegaly
   c) lymphocytosis
   d) lymphocyte atypia of more than 40%
   e) none of the above

229. The treatment of choice for uncomplicated acute infectious mononucleosis is:

   a) penicillin
   b) prednisone
   c) penicillin plus prednisone
   d) penicillin plus high dose ASA
   e) none of the above

CODE: (a:1, 2 and 3; b: 1 and 3; c: 2 and 4; d: 4 only; e: all of the above)

230. Which of the following signs commonly occur in acute infectious mononucleosis?

   1) palatine petechiae
   2) splenomegaly
   3) periorbital edema
   4) generalized lymphadenopathy

231. Which of the following are complications of acute infectious mononucleosis?

   1) pneumonitis
   2) pericarditis
   3) meningoencephalitis
   4) Bell's palsy

227. b) The following are the major clinical features of acute symptomatic infectious mononucleosis:
1) fever 98-100%
2) exudative tonsillitis 98-100%
3) generalized lymphadenopathy 98-100%
4) splenomegaly 75%
5) palatine petechiae 50%
6) periorbital edema 33%
7) hepatomegaly 20%

228. d) In one study, in patients with clinical evidence of infectious mononucleosis
and atypical lymphocytosis of more than 20%, 69% of patients had infectious
mononucleosis, 5% had toxoplasmosis, and 2% had cytomegalovirus infection. In 24%, a definitive diagnosis could not be made.

Lymphocyte atypia of 40% or greater is so specific for infectious mononucleosis that further serologic testing, including either a heterophil antibody or
a "spot test" for heterophil antibodies is unnecessary.

229. e) The treatment of choice for acute uncomplicated infectious mononucleosis
is symptomatic. This approach includes bed rest, the avoidance of strenuous
exercise because of the danger of splenic rupture (especially contact sports),
and aspirin or other analgesics. Antibiotics have no place in the treatment of
this condition. The treatment in infectious mononucleosis with ampicillin or
similar antibiotics results in a skin rash in most patients. Corticosteroids may
occasionally be useful in the treatment of pharyngeal swelling and severe
odynophagia.

230. e) All of the symptoms listed in this question occur in acute infectious
mononucleosis. See the critique of question #227.

231. e) The complications of acute infectious mononucleosis include meningoencephalitis, Guillain-Barré syndrome, Bell's palsy, pneumonitis, pericarditis, myocarditis, and the syndrome of inappropriate secretion of antidiuretic
hormone.

Reference

McSherry J. Diagnosing Infectious Mononucleosis. American Family Physician 1985; 32(4):
33-37, 129-132.

PROBLEM #33: A 40 YEAR OLD EXECUTIVE WHO SMOKES 3 PACKS OF CIGARETTES PER DAY

232. A 40 year old executive who smokes 3 packs of cigarettes/day presents for his routine health assessment. He wants more information on the association between cigarette smoking and coronary artery disease. You tell him that according to reliable estimates, the percentage of deaths from coronary heart disease that can be attributed to cigarette smoking is:

    a) less than 5%
    b) 10%
    c) 20%
    d) 25%
    e) 30%-40%

233. Which of the following malignancies is not associated with cigarette smoking?

    a) carcinoma of larynx
    b) carcinoma of esophagus
    c) carcinoma of bladder
    d) carcinoma of the colon
    e) carcinoma of the pancreas

234. With regard to "passive smoking" which of the following statements is FALSE?

    a) spouses of patients who smoke are not at an increased risk of carcinoma of the lung
    b) "sidestream smoke" contains more carbon monoxide than "mainstream smoke"
    c) infants of mothers who smoke absorb measurable amounts of their mothers' cigarette smoke
    d) children of parents who smoke have an increased incidence of bronchitis and pneumonia
    e) the most common symptom arising from exposure to passive smoking is eye irritation

CODE: (a: 1, 2 and 3; b: 1 and 3; c: 2 and 4; d: 4 only; e: all of the above)

235. Which of the following diseases is/are directly associated with cigarette smoking?

    1) peripheral arterial occlusive disease
    2) peptic ulcer
    3) oral cancer
    4) periodontal disease

236. Which of the following interventions have been shown to be successful in helping patients quit smoking?

 1) physician suggestion
 2) smoking cessation classes
 3) nicotine containing chewing gum
 4) a switch to very-low nicotine cigarettes

ANSWERS

232. e) According to reliable estimates, 30-40% of the deaths from coronary artery disease are directly attributable to smoking. Ten major cohort studies, accounting for over 20 million person-years of observation in several countries, each revealed an incidence of myocardial infarction and death from coronary heart disease-averaging 70% higher in cigarette smokers than in non-smokers.

233. d) The only cancer listed which is not associated with cigarette smoking is cancer of the colon.

 Cancer of the larnyx and cigarette smoking are directly linked. One case-control study estimated that 84% of all the laryngeal cancer among men could be attributed to smoking.

 Data from a number of case-control and cohort studies indicate that cigarette smoking is a major cause of esophageal cancer. Mortality ratios from case-control studies range from 1.3-11.1 among heavy smokers as compared to nonsmokers.

 The percentage of bladder cancers attributable to smoking in North America is estimated to be 40-60% in men and 25-35% in women. Smoking may also act synergistically with other carcinogens in some work settings.

 Both case-control and cohort studies through the years have demonstrated an association between smoking and pancreatic cancer, with the risk for a smoker approximately twice that for a non-smoker.

 Other cancers that are directly associated with cigarette smoking are lung cancer (which still accounts for 25% of all cancer deaths), oral cancer and kidney cancer.

234. a) Tobacco smoke in the environment is derived from two sources: "mainstream smoke" exhaled by a smoker, and "sidestream" smoke arising from the burning end of a cigarette. Sidestream smoke contains a higher concentration of potentially dangerous gas-phase constituents including carbon monoxide.

 Infants of mothers who smoke absorb measurable amounts of cigarette smoke. As well, several studies have reported a significant association between the prevalence of respiratory illnesses (bronchitis and pneumonia) in infants and children under the age of two and parental smoking habits.

The most common symptom arising from exposure to passive smoking is eye irritation. Other significant symptoms are headaches, nasal symptoms and cough. Exposure to tobacco smoke also precipitates or aggravates allergic attacks in persons with respiratory allergies.

Spouses of patients who smoke are at increased risk of developing lung cancer. In one cohort study, the relative risk of lung cancer in nonsmoking women whose husbands smoked one pack or less per day was 1.6, and in nonsmoking women whose husbands smoked more than one pack per day it was 2.1.

235. e) The diseases which have been directly linked to cigarette smoking are: (1) coronary heart disease, (2) peripheral arterial occlusive disease, (3) cerbrovascular disease, (4) lung cancer, (5) cancer of the larynx, (6) oral cancer, (7) cancer of the esophagus, (8) cancer of the bladder, (9) cancer of the pancreas, (10) chronic obstructive lung disease, (11) peptic ulcer disease and (12) periodontal disease.

236. a) The interventions which have been shown to be beneficial in helping patients quit smoking are physician recommendation (which increase smoking cessation by 1-5%); smoking cessation classes, which rely on behavioral techniques to augment the smoker's ability to resist the urge to smoke; and nicotine containing chewing gum, which can double the long-term abstinence rate.

A switch to low-tar cigarettes, rather than increasing the smoking cessation rate, actually results in greater intake to produce the same blood level of nicotine.

Reference

Fielding J. Smoking: Health effects and control. New England Journal of Medicine 1985; 313 (8/9) 491-496, 555-560.

PROBLEM #34: A 30 YEAR OLD FEMALE WITH A THYROID NODULE

237. A 30 year old female presents for a routine health assessment. On examination, you discover a thyroid nodule. Which of the following statements about thyroid nodules is INCORRECT?

    a) thryoid nodules are more common in men than in women
    b) the prevalence rate of palpable thryoid nodules is 4-7%
    c) solitary nodules are three times more common than multinodular goiter in clinically apparent (i.e. palpable) disease
    d) 50% of thyroid glands that are normal on palpation will harbour one or more nodules at autopsy
    e) the incidence of occult thyroid cancer in Canada is 6%

238. The most important risk factor for the development of thyroid cancer is:

    a) family history of thyroid cancer
    b) occupational exposure to benzene
    c) radiation to the area of the thyroid gland
    d) heavy cigarette smoking
    e) none of the above

239. The single most important test that should be performed in the evaluation of a thyroid nodule is:

    a) thyroglobulin antibody titre
    b) thyroxine and triiodothyronine levels
    c) diagnostic ultrasound
    d) radionuclide imaging
    e) fine needle aspiration biopsy

CODE: (a:1, 2 and 3; b: 1 and 3; c: 2 and 4; d: 4 only; e: all of the above)

240. Which of the following entities should be considered in the differential diagnosis of a thyroid nodule?

    1) a pyogenic infection
    2) a granulomatous infection
    3) a thyroid adenoma
    4) subacute thyroiditis

241. With regard to fine needle aspiration biopsy, which of the following statements is/are TRUE?

    1) fine needle biopsy has a specificity of 25% for the diagnosis of thyroid cancer
    2) fine needle biopsy has a sensitivity of 90% for the diagnosis of thyroid cancer
    3) significant bleeding is a common problem using this technique
    4) all suspicious thyroid lesions identified by fine needle biopsy should be excised

ANSWERS

237. a) Thyroid nodules are more common in women than in men. In the United States, clinically apparent nodules are present in 4-7% of the adult population.

    Solitary nodules are three times more common than multinodular goiter in clinically apparent (palpable) disease. In contrast, approximately one-half of the glands that are normal on the basis of palpation will have one or more nodules at autopsy. Moreover, in an autopsy study of glands that were normal to palpation, the incidence of occult thyroid cancer varied from 6% in Canada to 28.4% in Japan.

238. c) The single most important risk factor for the development of thyroid cancer is radiation exposure to the area of the head and neck. Radiation increases the incidence of both benign and malignant disease.

    A family history of thyroid cancer, occupational exposure to benzene and heavy cigarette smoking are not significantly correlated with the future development of thyroid cancer.

239. e) Fine needle aspiration biopsy is the single most important test that should be performed in the evaluation of a thyroid nodule. It is 90% sensitive and 70% specific for the diagnois of thyroid cancer.

    Neither scintigraphy nor ultrasound has sufficient specificity to distinguish benign from malignant nodules; therefore, these procedures should not be done routinely in the evaluation of a thyroid nodule. Detection of thyroid nodules on the basis of the history, physical examination, scintiscanning, and ultrasonography results in the detection of malignant disease in 10-20% of surgically excised nodules. Use of fine-needle aspiration biopsy has halved the number of patients who undergo operation and has doubled the incidence of malignant disease detected in surgically excised lesions.

    Thyroxine and triiodothyronine levels, along with thyroglobulin antibody titres are not useful in the diagnostic evaluation of a solitary thyroid nodule.

240. e) The differential diagnosis of a thyroid nodule includes (1) granulomatous, pyogenic and viral infections; (2) congenital anomalies such as unilateral lobe agenesis, cystic hygroma, dermoid cyst, and teratoma; (4) a prominent area of generalized thyroiditis such as subacute thyroiditis, Hashimoto's thyroiditis, and Riedel's stroma; and (5) a focal anatomical lesion such as a thyroid cyst, adenoma or carcinoma.

241. c) Fine needle aspiration biopsy is the diagnostic procedure of choice in the evaluation of a thyroid nodule. It is 90% sensitive and 70% specific for the diagnosis of thyroid cancer. Because of its high sensitivity and specificity all suspicious lesions identified should be surgically excised. Significant bleeding is not a problem.

Reference

Rojeski M, Gharib H. Nodular Thyroid Disease. New England Journal of Medicine 1985; 313(7): 428-434.

Obstetrics and Gynecology

PROBLEM #35: A 23 YEAR OLD FEMALE ON THE ORAL CONTRACEPTIVE PILL

242. A 23-year old female whom you put on the oral contraceptive pill 6 months ago comes in complaining of increasing acne since she began the pill. How would you change the oral contraceptive to hopefully improve the acne?

   a) decrease the estrogenic activity
   b) increase the androgenic activity
   c) increase the estrogenic activity
   d) increase the progestational activity
   e) make no change in the oral contraceptive and review in one year

243. A 25-year old female comes to your office complaining of anorexia and nausea since beginning the oral contraceptive pill 4 months previously. How would you change the oral contraceptive to hopefully improve the nausea?

   a) increase the estrogenic activity
   b) increase the progestational activity
   c) decrease the progestational activity
   d) decrease the estrogenic activity
   e) increase the androgenic activity

244. A 27-year old female comes into your office complaining of tender breasts, bloating, edema of the lower extremities, and weight gain since you started her on the oral contraceptive pill 7 months ago. How would you change the oral contraceptive to hopefully improve her symptoms?

   a) increase the estrogenic activity
   b) increase the progestational activity
   c) decrease the estrogenic activity
   d) decrease the progestational activity
   e) increase the androgenic activity

245. An 18-year old female whom you began on the oral contraceptive pill 4 months ago comes into the office with a complaint of regular spotting on days 7-10 of the menstrual cycle since she began the pill. How would you change the oral contraceptive to hopefully eliminate the spotting?

a) increase the estrogenic activity
b) increase the progestational activity
c) decrease the estrogenic activity
d) decrease the progestational activity
e) either a or b

246. A 23-year old patient who has been on the oral contraceptive pill for 10 months begins experiencing spotting on days 11-23 of the menstrual cycle. This has occurred for the past 3 cycles. How would you change the oral contraceptive to hopefully eliminate the spotting?

a) increase the estrogenic activity
b) increase the progestational activity
c) decrease the estrogenic activity
d) decrease the progestational activity
e) increase the androgenic activity

247. A 24-year old student, who is slightly overweight, presents for her first checkup since starting the oral contraceptive pill. On her previous examination her blood pressure was 120/82. Today, her blood pressure is 128/92 in both the supine and sitting positions. It does not change after a period of rest. How would you change the oral contraceptive pill to hopefully decrease her blood pressure?

a) decrease the progestational activity
b) increase the progestational activity
c) decrease the estrogenic activity
d) increase the estrogenic activity
e) increase the androgenic activity

248. An 18-year old female whom you started on the oral contraceptive pill 8 months ago comes into your office complaining of depression since beginning the pill. How would you change the oral contraceptive pill to hopefully eliminate her depression?

a) decrease the estrogenic activity
b) decrease the progestational activity
c) increase the estrogenic activity
d) decrease the androgenic activity
e) increase the androgenic activity

CODE: (a:1, 2 and 3; b: 1 and 3; c: 2 and 4; d: 4 only; e: all of the above)

249. Which of the following conditions are ABSOLUTE contraindications to the use of the oral contraceptive pill?

    1) history of thromboembolic disorder
    2) abnormal vaginal bleeding
    3) hypercholesterolemia
    4) impaired liver function

250. Which of the following conditions are RELATIVE contraindications to the use of the oral contraceptive pill?

    1) diabetes mellitus
    2) cigarette smoking
    3) migraine headaches
    4) age greater than 30

251. Which of the following drugs may interact with the oral contraceptive pill to decrease its efficacy?

    1) phenobarbitol
    2) clofibrate
    3) valium
    4) ampicillin

ANSWERS

242. c) Androgenic symptoms such as acne will improve most of the time if a switch is made to an OC with a higher estrogenic activity. The possibility that androgenic symptoms are the result of androgenic activity of the OC may be determined by switching to an OC with less androgenic activity, but equal estrogenic activity.

243. d) Nausea while taking the oral contraceptive pill may be relieved by taking the OC with food at bed time. If this is not effective, then switching to an OC with less estrogenic activity and following a diet low in refined carbohydrates may improve the situation.

244. c) Symptoms such as abdominal bloating and edema are usually due to sodium and water retention caused by excessive estrogen. Abdominal bloating may also be caused by a reduction in bowel peristalsis due to the smooth muscle relaxing effect of progestins. These symptoms may be improved by switching to an OC with lower estrogenic activity.

245. e) Bleeding which starts early in the cycle, before the tenth OC is taken, or never ceases completely after menstruation is due to insufficient estrogen activity. Therefore, therapy with an oral contraceptive which is higher in estrogenic activity is usually effective. OC's with higher progestational activity may also be used, as they usually are more biologically active.

246. b) Bleeding which starts in the latter half of the OC cycle, after the 10th OC is taken, is due to insufficient endometrial activity of the progestin component. Therapy is therefore directed at increasing the progestin dose or substituting a more biologically active progestin at the same or a lower dose.

247. a) Women who use OC's are 6 times more likely to develop hypertension than non-OC users. The probability of developing hypertension increase with age and duration of use. Hypertension is usually due to the progestin component, and therefore mild increases in blood pressure may be initially treated by switching to an OC with less progestin activity and, if possible, the same estrogen content. Three months should be allowed for a change to occur. If hypertension continues, the OC should be stopped and an alternative birth control method considered.

248. b) Symptoms of tiredness, weakness, and depression in OC users may be due to the progestin component and may be similar to the symptoms of mid and late pregnancy. Patients with a history of psychic depression should be carefully observed and the drug discontinued if depression worsens while taking OC's. Use of tricyclic antidepressants should be avoided because of their possible interaction with OC's causing a decrease in their efficacy. Vitamin B_6, 25 mg./day may cause improvement in some cases.

     Switching to an OC with a lower progestin dose may relieve symptoms of depression and should be considered as a primary treatment before discontinuing the oral contraceptive.

249. e) The absolute contraindications to the oral contraceptive pill are (1) thrombophlebitis or thromboembolic disorder or past history of same, (2) coronary artery or cerebrovascular disease, (3) undiagnosed abnormal vaginal bleeding, (4) known or suspected pregnancy, (5) markedly impaired liver function, (6) known or suspected carcinoma of the breast or uterus, and (7) Type II hyperlipidemia or hypercholesterolemia.

250. a) The relative contraindications to the oral contraceptive pill are (1) diabetes mellitus, (2) obesity, (3) cigarette smoking, (4) vascular or migraine headaches, (5) cardiac or renal dysfunction, (6) hypertension, (7) psychotic depression, (8) varicose veins, (9) sickle cell disease or trait, (10) history of cholestatic jaundice during pregnancy, (11) worsening of any chronic condition during pregnancy, (12) hepatitis or infectious mononucleosis during the past year, (13) asthma, (14) first order family history of fatal or non-fatal cardiovascular

disease before age 50, (15) ulcerative colitis, and (16) the use of drugs such as anticonvulsants, antibiotics, benzodiazepines, antidepressants and antipsychotics.

Age past 35, rather than 30, is also thought to be a relative contraindication.

251. e) The drugs which are known to interact with the OC and decrease its efficacy can be divided into 5 groups. They are:

1) the anticonvulsants — phenobarbitol, carbamazepin, primidone, phenytoin, and ethosuximide
2) the cholesterol lowering agents such as clofibrate
3) the antibiotics — rifampin, isoniazid, penicillin, ampicillin, metronidazole, tetracycline, neomycin, chloramphenicol, sulfonimides, and nitrofurantoin
4) sedatives, hypnotics, tricyclics, and antipsychotics — valium, chloral hydrate, elavil, largactil etc.
5) antacids

Reference

Dickey R. Managing contraceptive pill patients. Creative Infomatics (Canada) Inc. 4th edition, 1984.

PROBLEM #36: AN EXHAUSTED 25 YEAR OLD MOTHER IN THE SECOND STAGE OF LABOUR

252. A 25 year old primigravida in the second stage of labor has reached the point of exhaustion. You decide to apply prophylactic forceps. You recall that prophylactic forceps is the application of outlet forceps to facilitate delivery when the perineum and coccyx offer the only resistance to delivery. Which of the following is FALSE regarding prophylactic forceps?

a) an episiotomy should be done prior to the application of forceps
b) it is intended to spare the fetal head unpredictable stress
c) it may shorten the second stage of labour
d) it may prevent injury to the pelvic floor
e) may be performed before the fetal scalp has reached the introitus

253. Which of the following IS NOT an indication for forceps delivery?

a) maternal exhaustion
b) maternal cardiac or pulmonary dysfunction
c) fetal bradycardia
d) meconium stained amniotic fluid
e) early decelerations on the fetal heart tracing

254. The main advantage of the silastic vacuum extractor over the outlet forceps for vaginal delivery is:

a) it is easier to apply the vacuum correctly
b) the vacuum extractor may be applied at an earlier stage
c) it causes less intracranial compression
d) the fetal head can usually be delivered more quickly
e) the incidence of cephalohematoma is less with the vacuum extractor

CODE: (a:1, 2 and 3; b: 1 and 3; c: 2 and 4; d: 4 only; e: all of the above)

255. Which of the following conditions must be satisfied before the obstetrical forceps is/are applied?

1) The cervix must be fully dilated
2) The membranes must be ruptured
3) The head must be engaged to station +2
4) The bladder should be empty

256. Which of the following conditions satisfy the definition of outlet forceps?

   1) the scalp is or has been visible at the introitus without the need to separate the labia
   2) the skull has reached the pelvic floor
   3) the sagittal suture is in the anteroposterior diameter
   4) a significant caput should not be present

ANSWERS

252. e) By definition, the fetal scalp has reached the introitus before a forceps delivery can be referred to as "outlet". Descent of the fetal head is a condition for prophylactic forceps. An episiotomy should be done to facilitate delivery and decrease the intracranial pressure during delivery. Prophylactic forceps spares the fetal head unpredictable stress; especially compression against the perineum. Prophylactic forceps shortens the second stage of labor if performed correctly, and may prevent injury to the pelvic floor.

253. e) There are both maternal and fetal indications for outlet forceps. Maternal indications include maternal exhaustion, maternal cardiac or pulmonary problems and intercurrent debilitating illness. Fetal indications include fetal bradycardia, late deceleration patterns on the fetal monitor strip, excessive fetal movements as a possible sign of fetal distress, and the passage of meconium stained amniotic fluid. Early deceleration patterns on the fetal monitor strip are a sign of fetal head compression but not fetal distress.

254. c) The main advantage of the silastic vacuum extractor over the obstetrical forceps in terms of fetal morbidity is the lower intracranial pressure increase produced by the instrument. Studies have indicated an almost 10X greater increase in intracranial pressure with the obstetrical forceps. It is also true that it may be applied at a higher station but this is not its major advantage in terms of lower fetal morbidity. If the proper technique is used, the instruments are equally easy to apply. If anything, the fetal head can probably be delivered more quickly with the obstetrical forceps. Cephalohematoma is more common with the use of the vacuum extractor.

255. e) The use of forceps is permissible only when all of the following conditions prevail, regardless of the urgent need for delivery. (1) The cervix must be fully dilated. (2) The membranes must be ruptured. (3) The head must be engaged (preferably deeply engaged) to a station below +2. (4) The presenting part must be vertex or face with chin anterior. One may apply forceps to the aftercoming head in breech presentation provided the head is engaged and is in the occiput anterior position. (5) There must be no significant cephalopelvic disproportion and (6) the bladder must be empty.

256.   a) An oulet forceps is defined as the application of forceps when the scalp is or
has been visible at the introitus (without the need to separate the labia), the
skull has reached the pelvic floor, and the sagittal suture is in the anteroposterior diameter of the pelvis. (In outlet forceps, the perineum and coccyx offer
the only resistance to delivery). The presence of caput has no bearing on
whether or not forceps can be applied.

Reference

Danforth D. Operative Delivery. Current Obstetric and Gynecologic Diagnosis and Treatment, 5th edition. Benson R., editor. Lange Medical Publications 1984; 946-991.

PROBLEM #37: A 25 YEAR OLD PRIMIGRAVIDA WITH HYPERTENSION

257. A 25-year old primigravida is seen in your office at 32 weeks gestation. Her blood pressure, which has been normal up to now, is 160/95. Her urine shows 100 mg./dl protein and she has gained 60 lbs. The appropriate management in this case is to:

a) reassure the patient and see her in another 2 weeks
b) hospitalize the patient
c) inform the patient that her blood pressure is up and she is going to need more rest at home
d) begin therapy with hydrochlorothiazide 50 mg./day and reassess the patient in 1 week
e) begin therapy with alpha-methyldopa and reassess the patient in 1 weeks time

258. Which of the following statements regarding preeclampsia is FALSE?

a) blood pressure readings are characteristically labile
b) mild pre-eclampsia may very quickly become fulminant eclampsia
c) preeclampsia is defined as a blood pressure reading of 160/90 after the 20th week of gestation
d) a decreased intravascular volume seems to be the primary event that is responsible for the rise in blood pressure
e) abnormalities of the clotting system and liver function may occur in preeclampsia

259. Which of the following medications is ABSOLUTELY CONTRAINDI-CATED in pregnancy?

a) captopril
b) propranolol
c) alpha-methyldopa
d) hydralazine
e) nifedipine

260. A 34 year old primigravida is seen in the office for her first prenatal visit. She is 8 weeks gestation. On questioning, you discover that she is hypertensive and has been on propranolol (Inderal) for 6 years. On examination her blood pressure is 120/70. Which of the following courses of action would you now recommend?

a) discontinue the propranolol
b) discontinue the propranolol and substitute hydrochlorothiazide
c) continue the propranolol
d) discontinue the propranolol and substitute alpha-methyldopa
e) discontinue the propranolol and substitute captopril

CODE: (a:1, 2 and 3; b: 1 and 3; c: 2 and 4; d: 4 only; e: all of the above)

261. The classification of hypertensive disorders in pregnancy proposed by the American College of Obstetricians and Gynecologists includes:

    1) preeclampsia and eclampsia
    2) chronic hypertension
    3) chronic hypertension with superimposed preeclampsia
    4) transient or late hypertension

ANSWERS

257. b) Ambulatory treatment has no place in the management of pregnancy-induced or pregnancy-aggravated hypertension. Immediate hospitalization and absolute bed rest of this patient are indicated.

    At this point in time, therapy for the hypertension can be withheld. Diuretics would not be used in any case, as this would aggravate an already volume-contracted state. The drug of choice for the hypertension associated with severe preeclampsia (diastolic pressure greater than 105) is hydralazine.

    The treatment of choice for preeclampsia is delivery of the fetus, with the delivery date being dictated by the risk of the fetus remaining in utero compared to the risk of complications of prematurity.

258. c) Preeclampsia is defined as a blood pressure of 140/90 mm. Hg. or greater, or an increase in systolic of 30 mm. Hg. or 15 mm. Hg. diastolic over baseline values on at least 2 occasions 6 or more hours apart; plus proteinuria, or edema which is generalized and overt.

    The blood pressure readings are characteristically labile reflecting the intense sensitivity of the vasculature to endogenous pressor peptides and catecholamines.

    Mild preeclampsia may very quickly develop into fulminant eclampsia, and thus hospitalization of almost all patients is mandatory. Severe preeclampsia and eclampsia are associated with disorders of coagulation including disseminated intravascular coagulation, and hepatic dysfunction.

    A decreased intravascular volume seems to be the primary event that is responsible for the rise in blood pressure; (e.g., placental hypoperfusion may induce the release of a pressor substance from the uterus, or relative hypovolemia may result in excessive instead of compensatory secretion of catecholamines.)

259. a) Captopril is ABSOLUTELY contraindicated in pregnancy. Captopril has had disastrous effects on the fetusus of several species and should not be used.

    Propranolol, hydrochlorothiazide, alpha-methyldopa, and hydralazine may be safely used in pregnancy. It is recommended to keep a patient with chronic hypertension who is taking one of these drugs on her medication during pregnancy. If a patient is going to be started on antihypertensive medication during pregnancy, either alpha-methyldopa or propranolol are probably the best choices.

Nifedipine is a calcium-channel blocking agent that is finding increasing use as an antihypertensive in acute hypertensive emergencies in pregnancy.

260. c) (See the critique of question #259). The best course of action in this patient would be to keep her on the propranolol which she has been taking for the last 6 years.

261. e) The classification of hypertension in pregnancy purposed by the American College of Obstetricians and Gynecologists includes (1) preeclampsia and eclampsia, (2) chronic hypertension (of whatever cause), (3) chronic hypertension with superimposed preeclampsia and (4) late or transient hypertension.

Late or transient hypertension is hypertension which develops alone (without proteinuria) in the last trimester or in the immediate puerperium, and returns to normal within 10 days of delivery. The outcome of such pregnancies is almost always excellent.

References

Lindheimer M, Katz A. Hypertension in pregnancy. New England Journal of Medicine 1985; 313(11): 675-679.

Pritchard J, MacDonald P, Gant N. Williams Obstetrics, 17th edition. Appleton-Century-Crofts, Norwalk, 1985.

PROBLEM #38: A 30 YEAR OLD FEMALE WITH PREMENSTRUAL SYNDROME

262. A 30 year old female with a 6 month history of headache, irritability and depression beginning at ovulation and continuing until the onset of menstruation presents to your office. You suspect premenstrual tension syndrome and wish to begin treatment. Which of the following has NOT been advocated as a treatment for premenstrual syndrome?

    a) Vitamin E
    b) zinc sulfate
    c) progesterone
    d) spironolactone
    e) a high protein diet

263. The most important element in establishing a diagnosis of premenstrual syndrome is a good history. The most important information that can be obtained in the history is:

    a) the severity of symptoms
    b) the number of symptoms
    c) the timing of the symptoms in the menstrual cycle
    d) the presence and severity of the depression or anxiety
    e) all of the above symptoms are of equal importance

264. Many theories have been hypothesized to explain the premenstrual syndrome. Which of the following theories is currently felt to have the greatest support?

    a) the multiple hormonal etiology theory
    b) the endogenous opiate peptide theory
    c) the monoamine oxidase activity theory
    d) the psychogenic theory
    e) the water retention theory

CODE: (a:1, 2 and 3; b: 1 and 3; c: 2 and 4; d: 4 only; e: all of the above)

265. For the diagnosis of premenstrual syndrome to be made, which of the following criteria must be fulfilled?

    1) the symptoms must occur in three consecutive cycles
    2) the symptoms must be limited to the luteal phase
    3) there must be a complete absence of symptoms for at least one week in the postmenstrual period
    4) depression must be one of the symptoms

266. Progesterone therapy is currently one of the most popular forms of therapy for premenstrual syndrome. Which of the following are preferred progesterone regimes for the treatment of PMS?

   1) Provera 10 mg. p.o. starting at ovulation
   2) progesterone suppositories 400-1600 mg./day starting five days before the symptoms are expected
   3) Depo-Provera 150 mg. IM every month
   4) progesterone IM 25-100 mg./day starting 5 days before the symptoms are expected

ANSWERS

262. e) Many different forms of therapy have been advocated for the treatment of premenstrual syndrome. It is reasonable to look first at the disability that the syndrome is causing the individual rather than making a blanket statement about therapy.

   For PMS that does not interfere significantly with the patient's life, job or relationships, the appropriate treatment is education, understanding and reassurance. The patient should be advised to adjust her life to reduce stress, especially in the premenstral period, and the family should be educated about PMS. Mild PMS is essentially controlled by these measures and requires no medication.

   For PMS that interferes with the patient's lifestyle, discontinue the birth control pill, if the patient continues to have symptoms while taking it. Dietary management may be helpful. The woman should eat every three hours; complex carbohydrates are best. The patient should also limit fluid and sodium intake if water retention is a problem, and decrease caffeine intake if she suffers from irritability and palpitations. Lifestyle changes should include moderate exercise, stress reduction and extra rest in the premenstrual period.

   Analgesics and diuretics can be taken as required. The most effective diuretic is spironolactone 100 mg./day starting 5 days prior to the onset of symptoms.

   Pyridoxine 100-300 mg./day may be effective. This agent is a necessary co-factor in the synthesis of dopamine and serotonin in the brain.

   For PMS symptoms that are life-threatening or interfering significantly with the patient's relationships, job or life, the best treatment is natural progesterone and counselling.

   Vitamin E therapy has been advocated for the relief of breast tenderness that is not responsive to the decrease in caffeine intake. The dosage is 600 IU/day.

   Zinc sulfate in a dose of 135 mg./day is effective in patients in which acne is a component of PMS.

263. c) The most important single factor in providing a diagnosis of premenstrual syndrome is the relationship of the symptoms to the menstrual cycle. This is best established by the patient keeping a calendar for three months that correlates symptoms with the major events of the cycle. The number of symptoms including headache, breast tenderness, abdominal bloating, peripheral edema, fatigue, depression, tension, irritability, and increased appetite are of secondary importance. Also, the severity of symptoms and the presence or absence of depression are not diagnostic criteria.

264. a) The multiple hormonal etiology theory is currently thought to have the greatest support. This theory hypothesizes a relative or absolute deficiency of progesterone in the luteal phase of the menstrual cycle. The involvement of the sex hormone binding globulin (SHBG) is also thought to play a role. In this theory, the estrogen may be elevated above normal levels.

Other theories that have been put forward are the endogenous opiate peptide theory, that postulates the involvement of endorphins and their inhibitory effect on gonadotrophin secretion; the monoamine oxidase activity theory in which MAO levels are apparently high in the premenstrual period; the psychogenic theory and the water and sodium retention theory.

265. a) For the diagnosis of premenstrual syndrome to be made the following criteria have to be fulfilled:

   a) the charted symptoms must be present in three consecutive cycles
   b) the symptoms must be limited to the luteal phase
   c) there must be a complete absence of symptoms for at least one week in the postmenstruum

The presence or absence of depression is not a diagnostic criteria.

266. c) Natural progesterone is currently thought to be more effective for therapy than a synthetic progestin such as Provera. Natural progesterone suppositories 400 mg. o.d.-q.i.d. may be given starting 5 days before the onset of symptoms. If symptoms occur as early as ovulation, therapy may be begun 2 days prior to expected ovulation. Progesterone may also be administered intramuscularly in a dose of 25-100 mg. o.d. The starting time for this regime should be the same.

Therapy should be continued for at least 6-9 months. Women over 40 will likely need progesterone until menopause. Women under 25 will need it for six to nine months. For those women aged 25-40, the length of treatment will depend on other risk factors such as history of pre-eclampsia and post-natal depression, and individual response to medication.

References

Havens C. Premenstrual syndrome. Postgraduate Medicine 1985; 77(7): 32-37.
Simkin R. Premenstrual Syndrome: Approaches to Diagnosis and Treatment. Canadian Family Physician 1985; 77: 1959-1967.

PROBLEM #39: A 25 YEAR OLD NULLIPARA AT 8 WEEKS GESTATION WITH VAGINAL BLEEDING

267. A 25 year old female para 0 gravida 3 presents to your office at 8 weeks gestation with vaginal bleeding and mild cramping. Her previous two pregnancies ended in miscarriages at 9 weeks. On examination a moderate bright red flow is seen coming from the cervical os. The cervix is closed. Clinical palpation reveals an 8 week uterus. The diagnosis at this time is:

    a) threatened abortion
    b) inevitable abortion
    c) incomplete abortion
    d) habitual abortion
    e) complete abortion

268. Referring to the patient described in question #267, the flow increases slightly while the patient is in your office. She is now soaking through approximately 1 pad every 2 hours. You would recommend:

    a) observation at home and outpatient investigation
    b) observation in hospital and inpatient investigation
    c) outpatient observation only, no further investigations
    d) inpatient observation only, no further investigations
    e) it doesn't really matter

269. The patient described in question #267 goes on to abort the fetus 3 days later. On examination it appears that most of the placental tissue is present. You would now recommend:

    a) no further treatment
    b) ergonovine maleate to contract the uterus
    c) prophylactic antibiotics to prevent infection
    d) dilatation and curettage
    e) b and c

270. One week later the patient described in question #267 comes to your office tearful and depressed. She states that she lifted 3 heavy boxes the day before she began to bleed. She now feels sure that this caused the abortion. She asks you to confirm her suspicions. In couselling this patient you should explain that:

    a) yes, carrying the heavy boxes did probably cause the abortion, but not to worry; she can always get pregnant again
    b) yes, carrying the heavy boxes may have had an influence in causing the abortion but it probably won't happen again
    c) guilt is a universal response to grief and that is why she is wondering about carrying the boxes. However, there is no reason to believe that the carrying of the boxes had anything to do with the miscarriage

d) miscarriage is nature's way of dealing with bad chromosomes and if carrying the boxes had anything to do with the miscarriage then it probably was for the best
e) boxes or no boxes, the pregnancy was doomed to failure from the start

CODE: (a:1, 2 and 3; b: 1 and 3; c: 2 and 4; d: 4 only; e: all of the above)

271. Which of the following statements regarding chromosomal abnormalities in spontaneous abortions is/are TRUE:

1) most situations of a chromosomal abnormality in the fetus result from a chromosomal abnormality in one or both parents
2) structural abnormalities are much more common than abnormalities in the number of chromosomes
3) the most common chromosomal abnormality is 47 XX
4) 50-60% of early spontaneous abortions are associated with a chromosomal anomaly of the conceptus.

272. Which of the following statements is/are TRUE regarding habitual abortion?

1) habitual abortion is defined as three or more consecutive abortions
2) repeated spontaneous abortions are likely to be a chance phenomena in most cases
3) couples who have a history of habitual abortion should receive a complete chromosomal analysis
4) the probability of having a successful pregnancy after three consecutive spontaneous abortions is 70-85%.

ANSWERS

267. a) Threatened abortion is presumed when any bloody vaginal discharge or vaginal bleeding appears during the first half of pregnancy. A threatened abortion may or may not be accompanied by mild crampy pain resembling that of a menstrual period or by low backache.

Inevitable abortion refers to vaginal bleeding during the first half of pregnancy accompanied by cervical dilatation and rupture of the gestational sac.

Incomplete abortion refers to the incomplete evacuation of the products of conception during the abortion. It is often difficult to be sure all of the products of conception have been expelled without doing a dilatation and curettage.

Habitual abortion refers to three or more consecutive completed abortions. Complete abortion refers to the complete evacuation of the products of conception from the uterus during the first half of pregnancy.

268. b) In any patient with more than slight bleeding hospitalization is wise. With the associated cramping there is a very good probability that she will go on to abort the fetus. Investigations in hospital should include a beta HcG level and an obstetrical ultrasound, looking for a gestational sac with a fetal pole and fetal cardiac motion.

269. d) Unless all of the fetus and placenta can be positively identified, dilatation and curettage is indicated. It is often very difficult to be sure that an abortion is indeed complete.

Ergonovine maleate and prophylactic antibiotics are most useful when excessive bleeding occurs in the post-partum period and when that bleeding is unlikely to be due to retained products of conception.

270. c) Guilt is a universal response to a miscarriage. Women go back over their pregnancies and often find something to "blame" the event on. It is extremely important to establish that there is *nothing* the patient could have done to alter the outcome. This concept may have to be discussed repeatedly before it is finally accepted.

Although it is true that 50-60% of early spontaneous abortions are associated with a chromosomal abnormality, it is inappropriate to dismiss a miscarriage as "nature's way of dealing with bad chromosomes". The situation discussed calls for explanation about guilt feelings, time, and most of all empathy, on the part of the physician.

271. d) It is now appreciated that chromosomal abnormalities are common among embryos and early fetuses that are aborted spontaneously and account for most early pregnancy wastage. From several studies it is apparent that 50-60% of early spontaneous abortions are associated with a chromosomal anomaly of the conceptus.

Abnormalities in the number of chromosomes are much more common than are structural abnormalities of chromosomes. Structural abnormalities can be transmitted by one of the parents who is a balanced chromosome carrier or the structural abnormality can arise denovo.

Parents of fetuses with chromosomal abnormalities most often have normal chromosome complements themselves. Numerical abnormalities include monosomies, trisomies and polyploidies with the most common being the monosomy 45X.

Pregnancies destined to abort because of a chromosomally abnormal zygote may, on the one hand, go unrecognized because the products of conception are aborted with little or no delay in the onset of menstruation, or on the other, may continue for some time after the embryo or early fetus has died.

272. e) Habitual abortion is defined as three or more consecutive spontaneous abortions. Repeated spontaneous abortions are likely to be a chance phenomenon in the majority of cases. The spontaneous pregnancy rate after as many as three consecutive spontaneous abortions will range from 70-85%.

Several investigators now recommend karyotyping the parents after they have experienced two or three spontaneous abortions. When karyotyping is performed, chromosomal banding techniques should be applied.

Reference

Pritchard J, MacDonald P and Gant N., editors. Williams Obstetrics, seventeenth edition. Appleton-Century-Crofts, Norwalk: 1985; pages 467-475.

PROBLEM #40: A 30 YEAR OLD FEMALE WITH AMENORRHEA

273. A 30 year old female with a 4 year history of amenorrhea presents for evaluation of infertility. Her physical examination is normal. Serum thyroxine and prolactin are normal, and a pregnancy test is negative. The next step in the investigation should be:

a) a pelvic ultrasound
b) a CT scan of the pituitary gland
c) a hysterosalpingogram
d) a progestin challenge test
e) an estrogen challenge test

274. The two most important assays to perform in a woman with amenorrhea and symptoms of androgen excess are:

a) dihydrotestosterone and dehydroepiandrosterone sulfate
b) dihydrotestosterone and testosterone
c) androstenedione and testosterone
d) dehydroepiandrosterone sulfate and androstenedione
e) dehydroepiandrosterone sulfate and testosterone

275. Which of the following statements about a patient who bleeds following a progestin challenge test is CORRECT?

a) this is a negative test result and suggests endometrial pathology
b) this is a positive test result and suggests endometrial pathology
c) this is a positive test result and suggests anovulation
d) this is a negative test result and suggests anovulation
e) this result is too nonspecific to suggest anything

276. A 30 year old woman with a 1 year history of amenorrhea and hirsutism presents to your office. Her physical examination reveals excessive facial hair. Her serum testosterone level is twice normal (3.0 ng./dl). Her dehydroepiandrosterone sulfate level is normal. The most likely diagnosis in this patient is:

a) ovarian neoplasm
b) virilizing adrenal neoplasm
c) Cushing's syndrome
d) polycystic ovary syndrome
e) congenital virilizing adrenal hyperplasia

277. Assuming that other investigations confirm your diagnosis, the treatment of choice for the patient described in question #276 is:

   a) bromocriptine
   b) danazol
   c) the oral contraceptive
   d) electrolysis
   e) diethylstilbesterol

CODE: (a:1, 2 and 3; b: 1 and 3; c: 2 and 4; d: 4 only; e: all of the above)

278. A 35 year old patient presents with a 2 month history of amenorrhea along with hot flushes, sweating and palpitations. Her physical examination is normal. Her progesterone challenge test is negative. The next step(s) in her evaluation should include:

   1) determination of serum LH
   2) estrogen/progesterone challenge tests
   3) determination of serum FSH
   4) CT scan of the pituitary gland

ANSWERS

273. d) Having ascertained that the amenorrheic patient is not pregnant, the questions that remain are: 1) Does she produce a biologically significant amount of estrogen? 2) Is her endometrium capable of bleeding? and 3) If she is not estrogenized, is it because her ovaries are incapable of responding to gonadotrophin stimulation or because gonadotrophin release is impaired? One can address the first two questions by administering a progestational agent — the so-called progesterone challenge test. Oral medroxyprogesterone acetate 5-10 mg./day is given for 5 days. Several days after instituting the regime the woman who produces adequate estrogen and has a normal endometrium will experience uterine bleeding. The test reliably distinguishes between estrogenized and non-estrogenized women. Most amenorrheic women who bleed after receiving a progestin challenge test have anovulation as the cause for their amenorrhea. At this stage it would also be reasonable to check the serum prolactin level to rule out a prolactinoma.

274. e) The two most important assays to perform in a woman with amenorrhea and symptoms of androgen excess are dehydroepiandrosterone sulfate and testosterone. Dehydroepiandrosterone sulfate uniquely reflects adrenal androgenesis. Unfortunately, no counterpart of DS is a unique product of ovarian androgenesis. Nevertheless, most endocrinologists interpret the serum testosterone concentration to be largely an indicator of ovarian androgen production.

275. c) The rationale for the progestin challenge test has been explained in the critique of question #273. If the patient bleeds following 5-10 mg./day of oral medroxyprogesterone acetate for 5 days she is producing adequate estrogen and the most likely reason for her amenorrhea is anovulation. The test result is then positive. If she does not bleed the test result is negative and she is not producing adequate estrogen. In this case the investigation for the amenorrhea must be continued with an estrogen/progesterone challenge test. If the patient fails to bleed following the adminstration of both estrogen and progesterone, uterine pathology such as Ashermann's syndrome or granulomatous endometritis must be considered.

276. d) The two most common causes of hirsutism are constitutional hirsutism and polycystic ovary syndrome. An elevated serum testosterone and normal dehydroepiandrosterone sulfate mean the androgen excess is from the ovary, making virilizing adrenal neoplasia and congenital virilizing adrenal hyperplasia extremely unlikely. Although an ovarian neoplasm is a possibility that obviously must be ruled out by ultrasound, polycystic ovary syndrome is much more likely.

    Cushing's syndrome, although sometimes associated with virilizing features would present with many other symptoms of glucocorticoid excess.

277. c) The treatment of choice for polycystic ovary syndrome is the oral contraceptive pill. Preferably, this should be an oral contraceptive with a weak progestational and androgenic component. This will decrease serum testosterone production from the ovary. As well, this treatment should regulate the menstrual cycle. If the patient wanted to become pregnant then clomiphene citrate would be the treatment of choice.

    Bromocriptine is a dopamine agonist/prolactin inhibitor and is therefore not indicated in treatment of polycystic ovary syndrome. Danazol is a gonadotrophin inhibitor with mild androgenic effects that may possibly increase the hirsutism. Diethylstilbesterol is only indicated for use as adjuvant therapy in advanced prostatic cancer. Electrolysis may decrease the hair already present on the body but will not effect hair production.

278. a) This lady's history is suspicious of premature ovarian failure. As well as serum LH and FSH, she should have an estrogen/progesterone challenge test to prove that her endometrium can be stimulated and be shed. For this test, Premarin 2.5 mg. daily is given on days 1-25 with Provera 5-10 mg. daily on days 21-25. If the test is positive and she bleeds, and if the LH/FSH levels are elevated she has primary premature ovarian failure. A pelvic CT scan would not be of any assistance in this case.

Reference

Siwek J, editor. American Academy of Family Physicians Home Study Self Assessment — Office Gynecology I, Monograph 73. Kansas City: 1985, pages 28-36.

PROBLEM #41: A 17 YEAR OLD PRIMIGRAVIDA WITH A SMALL BABY

279. A 17 year old nulliparous female with pre-eclampsia is being followed for possible intrauterine growth retardation. She is presently at 34 weeks gestation. She has noticed decreased fetal movements for the past 2 days. A biophysical profile gives her a score of 4 out of 10. In addition deep decelerations are seen in response to an oxytocin challenge test. Her blood pressure is 170/100. The immediate course of action should be to:

   a) lower the diastolic blood pressure to 80 mm.Hg. and reassess the situation
   b) immediate caesarian section
   c) immediate induction of labor with prostaglandin gel
   d) bed rest, antihypertensive agents and reassessment in 24 hours
   e) immediate induction of labor with syntocinon.

280. The leading cause of stillbirth in intrauterine growth retarded fetuses is:

   a) intrauterine asphyxia
   b) pre-eclampsia in the mother
   c) diabetes in the mother
   d) meconium aspiration
   e) none of the above

281. The biophysical profile has become a standard for the assessment of fetusus at risk for intrauterine growth retardation (IUGR). Which of the following parameters IS NOT a part of the biophysical profile?

   a) fetal cardiac reactivity
   b) fetal posture and tone
   c) the ratio of the biparietal diameter to the abdominal circumference
   d) fetal limb movements
   e) amniotic fluid volume

CODE: (a:1, 2 and 3; b: 1 and 3; c: 2 and 4; d: 4 only; e: all of the above)

282. Intrauterine growth retardation can be divided into symmetrical and asymmetrical. Symmetrical IUGR refers to impairment of growth with reduced birth weight, length, and head circumference. Asymmetrical IUGR, on the other hand, is associated with a normal head circumference and is widely believed to spare brain growth. Which of the following is/are causes of asymmetric IUGR?

   1) congenital malformations, including dysmorphic syndromes
   2) preeclampsia
   3) chromosomal abnormalities
   4) cigarette smoking

283. Which of the following statements regarding the diagnosis of IUGR is/are CORRECT?

   1) Thirty to fifty percent of growth retarded babies remain undetected by clinical examination.
   2) Abdominal palpation is unreliable for the assessment of fetal weight.
   3) Ultrasonic measurement of biparietal diameter detects only 50-60% of growth retarded fetuses.
   4) Serial plotting of symphysis-fundal height is a reliable indicator of uterine growth in almost all cases.

ANSWERS

279. b) The only course of action that is reasonable in this situation is immediate caesarian section. The fetus has not been moving well for the past two days, has a poor biophysical profile score and has a positive contraction stress test. This indicates acute fetal distress and immediate delivery is indicated.

   Induction of labor will delay delivery and stress an already compromised uteroplacental blood flow. To bring the blood pressure down to 80 mm. Hg. is an unnecessary waste of time. To observe this fetus in utero for 24 hours will quite probably result in the death of the baby.

280. a) The leading cause of stillbirth in intrauterine growth-retarded fetuses is intrauterine asphyxia. Not only is placental gaseous exchange compromised but the growth-retarded fetus has low reserves of cardiac glycogen and this makes them intolerant to asphyxia compared with fetuses experiencing normal growth. A growth-retarded fetus living on the brink of asphyxia is at special risk during labour, when uteroplacental flow is further restricted.

   Preeclampsia in the mother and diabetes in the mother may cause intrauterine asphyxia by their deleterious effect on utero-placental blood flow. Meconium staining is a sign of potential fetal distress and intrauterine asphyxia.

281. c) The biophysical profile incorporates five parameters into fetal assessment. They are (1) cardiac reactivity; (2) fetal posture; (3) fetal limb movements; (4) fetal breathing movements; and (5) amniotic fluid volume. Each of these has been shown to be an independant predictor of fetal health and well-being; therefore a combination of the five variables should theoretically be a better predictor than a single variable. Each of the 5 components is given a score of "0-2" for a possible score of 10 points. A comparison of biparietal to abdominal circumference will predict asymmetrical IUGR but is not part of the biophysical profile.

282. c) The underlying pathogenic factor in asymmetrical IUGR is uteroplacental insufficiency. In some cases there is an underlying maternal disorder including preeclampsia, recurrent antepartum hemorrhage, chronic hypertension,

147

renal disease, diabetes with microvascular changes, sickle cell disease, cyanotic congenital heart disease, malnutrition, alcohol and cigarette smoking. In about 30% of cases, no risk factor is apparent; such cases are referred to as idiopathic IUGR.

Causes of symmetrical growth retardation include congenital malformations, including dysmorphic syndromes; chromosomal abnormalities; and congenital viral infections, with the most common being cytomegalovirus.

283. a) Aside from specific maternal medical conditions the risk factors associated with an increased incidence of intrauterine growth retardation include a history of intrauterine growth retardation, low weight before pregnancy, low weight gain during pregnancy, multiple pregnancy and smoking. About 30-50% of growth retarded fetuses remain undetected by clinical examination. Abdominal palpation is notoriously unreliable for the assessment of fetal weight, and serial examinations carried out at weekly intervals will detect only the most severe examples of growth retardation. Serial plotting of symphysis-fundal height is a useful screening test for intrauterine growth retardation according to some observers, but not everyone agrees. It is certainly of little value in multiple pregnancy, polyhydramanios, transverse lie, or extreme maternal obesity.

Ultrasound measurements are used singly or in formulations to monitor fetal growth or predict fetal weight. Measurement of the biparietal diameter identifies only 50-60% of growth-retarded fetuses, while over half of those suspected of being growth retarded prove to be normally grown at birth. Limitations arise because of variations in the shape of the head, and because the size of the head is spared or compromised only late in asymmetrical intrauterine growth retardation.

Reference

Chiswick M. Intrauterine Growth Retardation. British Medical Journal 1985; 291: 845-847.

PROBLEM #42: AN 18 YEAR OLD FEMALE WITH AN ABNORMAL PAP SMEAR

284. An 18 year old female presents for her annual physical examination. On pelvic examination, a foul-smelling vaginal discharge is present. The wet mount is positive for Trichomonas vaginalis. A pap smear is taken and comes back as mild dysplasia (Class II). Your next step should be to:

    a) repeat the Pap smear in 1 year
    b) repeat the Pap smear in 6 months
    c) refer the patient for cone biopsy
    d) refer the patient for colposcopy
    e) treat the infection and repeat the Pap smear

285. A 25 year old female presents for her annual physical examination. Pelvic examination is normal and the cervix looks healthy. There is no vaginal or cervical discharge. However, the Pap smear comes back as Class II (mild dysplasia). Your next step should be to:

    a) repeat the Pap smear in 1 year
    b) repeat the Pap smear in 6 months
    c) repeat the Pap smear in 3 months
    d) refer the patient for colposcopy
    e) refer the patient for cone biopsy

Questions 286-289 are TRUE and FALSE questions. If the statement is TRUE mark "a", if it is FALSE mark "b".

286. The incidence of C.I.S. (carcinoma-in-situ) is rising in the North American population.

287. The time it takes for cervical intraepithelial neoplasia (C.I.N.) to progress to invasive cancer is believed to be relatively long, on average 10-15 years.

288. The false-negative rate of the Pap smear is currently thought to be about 33%.

289. There is a clear association between C.I.N. and human papillomavirus.

CODE: (a:1, 2 and 3; b: 1 and 3; c: 2 and 4; d: 4 only; e: all of the above)

290. A recent North American study indicated that up to 90% of the young women under 35 were at high risk for cervical intraepithelial neoplasia. Which of the following factor(s) is/are considered high risk factors for this condition?

    1) multiple sexual partners
    2) cigarette smoking
    3) first sexual intercourse before age 20
    4) low socioeconomic status

ANSWERS

284. e) Infections are notorious for changing normal cervical epithelia to inflammed epithelia with mild atypical features. Once the infection is treated, the epithelium will often return to normal. Therefore, once the infection has cleared the Pap smear should be repeated. If it is still abnormal referral for colposcopy is mandatory. If it is normal another Pap smear should be arranged within 1 year.

285. d) An abnormal Pap smear in the absence of vaginal or cervical infection should be assessed by colposcopy. As discussed earlier, there is a certain subset of lesions that may progress through the stages of intraepithelial neoplasia rather quickly, making delineation and assessment of the lesion mandatory. Dysplasias are usually treated by cryotherapy and laser therapy, and cone biopsy is much less common than it used to be.

286. a) TRUE. The incidence of C.I.S. is rising in the North American population. Since 1970 there has been a dramatic increase in the number of cases of in-situ carcinoma. This may be due to new trends in sexual promiscuity, with an increase in the number of sexual partners and a decrease in the mean age of first intercourse.

287. a) TRUE. The time it takes for cervical intraepithelial neoplasia (C.I.N.) to progress to invasive cancer is believed to be relatively long, on average 10-15 years, and according to some, less than half of the most undifferientated precursor forms (C.I.N. grade II or carcinoma-in-situ) progress to invasive cancer. However, there seems to be a small subset of patients with grade III C.I.N., perhaps 5%, who progress to invasive cancer in less than 3 years. Another estimate suggests that 4% of grade III C.I.N. lesions will progress to occult invasive carcinoma in one year.

   Unfortunately, as of today, no means other than frequent cytologic screening exist to detect early, rapidly growing cervical cancer precursors. This brings into serious question the recommendation put forward by the Canadian Task Force on the Periodic Health Examination and endorsed by the American Cancer Society that screening be done only every 3 years after 2 negative Pap smears. The American Society of Obstetricians and Gynecologists recommends that at this time we continue with yearly screening.

288. a) TRUE. The false negative rate of the Pap smear is generally thought to be about 33% in everyday clinical practice. False negative rates are comparatively higher in the early and generally smaller grade I C.I.N. lesions than in their long-standing well-established grade 3 counterparts. As a result, the chances are greater to have an even larger number of early lesions missed with the Pap smear. False negative rates can be considerably decreased by aspirating the outer portion of the endocervical canal as well as sampling the squamous columnar junction of the exocervical transformation zone epithe-

lium. The combination technique, (i.e.) endocervical canal aspiration followed by exocervical scraping not only produces a better yield (as low as 2-3% false-negative rates) for squamous lesions but may also detect asymptomatic adenocarcinoma located in the endocervical canal or endometrium.

289. a) TRUE. Cervical intraepithelial neoplasia is now regarded as a sexually transmitted disease. Recent epidemiologic, morphologic and immunologic data suggest a close relationship between human papillomavirus types 16, 18, and 31 and lower female genital tract carcinogenesis. Up to now, cytology is the only meaningful means to detect HPV infection of the lower female genital tract in the form of koilocytotic atypia of the exfoliated epithelial cells.

290. a) Risk factors for cervical intraepithelial neoplasia include multiple sexual partners, and/or first sexual intercourse before age 20. This is associated with transmission of the human papillomavirus to susceptible cervical cells. As well, recent epidemiologic investigations have shown a strong association between cigarette smoking and invasive and noninvasive squamous cell carcinoma of the uterine cervix. The smoking association was independent of other variables and co-variables of cervical cancer. It is particulary strong (17 fold) in women aged 20-29 years.

No association between socio-economic status and cervical intraepithelial neoplasia has been shown.

Reference

Ferenczy A. Screening strategies for cervical cancer in today's practice. Contemporary OB/GYN 1985; Sept/Oct: 27-33.

PROBLEM #43: A 23 YEAR OLD FEMALE WITH PELVIC PAIN AND VAGINAL DISCHARGE

291. A 23 year old female presents to the office with a 3 day history of fever, chills, abdominal pain and increased vaginal discharge. You suspect pelvic inflammatory disease. The most common sexually-transmitted infection in North America today is infection with:

    a) gonorrhea
    b) herpes hominis
    c) chlamydia
    d) syphillis
    e) gardnerella

292. The intrauterine device has been implicated as a cause of pelvic inflammatory disease. Which of the following statements regarding the IUD and PID is FALSE?

    a) the IUD is associated with a four-to-six fold increase in the incidence of pelvic inflammatory disease
    b) the IUD carries a greater risk of PID in a young nulliparous woman than in an older woman
    c) the multifilamentous tail of the IUD may act as a wick whereby bacteria ascend to the endometrium
    d) the Dalkon Shield which is no longer manufactured has a particularly high incidence of PID
    e) pelvic inflammatory disease associated with the IUD is frequently due to Actinomyces

293. Which of the following investigations is the most sensitive diagnostic test for pelvic inflammatory disease?

    a) elevated ESR
    b) elevated WBC count
    c) culdocentesis
    d) laparoscopy
    e) cervical culture

CODE: (a:1, 2 and 3; b: 1 and 3; c: 2 and 4; d: 4 only; e: all of the above)

294. Which of the following signs/symptoms may be seen in patients with pelvic inflammatory disease?

    1) guarding and rebound tenderness
    2) tenderness on cervical motion
    3) beginning of symptomatology following the menstrual period
    4) dysuria

295. Regarding the incidence in infertility after pelvic inflammatory disease, which of the following statements is/are TRUE?

    1) the incidence of infertility after one episode of PID is 12-15%
    2) the incidence of infertility after two episodes of PID is 35%
    3) the incidence of infertility after three episodes of PID is 75%
    4) the incidence of PID following a chlamydial infection is less than following a gonococcal infection

296. The initial treatment of pelvic inflammatory disease should include which of the following antibiotics?

    1) penicillin G
    2) gentamicin
    3) tetracycline
    4) chloramphenicol

ANSWERS

291. c) Chlamydial infection is now the most common sexually transmitted disease in the United States, surpassing gonorrhea. Many physicians fail to recognize chlamydial infection, which is often a diagnosis of exclusion. Chlamydia is not evident on Gram stain and is difficult to culture. It is an obligatory intracellular parasite and like a virus must be grown on tissue culture.

292. e) IUD's are associated with a four-to-six fold increase in the incidence of pelvic inflammatory disease. This effect, which is most marked in single, nulliparous women, may be a result of multiple sexual partners and, consequently, greater potential exposure to infectious agents. The multifilamentous tail of the IUD may act as a wick by which bacteria ascend to the endometrium. The shape of the IUD may also be a factor; the Dalkon Shield which is no longer manufactured was associated with a particularly high incidence of pelvic inflammatory disease. Any woman who still has a Dalkon Sheild in place should have it removed immediately.

    Actinomyces which may be associated with long term use of an IUD is a very uncommon cause of acute PID.

293. d) Pelvic inflammatory disease is often manifested by an elevated white blood cell count (in 30-50% of cases) or an elevated ESR (especially in chronic disease). These tests, however, are very non-specific.

    A cervical culture is useful if positive, but it has a low sensitivity especially in cases involving Chlamydia or Mycoplasma.

    Culdocentesis may be performed to distinguish ectopic pregnancy from PID. In patients with PID, turbid fluid containing many white blood cells may be recovered from the cul-de-dac and sent for a gram stain and culture.

    Laparoscopy is the most sensitive test for the diagnosis of PID. In Sweden, all patients with possible pelvic inflammatory disease undergo laparoscopy. However, in the United States, this costly procedure is reserved for patients who present a diagnostic dilemma. In pelvic infections, the fallopian tubes may appear edematous and erythematous, with some fibrinous exudate. Tubal material and peritoneal fluid may be obtained for culture. Laparoscopic studies suggest that the diagnosis of pelvic inflammatory disease strictly on clinical grounds may be erroneous in 25-30% of patients.

294. e) The following signs and symptoms occur with pelvic inflammatory disease:
  1) lower abdominal and pelvic pain
  2) nausea and vomiting
  3) dysuria, especially if there is an associated urethritis caused by Mycoplasma or Ureaplasma
  4) beginning of symptoms after the menses
  5) vaginal discharge-purulent with gonorrhea
  6) fever and/or chills
  7) tenderness in one or both adnexa and tenderness on cervical motion
  8) guarding and rebound tenderness which suggest peritoneal inflammation

295. a) The estimated incidence of infertility following one episode of pelvic inflammatory disease is 12-15%. The incidence increases with subsequent episodes, rising to 35% after two episodes and 75% after three episodes.

   Other complications of pelvic inflammatory disease include ectopic pregnancy, the incidence of which has risen dramatically in recent years; chronic pelvic infections; abscess formation; peritonitis; and perihepatitis with the formation of adhesions around the liver.

   The incidence of PID following a chlamydial infection is just as great as following a gonococcal infection.

296. b) Initial treatment of pelvic inflammatory disease should include agents that are active against both gonorrhea and chlamydia. Thus, penicillin (or amoxicillin) plus probenecid for gonorrhea and tetracycline for chlamydia is a reasonable regime. A usual outpatient dose would be 3.0 grams of amoxicillin or 4.8 million units of penicillin plus 1 gram of probenecid as a stat dose with 500 mg. of tetracycline q.i.d. for 10 days. Some authorities recommend that all patients with PID be treated in hospital with IV antibiotics for the first 48-72 hours. In this case IV penicillin G and tetracycline would be a reasonable combination.

   Gentamicin is usually not indicated in the treatment of PID because its spectrum of activity is mainly against gram negative organisms which do not play a major role in PID.

   Metronidazole is sometimes used to treat the anaerobic component of PID. It can be used in both the IV and the oral form.

   Chloramphenicol does not have any role to play in the treatment of pelvic inflammatory disease.

Reference

Swinker M. Salpingitis and Pelvic Inflammatory Disease. American Family Physician 1985; 31(1): 143-149, 33-37.

PROBLEM #44: AN 18 YEAR OLD FEMALE WITH LOWER ABDOMINAL PAIN RELATED TO THE MENSTRUAL CYCLE

297. An 18 year old female presents to your office with a dull, lower abdominal ache beginning two days prior to menstruation, with the most severe pain occurring on the first day of menstruation. The pain usually continues for the first three days of the menstrual period. Based on the history, the most likely diagnosis is:

   a) primary dysmenorrhea
   b) pelvic inflammatory disease
   c) secondary dysmenorrhea
   d) endometriosis
   e) psychogenic abdominal pain

298. Which of the following is currently felt to be the most likely cause of primary dysmenorrhea?

   a) a psychologic or personality factor in the individual
   b) neuromuscular activity of the uterus
   c) the production of prostaglandins
   d) spasmodic uterine activity independent of neuronal control
   e) the premenstrual tension syndrome

CODE: (a:1, 2 and 3; b: 1 and 3; c: 2 and 4; d: 4 only; e: all of the above)

299. Which of the following is/are primary treatment(s) for primary dysmenorrhea?

   1) danazol
   2) prostaglandin synthetase inhibitors
   3) narcotic analgesics
   4) low dose oral contraceptives

300. Which of the following is/are common symptoms of primary dysmenorrhea?

   1) nausea and vomiting
   2) diarrhea
   3) breast tenderness
   4) dull, lower abdominal ache and cramping

301. The cause(s) of secondary dysmenorrhea include:

   1) endometriosis
   2) the intrauterine device
   3) pelvic inflammatory disease
   4) uterine fibroids

ANSWERS

297. a) Primary dysmenorrhea is menstrual pain which is not associated with pelvic pathology and which is severe enough to limit activity or require medical attention. The pain usually begins with the onset of ovulatory cycles, typically a few hours before or coincident with menstruation. Primary dysmenorrhea is more common in young women in their late teens and early twenties and declines thereafter. Primary dysmenorrhea is more common in nulliparous and obese women.

Primary dysmenorrhea characteristically presents as a dull, lower abdominal ache or cramping, generally occurring with ovulatory menstruation. The pain tends to be spasmodic and cyclic and may radiate to the back or the inner aspects of the thighs. Some discomfort may begin up to two days before the onset of menses, with the most severe pain occuring on the first day of menstruation. Pain lasts from several hours to three days and is sometimes accompanied by increased menstrual flow.

Other symptoms have also been associated with dysmenorrhea. Gastrointestinal problems such as nausea, vomiting, and diarrhea are among the common complaints. In addition headache, breast tenderness and fatigue are often reported; in severe cases syncope or collapse may occur.

Secondary dysmenorrhea is dysmenorrhea that is associated with pelvic pathology. Pelvic inflammatory disease and endometriosis are the two primary causes of secondary dysmenorrhea.

Psychogenic factors, although thought by some to be a cause of dysmenorrhea, are unlikely to be responsible for the continuing cyclic problems.

298. c) Although the literature concerning the etiology of dysmenorrhea has traditionally emphasized the role of psychosocial factors current evidence suggests that the production of prostaglandins by the endometrium and their subsequent effect on uterine contractility is the primary cause. The spasmodic uterine activity that is associated with dysmenorrhea appears to be under local endometrial control, rather than central neuronal control.

The premenstrual tension syndrome, rather than being a cause of dysmenorrhea, is often a confusing diagnostic dilemma. Symptoms such as headache, breast tenderness and irritibility can be common to both syndromes. As well, a woman may have both conditions. In general, the symptoms of premenstrual tension occur earlier in the cycle, and the pain of menstruation is not as disabling as it is with dysmenorrhea.

299. c) Low dose oral contraceptives are the treatment of choice for primary dysmenorrhea. These agents work by presumably decreasing the synthesis of prostaglandins by the endometrium, and thus alleviating the symptoms. For those women who cannot take oral contraceptives or who prefer not to, prostaglandin synthetase inhibitors such as mefenamic acid, naproxen sodium, ibuprofen and acetylsalicylic acid are appropriate.

The antigonadotrophic agent danazol is useful in the treatment of secondary dysmenorrhea, but has no role to play in primary dysmenorrhea. Narcotic analgesics, especially when used for long periods of time, are potentially addictive and should not be used.

300. e) See critique of question #297.

301. e) Secondary dysmenorrhea is defined as dysmenorrhea that is secondary to pelvic pathology. The two most common causes of secondary dysmenorrhea are endometriosis and chronic pelvic inflammatory disease. Other causes include the intrauterine device, congenital malformations of the genital tract, adenomyosis, myomas, endometrial polyps, uterine fibroids, adhesions, ovarian cysts, pelvic congestion syndrome and cervical stricture.

Reference

Jay M, Durant R. The patient with dysmenorrhea. Postgraduate Medicine 1983; 73(4): 103-111.

PROBLEM #45: AN INFERTILE COUPLE

302. A 22 year old female with previous severe pelvic inflammatory disease who has been trying to get pregnant for 2 years becomes pregnant with an ectopic pregnancy in the left tube. The right tube is badly scarred with multiple adhesions. The entire left tube is removed at surgery. A methylene blue dye test done at the same time shows no flow through the right tube. The couple desperately wants a child. As the family physician you should:

   a) tell the couple the outlook is hopeless and ask them to contact the adoption agency
   b) refer the couple back to the gynecologist to break the news
   c) discuss in-vitro fertilization and tubal reconstruction and at the same time encourage the couple to begin looking into adoption
   d) begin the wife on clomiphene citrate
   e) refer the couple to a psychiatrist

303. Infertility affects approximately what percentage of married couples in North America?

   a) <1%
   b) 1-5%
   c) 6-9%
   d) 10-15%
   e) 20-22%

304. In what percentage of infertility problems is the problem due to a male factor?

   a) 10%
   b) 25%
   c) 40%
   d) 50%
   e) 60%

305. Which one of the following statements regarding the occurrence of ovulation is TRUE?

   a) the female partner should keep at least 6 months of basal body temperature charts before ovulation can be precisely determined
   b) a woman who has a menstrual period every 6 months may still be ovulating on a monthly basis
   c) if a woman has regular cycles associated with cyclical premenstrual sensations or symptoms (molimina), then she is almost certainly ovulating
   d) the only accurate method of determining ovulation is by endometrial biopsy
   e) if a woman has been anovulatory for a period of greater than 1 year, it is unlikely that she will ever ovulate again

306. A semen analysis submitted by a male patient shows the following:

Sperm — count $10 \times 10^6/$ml
        — motility $>45\%$ show forward progression
        — viability 65%
        — morphology 60% normal forms
Semen — $<4.0 \times 10^6/$ml
  leukocytes

Which of the preceeding variables is ABNORMAL?

a) the sperm count
b) the sperm motility
c) the sperm viability
d) the sperm morphology
e) the semen leukocytes

307. A couple is currently undergoing investigation for infertility. The results of physical examinations on both partners has been normal. Regular ovulation has been documented in the wife and the seminal analysis is completely normal in the husband. The post-coital test shows 15 motile sperm/HPF. The next step in the investigation should be:

a) endometrial biopsy to investigate a possible luteal phase defect
b) serum prolactin measurement on the wife
c) evaluation of cervical bacteriology (esp. for T-strain mycoplasma)
d) evaluation of the structural integrity of the uterus and tubes
e) immunological testing for sperm-agglutinating antibodies and sperm-immobilizing antibodies.

CODE: (a:1, 2 and 3; b: 1 and 3; c: 2 and 4; d: 4 only; e: all of the above)

308. Which of the following statements regarding the post-coital test is/are CORRECT?

1. the ideal time for performing the post-coital test is two days prior to ovulation
2. the most common cause of an abnormal result is improper timing
3. for a post-coital test to be considered normal there must be approximately 10 highly motile sperm in the cervical mucus/HPF
4. the wife should be examined within 3 hours of intercourse without having bathed or douched

309. A young couple is currently undergoing infertility investigations. The results of the physical examination and investigations performed so far are listed below.

Husband: 1) history and physical examination-normal except varicocele of left pampiniform plexus noted
2) laboratory — semen analysis shows:
count — 10×10^6/ml
motility — 20%
viability — >60%
morphology — >70% normal forms

Wife: 1) history: irregular menstrual cycles — last cycle six months ago. Basal body temperature charting suggests anovulatory cycles
2) physical examination — normal
3) laboratory — serum prolactin 10 μg./L (normal <25 μg./L)

Based on these findings, which of the following courses of action should be undertaken:

1) correction of the husband's varicocele
2) continuation of basal body temperature charting in the wife
3) induction of ovulation in the wife with clomiphene citrate
4) glucose tolerance tests in both husband and wife

ANSWERS

302. c) The emotional impact of infertility can be devastating to a young couple. The family physician should take the time to discuss all possible options with the couple. Referral back to the gynecologist or a psychiatrist as you are the family physician in charge is inappropriate. Likewise, to dismiss the outlook as hopeless and to advise referral to an adoption agency is also inappropriate.

Beginning this patient on clomiphene is also inappropriate as the problem lies at the level of the tube. The woman in this case has what appears to be irreversible tubal damage. Tubal reconstruction and in-vitro fertilization are really the only two options remaining for this couple in terms of a natural family. Both options, along with their limitations, should be discussed. As well, the possibility of adoption should be discussed in an open, frank manner with attention given to the long waiting period.

303. d) Infertility affects approximately 10-15% of married couples in North America. The etiology of infertility can be considered under four major headings:

1) problems affecting the female partner
2) problems affecting the male partner
3) problems affecting both partners

4) a fertility problem for which no cause can be discovered

The proportion of cases belonging to each of these categories varies in different studies. On average, a male factor is identified in approximately 40% of couples and no explanation for infertility can be found in only 3-10% of couples. In approximately 90% of cases in which the cause of infertility is known, it is attributable either to a male factor, to an abnormality of the fallopian tubes or to ovulatory disturbances.

304. c) See critique of question #303.

305. c) If a woman has regular menstrual cycles associated with cyclical premenstrual sensations or symptoms (molimina) then she is almost certainly ovulating. A woman who is menstruating regularly does not have to keep taking her basal body temperature for 6 months; to do so is both unnecessary and anxiety provoking. On the other hand, a woman who has a menstrual period only every 6 months is almost surely not ovulating.

Ovulation is most easily assessed by a history of regular cyclical menses; endometrial biopsy is rarely necessary. Many women who are anovulatory for long periods can have ovulation induced with clomiphene; therefore a one year history of anovulation is not at all hopeless.

306. a) the normal sperm count is $>20 \times 10^6$. The other important values are: 1) motility $>40\%$ showing forward progression; 2) viability $>60\%$; 3) morphology $>60\%$ normal forms. As well, the normal value of semen leukocytes is $<4.7 \times 10^6$.

307. d) Endometrial biopsy for the diagnosis of luteal phase defects, serum prolactin levels to rule out prolactinoma in the female, evaluation of cervical bacteriology and immunological testing for sperm-aggulutinating and sperm immobilizing antibodies are all important subsequent investigations; however, the next step should be evaluation of the structural integrity of the tubes and ovaries by hysterosalpinography. This follows from the methodical series of steps that is part of every infertility investigation and which includes:

1) determination of the occurrence of ovulation
2) semen analysis
3) post-coital testing
4) evaluation of the structural integrity of the uterus and tubes

308. e) Interaction between the sperm and the cervical mucus is determined approximately 2 days prior to the expected time of ovulation. The wife is instructed to remain in the supine position for half an hour after intercourse. She should be examined within 3 hours of intercourse without having bathed or douched during the interval. For a post-coital test to be considered normal there must be approximately 10 highly motile sperm in the cervical mucus per high power field. Should the result of this test be repeatedly abnormal, more

specific tests are planned to determine the exact cause of the abnormality. These include in-vitro testing of sperm and mucus, cervical cultures and sperm—immobilizing and sperm—, and agglutinating antibody tests. However, the most common cause of an abnormal post-coital test is still improper timing.

309.   b) The two reasons for potential infertility in this couple are (1) a varicocele in the husband with an associated low sperm count and (2) anovulation in the wife.

   To continue with basal body temperature charting is both non-productive and anxiety provoking. To subject both partners to 3-hour glucose tolerance tests is neither fruitful nor reasonable.

   It is reasonable to attack both potential problems at once. The husband should be referred to a urologist for correction of his varicocele at the earliest opportunity. At the same time, induction of ovulation, starting with clomiphene citrate 50 mg./day on day 5 of the menstrual cycle should be undertaken in the wife. The goal in infertility investigation and treatment is to complete the study with a successful treatment as soon as possible.

Reference

Current status of the investigation of infertility. Bulletin of the Society of Obstetricians and Gynaecologists of Canada 1982; IV(4): 1-3.

PROBLEM #46: A 42 YEAR OLD FEMALE WITH MENORRHAGIA

310. A 42 year old female presents to your office with a chief complaint of menorrhagia (with clots) present for the last six months. Physical examination is normal. A diagnostic curettage and hysteroscopy is normal. You make the diagnosis of dysfunctional uterine bleeding. You elect to start her on a medication. Your first choice would be:

a) a low dose oral contraceptive pill
b) depo-progesterone by IM injection
c) a non-steroidal anti-inflammatory drug
d) aminocaproic acid
e) danazol

Questions 311-313 are TRUE and FALSE questions. If the statement is TRUE, mark "a"; if it is FALSE, mark "b".

311. Ovulatory dysfunctional uterine bleeding is most common in parous women aged 30-45.

312. Anovulatory dysfunctional uterine bleeding may occur at any age and is physiologic in the first year or two after menarche and for several years before menopause.

313. Dysfunctional uterine bleeding appears to be mediated by excess prostaglandins, particularly prostacyclin.

CODE: (a:1, 2 and 3; b: 1 and 3; c: 2 and 4; d: 4 only; e: all of the above)

314. Which of the following medications have been successfully used in the treatment of dysfunctional uterine bleeding?

1) low dose oral contraceptives
2) medroxyprogesterone acetate 10 mg./day in the luteal phase of the cycle
3) depo-progesterone 100 mg. IM every month
4) danazol

ANSWERS

310. c) The pathophysiology of dysfunctional uterine bleeding is thought to originate in the excess production of the prostaglandin prostacyclin. A medication that inhibits the production of prostaglandins should, theoretically, produce a decrease in bleeding. Therefore, the group of drugs known as non-steroidal anti-inflammatory drugs are the agents of choice. This group of drugs includes

naproxen, mefenamic acid and ibuprofen. As an example, naproxen in a dose of 1275 mg./day will decrease blood flow from greater than 200 mls./cycle to less than 80 mls./cycle.

A low dose oral contraceptive which also works by decreasing the synthesis of prostaglandins would be appropriate therapy for a woman under the age of 35 but is contraindicated in a woman over the age of 40. Depo-progesterone by IM injection, as well as oral medroxyprogesterone acetate work by producing endometrial atrophy. They are the second choice agents after non-steroidal anti-inflammatory drugs and low dose oral contraceptives.

Danazol (an anti-gonadotrophin that works by creating a pseudomenopause) and aminocaproic acid are agents that can be tried when everything else has failed; they both have significant side effects.

311. a) TRUE. Ovulatory dysfunctional uterine bleeding is most prevalent in parous women between the ages of 30 and 45 years. The cycle intervals are regular and predictable for the woman. Molimina (breast soreness, mood or energy changes, and pelvic discomfort) herald each flow. The amount, rapidity and duration of bleeding account for hypochromic, microcytic anemia.

312. a) TRUE. Anovulatory dysfunctional uterine bleeding can occur at any age and is physiologic in the first year or two after menarche and in the several years before the menopause. Anovulatory cycles are characterized by irregular length, bleeding patterns that vary in amount or duration and menstrual flows that are not associated with molimina. Specific causes of anovulatory bleeding such as hyperprolactinemia, thyroid dysfunction, androgen excess, obesity, and excessive exercise are investigated and treated appropriately.

313. a) TRUE. Dysfunctional uterine bleeding appears to be mediated by excess prostaglandins, particularly prostacyclin. The properties of prostacyclin make it a likely cause of ovulatory menorrhagia. It is locally produced within the intima of vessels, is a powerful vasodilator, and is an effective inhibitor of platelet aggregation. These actions of prostacyclin are opposite to the effects of the platelet-produced thromboxanes. Prostaglandin excess best explains both the mechanisms for dysfunctional uterine bleeding and why non-steroidal anti-inflammatory drugs should be effective.

314. e) The management of dysfunctional uterine bleeding after the exlusion of pathology in the genital tract includes:

1) reduction in activity during the days of heavy flow
2) the avoidance of aspirin during the week before and on the days of the flow
3) non-steroidal anti-inflammatory drugs
4) low dose oral contraceptives
5) danazol
6) depo-progesterone or oral medroxyprogesterone acetate
7) aminocaproic acid
8) hysterectomy (when everything else fails)

Reference

Strickler R. Dysfunctional uterine bleeding in ovulatory women. Postgraduate Medicine 1985; 77(1): 235-246.

PROBLEM #47: A 55 YEAR OLD PERIMENOPAUSAL FEMALE AT RISK FOR OSTEOPOROSIS

315. A 55 year old female who is currently on estrogen replacement therapy presents to your office seeking information on the relationship between estrogen therapy and endometrial cancer. Which of the following statements regarding the use of post-menopausal estrogens and the risk of endometrial carcinoma is FALSE?

a) women using estrogens are not at increased risk of death from any cause
b) the risk of developing endometrial carcinoma is 3-4X higher among estrogen users than among non-users
c) the risk of developing endometrial carcinoma is not significant at daily doses below 1 mg. of conjugated estrogens
d) estrogen-related endometrial carcinomas occur at an earlier stage, usually are well-differentiated and display minimal myometrial invasion
e) the risk of developing endometrial carcinoma while on estrogen therapy cannot be altered by the concomittant use of progesterone

316. The daily dose equivalent of conjugated estrogen that is needed to relieve both hot flushing and prevent osteoporosis is:

a) 0.125 mg
b) 0.3 mg
c) 0.625 mg
d) 1.25 mg
e) 2.5 mg

317. Which of the following statements regarding osteoporosis is FALSE?

a) estrogen retards the post-menopausal decrease in bone density
b) a dietary calcium intake of 1000 mg./day is suggested for post-menopausal women at risk for osteoporosis
c) estrogen therapy should be used for at least 10 years in patients who are at high risk for osteoporosis
d) the evidence that estrogen prevents later morbidity and mortality due to osteoporotic fractures is unequivocal
e) exercise decreases the risk of osteoporosis

318. Which of the following treatment regimes is the recommended method of giving estrogen for menopausal symptoms, such as hot flushes, or for the prevention of post-menopausal osteoporosis?

    a) conjugated estrogen 0.3 mg. daily continuously
    b) conjugated estrogen 0.625 mg. daily continuously
    c) conjugated estrogen 0.3 mg. daily on day 1-25 of each calendar month
    d) conjugated estrogen 0.625 mg. daily on day 1-25 on each calendar month
    e) conjugated estrogen 0.625 mg. daily on day 1-25 of each calendar month plus medroxyprogesterone acetate 5-10 mg. daily on day 16-25 of every third or fourth calendar month

319. The recommended length of treatment with estrogen for vasomotor symptoms such as hot flushes is:

    a) 6 months
    b) 1 year
    c) 2 years
    d) 5 years
    e) 10 years

CODE: (a:1, 2 and 3; b: 1 and 3; c: 2 and 4; d: 4 only; e: all of the above)

320. Which of the following is/are documented risk factors for the development of osteoporosis?

    1) slender build
    2) female sex
    3) Northern European ancestry
    4) cigarette smoking

ANSWERS

315. e) Evidence that estrogen use may be associated with endometrial cancer has accumulated in more than twenty case control studies during the last decade. In two Canadian studies which used different control groups, the risk of developing endometrial carcinoma was three to four times higher for estrogen users than for non-users.

    While no risk can be discounted entirely, the current evidence indicates that estrogen users are not at increased risk of death from any cause, and that morbidity can be reduced to a minimal level by appropriate prescribing habits. The risk becomes apparent after three to five years of estrogen use, and diminshes one year after the drug is discontinued. The risk of endometrial carcinoma increases with higher doses, and is not significant at daily doses below 1 mg. of conjugated estrogen.

Although estrogen use appears to increase the occurrence of endometrial carcinoma, women who develop estrogen-associated tumors are not at increased risk of death. Estrogen-related endometrial cancers occur at an earlier stage, usually are well-differentiated and display minimal myometrial invasion. Women with estrogen-related endometrial cancer have a survival rate that is similar to the age-adjusted survival of women in the general population. Several reports now agree that the use of progesterone reduces the incidence of estrogen-related hyperplasias. In 1983, however, less than 10% of the estrogen prescriptions in North American included progesterone.

316. c) The daily dose equivalent of conjugated estrogen that is needed to relieve both hot flushing and prevent osteoporosis is 0.625 mg./day. Lesser amounts are ineffective, particularly in the prevention of osteoporosis. Greater doses do not increase the response, but do increase the risk of endometrial carcinoma.

317. d) A series of high quality studies have shown the benefits of estrogen therapy in the short-term (up to 10 years) prevention of calcium loss from bone. After 10 years, while the bone mineral of the estrogen-treated group declines, their bone density remains significantly higher than in placebo treated women. However, the follow-up in these studies is not yet long enough to demonstrate conclusively that estrogen also protects against later morbidity and mortality which may occur more than twenty years after the menopause.

A calcium intake of 1000 mg./day is recommended for post-menopausal women at risk for osteoporosis. Most women in this age group would not take in this amount of calcium in their diets, and a calcium supplement necessary.

Exercise and maintained mobility has been shown to be very important in the prevention of "disuse" osteoporosis.

318. e) Current evidence indicates that estrogen should be given cyclically, with a period of time off during each month. As well, it has been shown that the correct dose of conjugated estrogen is probably 0.625 mg./day. This will treat vasomotor symptoms as well as prevent post-menopausal osteoporosis. A reasonable regime is 0.625 mg. conjugated estrogen on days 1-25 of the calendar month.

As discussed previously, the addition of progesterone will probably prevent estrogen-induced hyperplasia which could lead to endometrial carcinoma. However, giving post-menopausal women monthly progesterone will definately lead to withdrawal bleeding, which can be a very distressing symptom. Therefore, a compromise of giving medroxyprogesterone acetate 5-10 mg. in every third or fourth cycle from day 16-25 is reasonable. It will restrict withdrawal bleeding to every fourth cycle and yet will protect the endometrium from endometrial hyperplasia.

319. c) The recommended length of treatment for women with vasomotor symptoms is two years. Although 82% of the women who experience hot flushes

continue to have symptoms for more than one year, the symptoms persist for five years in only 25-50% of women.

During the subsequent drug free period, the patient should be assessed to decide whether to continue the therapy. Women who cannot tolerate their symptoms should receive therapy for two more years with a similar re-assessment at the end of that time.

For the prevention of post-menopausal osteoporosis, the recommended length of treatment is at least 10 years.

For women who require estrogens for vulvovaginal atrophy, prolonged therapy is necessary. In this case, estrogen vaginal cream can be used in place of oral conjugated estrogen. The vaginal dose can be titrated against symptoms by reducing the amount of hormone-containing cream in the applicator. A dose of 2-4 grams intravaginally daily in a cyclical manner will usually cause pronounced improvement in the symptoms.

320. e) Risk factors for the development of osteoporosis include northern European ancestry, slender build, cigarette smoking, alcohol, diets low in calcium, family history of osteoporosis and corticosteroid therapy.

Reference

Collins J. Estrogen replacement therapy: How to. Contemporary OBS/GYN 1985; Sept-Oct: 35-43.

PROBLEM #48: A 21 YEAR OLD FEMALE WITH A VAGINAL DISCHARGE

321. A 21 year old female presents to the office with a pruritic discharge that has the appearance of cottage cheese. You suspect monilial vaginitis. Which of the following IS NOT a characteristic of the discharge of Candida albicans vaginitis?

   a) white color
   b) high viscosity
   c) floccular consistency
   d) pH > 4.5
   e) absence of white blood cells

322. Which of the following IS NOT a risk factor for recurrent Candida vaginitis?

   a) diabetes mellitus
   b) broad spectrum antibiotics
   c) pregnancy
   d) oral contraceptives
   e) failure to treat the sexual partner

323. Which of the following IS NOT a characteristic of the discharge of Trichomonas vaginitis?

   a) yellow-gray color
   b) homogenous consistency
   c) absence of white blood cells
   d) pH > 4.5
   e) presence of amine odor on exposure to KOH.

324. The "clue cell" is most commonly seen in:

   a) trichomoniasis
   b) Gardnerella vaginitis
   c) candidiasis
   d) physiologic vaginal discharge

325. Which one of the following IS NOT a characteristic of the vaginal discharge of Gardnerella vaginitis (non-specific vaginitis)?

   a) presence of white blood cells
   b) homogenous consistency
   c) pH > 4.5
   d) low viscosity
   e) presence of amine odor on exposure to KOH

326. Which of the following treatment regimes is the treatment of choice for Gardnerella vaginitis?

    a) metronidazole 500 mg. b.i.d. for 7 days
    b) metronidazole 2 gram single dose
    c) ampicillin 500 mg. q.i.d. for 7 days
    d) triple sulfa vaginal cream
    e) ampicillin 3.5 gram single dose with 1.0 gram probenecid

CODE: (a:1, 2 and 3; b: 1 and 3; c: 2 and 4; d: 4 only; e: all of the above)

327. Which of the following organisms can be part of the normal vaginal flora of asymptomatic women?

    1) Beta-hemolytic streptococcus
    2) Candida albicans
    3) peptostreptococcus
    4) Gardnerella vaginalis

ANSWERS

321. d) The discharge of Candida albicans vaginitis is characterized by the absence of discharge at the introitus, a white color, high viscosity, floccular consistency and adherence of the discharge to the vaginal wall. As well, the discharge usually has a pH of less than 4.5, and white blood cells are absent. On exposure to KOH an amine odor is not produced.

    Traditionally, 100,000 units of nystatin in a vaginal suppository or a cream form was inserted intravaginally twice a day for 10 days. However, more active antifungal agents are now available. Miconazole, clotrimazole and boric acid capsules have all successfully treated candidiasis. Clinical or micro-biological cures have occurred among 50-80% of women treated with nystatin and 85-95% of women treated with the last three agents. Miconazole or clotrimazole can be administered as a suppository or cream preparation either twice a day for 3 1/2 days or once nightly for 7 nights.

322. d) Risk factors for persistent or frequently recurrent cadidiasis include diabetes mellitus, broad spectrum antibiotics, immunosuppressive drugs, failure to use the most active antifungal agents, untreated sexual partners, untreated vulvar candidiasis and pregnancy.

    Despite alterations of carbohydrate metabolism among women receiving oral contraceptives and early reports of a high rate of candidiasis most controlled studies have demonstrated that oral contraceptive use does not predispose to candidiasis. Asymptomatic candida may be isolated more commonly among women using the oral contraceptive pill, but infections are not more common.

323. c) Trichomonas vaginitis is characterized by discharge present at the introitus, a yellow-gray color, a low viscosity, homogenous consistency, and adherence of the discharge to the vaginal walls. The pH is greater than 4.5, white blood cells are present in the discharge and an amine odor is evident on exposure to KOH.

The amine odor is caused by the presence of diamines that become volitilized by alkalinization; putrescine and cadaverine are the diamines present in the highest concentration. A less prominent odor is present among women with trichomoniasis than among women with Gardnerella vaginitis.

The preferred treatment for trichomoniasis is a single 2.0 gram dose of metronidazole. It is preferred over an extended 250 mg. t.i.d. dose for 7 days because of increased compliance, less expense and the same effectiveness as the extended dose. Simultaneous therapy is recommended for the male partner. More than 90% of patients will be cured with a single regimen of treatment.

324. b) The "clue cell" is most commonly seen with Gardnerella vaginitis. The clue cell is a vaginal epithelial cell to which such a large number of organisms attach that the entire cell border is obscured. Among women with Gardnerella vaginitis 2-50% of the vaginal epithelial cells are clue cells. Trichomoniasis may also be seen together with clue cells, and thus the correlation is not specific.

325. a) The discharge of Gardnerella vaginalis is characterized by the presence of a discharge at the introitus, a gray color, low viscosity, homogenous consistency, adherence of the discharge to the vaginal walls, pH > 4.5, the presence of an amine odor on exposure of the discharge to KOH and the ABSENCE of white blood cells. As well, as mentioned previously, 2-50% of the vaginal epithelial cells are "clue cells".

326. a) The treatment of choice for Gardnerella vaginalis vaginitis is metronidazole 500 mg. b.i.d. for 7 days. This regime produces a cure rate of greater than 85%. A single 2.0 gram dose of metronidazole is effective in only 70% of cases. Ampicillin, in a dose of 500 mg. q.i.d. is only 60-65% effective. Triple sulfa vaginal cream has been reported to cure only 15-60% of patients. A single 3.5 gram dose of ampicillin with 1.0 gram probenecid is not recommended treatment.

327. e) The vaginal flora of asymptomatic women contain a large number of organisms. The most prevalent facultative organisms include species of lacto-bacilli, corynebacteria, Beta-hemolytic and Group D streptococci, Staphylococcous epidermidis and Gardnerella vaginalis. Common gram-negative organisms include E.coli and Klebsiella species. The most frequent anaerobic organisms include Peptococcus, Peptostreptococcus, bacteroides, fusobacterium, Clostridium, Eubacteria and Veillonella. As well, Candida albicans is recovered from 5-10% of asymptomatic women. Mycoplasma hominis can be recovered from 20-50% and Ureaplasma urealyticum from 50-70% of sexually active asymptomatic women.

Reference

Eschenbach D. Vaginal Infection. Clinical Obstetrics and Gynecology 1983; 26(1): 186-200.

PROBLEM #49: A 21 YEAR OLD FEMALE WHO BECOMES DEPRESSED ONE WEEK AFTER DELIVERY

A 21 year old female who delivered her first baby one week ago is seen in the office in a tearful, upset state. She states that she cannot handle being a mother. You suspect postpartum depression.

Each of the following statements regarding postpartum depression is either TRUE or FALSE. If the statement is TRUE, mark "a"; if it is FALSE, mark "b".

328. Data from studies of normal pregnant women indicate that from 20-40% of women report emotional disturbance or cognitive dysfunction, or both, in the early postpartum period.

329. Psychodynamic studies of postpartum mental illness point to conflicting feelings within the mother with regard to her mothering experience or instincts.

330. Symptoms of postpartum depression are almost always noted before the third postpartum day.

331. The most common depressive syndrome seen in the postpartum period is depressive neurosis.

332. Tricyclic antidepressants are contraindicated in the postpartum period if the mother is breast-feeding.

ANSWERS

328. a) TRUE. Data from studies of normal pregnant women indicate that 20-40% of women report emotional disturbance or cognitive dysfunction, or both, in the early postpartum period; this is referred to as "postpartum blues". One study suggested that 65% of mothers described depression postpartum, with 25% of these women reporting symptoms continuing longer than a few weeks. Questionnaires exploring psychiatric symptoms in an unselected sample of women up to 1 year after childbirth revealed that 25% had more than six symptoms that had apparently arisen postpartum. The most common symptoms were fatigue, irritability, tension and anxiety. Psychotic disturbances occur at a frequency of 1-2 per 1,000 deliveries.

329. a) TRUE. Psychodynamic studies of postpartum mental illness point to conflicting feelings within the mother with regard to her mothering experience or instincts, her new baby, her husband, and herself. The observation of hostility during pregnancy and after parturition is reported by many authorities.

330. b) FALSE. One of the outstanding features of post-partum depression relates to the time of onset of illness. Symptoms are almost never noted before the third day postpartum. Symptoms usually occur from the third to the seventh day. The 3-day latent period may be the period during which some kind of chemical hormonal development related to the child-bearing process takes place and leads to later manifestations of illness. Prodromal symptoms include insomnia, restlessness, feelings of fatigue, depression, irritibility, headache and lability of mood.

The clinical symptoms center on the patient's relationship to her baby and the maternal role. Depressed patients may show excessive concern about the baby's health or welfare or express guilt about their lack of love for the baby or lack of interest in caring for the baby. They may have feelings of inadequacy about caring for the baby and their ability to cope.

331. a) TRUE. Depressive neurosis seems to be the most common occurrence seen in these patients. Functional psychosis (schizophrenia or episodic affective disorders) are less common, but more often result in extensive hospitalization. These illnesses are largely related to the ambivalent feelings about motherhood and its attendant child care responsibilities.

332. b) FALSE. Tricyclic antidepressants are not contraindicated in the treatment of post-partum depression if the mother is breast feeding, although they should be used with caution. The drug and its metabolites do appear in the breast milk, but in insignificant amounts. Tricyclic antidepressants are the treatment of choice in patients with significant symptoms who are not effectively treated with psychotherapy alone.

Reference

Kaplan H and Sadock B, editors. Modern Synopsis of Comprehensive Textbook of Psychiatry III, 3rd edition; Williams and Wilkins, Baltimore: 1981; pages 380-383.

Pediatrics

PROBLEM #50: A CHILD WITH A HEART MURMUR

333. A 3 year old child is found to have a low-grade systolic heart murmur during a routine health assessment. Which of the following features IS NOT a characteristic of an innocent cardiac murmur?

a) low frequency
b) an associated thrill
c) short ejection systolic
d) grade I or II
e) increases with increasing heart rate

334. The frequency of cardiac murmurs in childhood is:

a) 10%
b) 20%
c) 30%
d) 40%
e) 50%

335. The most common congenital heart lesion in childhood is:

a) atrial septal defect
b) tetralogy of Fallot
c) ventricular septal defect
d) transposition of the great arteries
e) aortic stenosis

CODE: (a:1, 2 and 3; b: 1 and 3; c: 2 and 4; d: 4 only; e: all of the above)

336. A 6 month old child presents with a Grade III/VI systolic heart murmur present along the left sternal edge. There is no associated thrill or symptoms. Which of the following should be done at this time?

    1) reassure the mother that this is an innocent murmur and it will disappear with time
    2) chest X-ray
    3) echocardiogram
    4) electrocardiogram

337. An 18 month old child presents with a Grade IV/VI systolic heart murmur present along the left sternal edge. There is no associated thrill or symptoms. Which of the following should be done at this time?

    1) chest X-ray
    2) electrocardiogram
    3) referral of the child to a cardiologist
    4) reassure the mother that this is an innocent murmur and it will disappear with time

ANSWERS

333. b) The characteristics of an innocent cardiac murmur are (1) low frequency, (2) short systolic ejection murmur, (3) localized murmur and (4) accentuation with heart rate. An innocent cardiac murmur is never associated with a thrill.

334. e) The frequency of cardiac murmurs in children is nearly 50%. The majority of these are "innocent murmurs" which family physicians frequently refrain from mentioning to parents because experience has shown that such murmurs often disappear with time. This approach, however, is not recommended. The parents of a child with a murmur should be told that their child has a murmur. Failure to do so will probably effect the family physician's credibility.

335. c) The most common organic cardiac murmur in childhood is a ventricular septal defect. This represents 28% of all organic murmurs in the childhood period. Ventricular septal defects are silent at birth because the ventricular pressures are equal and there is no net shunt to produce flow turbulence. They are often picked up on the discharge examination or at the first well-baby checkup.

336. c) A child in the period newborn-1 year with a heart murmur greater than 2/6, and with no thrill or associated symptoms, should have a chest X-ray and an electrocardiogram performed. If these are normal the family physician need not order any further investigations. The child should be reviewed in 6 months time. Reassurance that this is an innocent cardiac murmur would probably be premature, as the grade of the murmur was greater than two.

337. a) A child older than 1 year with a heart murmur greater than 2/6 should, in addition to having a chest X-ray and an electrocardiogram, be referred to a cardiologist. It is quite likely that the murmur is organic in nature, and thus the parents should not be informed that it is innocent.

Reference

Duncan W. Childhood Cardiac Murmurs: Innocent or Not? Canadian Family Physician 1985; 31: 1047-1049.

PROBLEM #51: A 3 WEEK OLD INFANT WITH COLIC

338. An anxious mother presents with her 3 week old baby. She states that he is constantly crying. On examination he is gaining weight well. You suspect infantile colic. Which of the following HAS NOT been shown to be an etiological factor in infantile colic?

a) emotional stress in the family
b) breast feeding
c) aerophagia in the infant
d) primiparous mother
e) the ingestion of iron supplements

339. With regard to infant feeding practices and the incidence of infantile colic, which of the following statements is INCORRECT?

a) the incidence of colic in breast and bottle fed babies is the same
b) infantile colic may be alleviated by discontinuing cow's milk in the diet of the mother
c) soy-based formulas have been implicated as a cause of colic in some infants
d) iron supplementation appears to increase the incidence of colic
e) a hydrolyzed casein formula appears to be associated with a lower rate of infantile colic than other formulas

340. Which of the following medications have been shown to be of significant benefit in the treatment of infantile colic?

a) antihistamines
b) antispasmodics
c) acetaminophen
d) phenobarbitol
e) none of the above

CODE: (a:1, 2 and 3; b: 1 and 3; c: 2 and 4; d: 4 only; e: all of the above)

341. Which of the following conditions must be considered in the differential diagnosis of infantile colic?

1) urinary tract infection
2) intussusception
3) gastroesophageal reflux
4) milk allergy

342. Which of the following should be used in the treatment of a child with infantile colic?

1) involvement of all family members
2) application of heat or motion
3) instruction in feeding practices
4) medications including antispasmotics or antihistamines

ANSWERS

338. b) Factors which have been implicated in the causation of infantile colic include:

1) family stress
2) aerophagia (air swallowing) from the infant crying while eating, use of a poorly shaped or poorly fitted nipple, infrequent burping or improper burping techniques during meals, and frequent attachment of and detachment from the breast or bottle
3) delivery by a primiparous mother with a long labor
4) cow's milk and soy-based protein
5) iron supplementation

339. a) Feeding practices have been strongly implicated in the causation of infantile colic. Formula-fed babies, including soy-based formula fed babies, have a higher incidence of colic than breast fed babies. A hydrolyzed casein base formula seems to have a lower association with colic than any other formula.

The elimination of cow's milk from the mother's diet has also been positively correlated with a reduced incidence of colic in the infant.

Iron supplementation, in some studies, has been shown to increase the incidence of colic in infants.

340. e) No medication has been shown to be effective in the treatment of colic. It is strongly suspected that the major effect of all the medications listed, and many others, is placebo.

341. e) The differential diagnosis of infantile colic includes the following conditions:

1) any infection, but especially urinary tract
2) infantile seizures
3) abdominal obstruction including intussusception and volvulus
4) acute appendicitis
5) gastroesophageal reflux
6) milk allergy
7) lactose intolerance
8) constipation

342. a) An important point about therapy is that it probably should be delivered to the entire family. Therapy prescribed for the infant alone or for the infant's primary caretaker alone excludes other family members and leads to an uneven distribution of responsibility regarding the baby's care.

An assessment of the feeding technique should be done, with special attention to how the formula is prepared when the infant is a bottle fed baby, and whether the infant is crying while eating. A baby who cries while feeding is likely to swallow air.

The infant with colic may benefit from simple prescriptions such as a water bottle placed under the infant while it is lying prone. Swaddling babies in blankets or bathing them in warm water helps, as do car rides and automatic swings.

Elimination of cow's milk from the mother's diet will often help. As well, the formula can be changed to one that contains less iron. Another choice is to change the baby's formula from a cow's milk base to a soy-milk base, or even to a hydrolyzed casein formula.

Medications including antihistamines, antispasmodics, phenobarbitol, acetaminophen and many others have not been shown to be helpful. It is strongly suspected that their major effect is placebo.

Parents should be encouraged to take some time for themselves. Just getting out of the house for a short period of time, on a regular basis, seems to dramatically increase their ability to cope with this problem.

Reference

Karofsky P. Infantile Colic. Journal of Family Practice 1984; 19(1): 107-116.

PROBLEM #52: A 6 YEAR OLD CHILD WITH ENURESIS

343. A mother presents to the office with her 6-year-old enuretic boy. She demands that something be done to cure her child. With respect to enuresis, which of the following statements is FALSE?

a) at age 6 years 10% of children are enuretic
b) enuresis is more common in children in whom one or both parents were enuretic
c) the functional bladder capacity in enuretic children is significantly less than normal
d) enuresis usually implies significant psychopathology in the child
e) urethral valves, neurogenic bladder, and ectopic ureter may be associated with enuresis

344. Which of the following investigations is the MOST IMPORTANT in a child with enuresis?

a) urinalysis
b) urine culture
c) complete blood count
d) complete cystometric evaluation
e) intravenous pyelogram

345. Pharmacologic treatment is often effective in treating enuresis that is not improved with supportive counselling. Which of the following medications is the treatment of choice in this condition?

a) alprazolam
b) imipramine
c) chlorpheniramine
d) diazepam
e) hydroxyzine

CODE: (a:1, 2 and 3; b: 1 and 3; c: 2 and 4; d: 4 only; e: all of the above)

346. In supportive counselling of parents of children with enuresis, which of the following approaches is/are suggested?

1) provide information about the high prevalence rate
2) provide information about the high spontaneous cure rate
3) provide information about the unconscious nature of enuresis
4) encourage journal or chart-keeping by the child

347. In the treatment of enuresis, which of the following may be beneficial?

    1) alarm conditioning
    2) treatment with antidepressant agents
    3) supportive counselling
    4) confrontation therapy

ANSWERS

343. d) Enuresis is defined as nocturnal if it only occurs at night and diurnal if it occurs both during the day and night. It is defined as 'primary' if the child has never been dry and 'secondary' if the child has had at least one 3-month period of dryness. The prevalence of enuresis is 12-25% at 4 years, 10-13% at 6 years, 7-10% at 8 years, 3-5% at 10 years, 2-3% at 12 years, and 1-3% at 14 years.

    Enuresis is more common in children in which one or both parents were enuretic. If both parents were enuretic the incidence is 77%; if the mother was inuretic the incidence is 44% in the child; if the father was enuretic the incidence is 33%.

    It is hypothesized that children who are enuretic have a developmental immaturity leading to decreased functional bladder capacity. Other studies have shown a consistent decrement in average height and a lower mean bone age among enuretic children than non-enuretic children.

    Uropathies of all types probably account for 2-4% of the enuretics in a general pediatric setting. Lesions include urethral valves, neurogenic bladder, and ectopic ureter. Urinary tract infections are a more common organic cause of enuresis, especially of secondary enuresis in girls. Both anatomic and infectious urologic disorders are frequently associated with dirunal as well as nocturnal enuresis and with pain, urgency, or dribbling in urination.

    Although psychological factors have been implicated as a cause of enuresis in some children, there does not appear to be a cause and effect relationship between enuresis and various forms of serious psychopathology in children.

344. a) The only laboratory evaluation which is mandatory in every enuretic child is a urinalysis. Low specific gravity in diabetes insipidus, proteinuria or hematuria in kidney disease, glycouria in diabetes mellitus, and white cells in the urinary tract infections are important abnormalities that may be associated with enuresis. Urine culture, complete blood count, intravenous pyelogram and cystometric evaluation should be pursued on the basis of specific indications from the history or physical examination.

345. b) Although a number of drugs have been tried in the therapy of enuresis, only tricyclic antidepressants have been consistently more effective than placebo or the spontaneous cure rate. Imipramine is the most widely used, but other tricyclics (most notably desipramine) have been successfully employed.

The peripheral anticholinergic properties of imipramine first led to its trial in enuresis, but well-controlled trials of purely anticholinergic drugs such as methscopolamine have not shown them to be more effective than placebo. The rapid onset of improvement at lower doses without marked changes in mood or behaviour suggests a different mechanism in enuresis compared with the central psychotropic action of imipramine in depression.

The usual dosage range is 1-2.5 mg./kg./day. Overall, 20-40% of patients will be greatly improved after a trial of 6 months with imipramine. Relapse rates are quoted at 40%.

346. e) Supportive counselling of parents with enuretic children is often the only form of therapy needed. Supportive approaches should include the following:

1) provide information to parents about the high prevalence of enuresis (reduce guilt), the high spontaneous cure rate (instill hope), and the unconscious nature of enuresis (decrease control struggle).
2) advise parents to avoid shaming, punishment, and overemphasis on the problem
3) encourage a journal or chart-keeping by the child
4) reduce fluids prior to bedtime
5) awaken the child to void after several hours of sleep
6) reinforce effort and improvement

347. a) Treatment approaches that may be effective in the treatment of enuresis include alarm conditioning, supportive counselling and antidepressant drugs. The latter two have been dealt with in questions 3 and 4.

Alarm conditioning using a bell and pad method, whereby the first drops of urine touching a pad on which the child is sleeping complete an electrical circuit and cause an alarm to sound is common treatment for enuresis. If this method is employed, support of the child is essential. Success rates have variously been reported at 25-75%, with males responding better than females. Duration of treatment is 5-12 weeks. Relapse rates are quoted at 40%.

Confrontation therapy has no place in the treatment of enuresis. Without the co-operation of the child, all treatments are doomed to failure.

Reference

Fritz G, Armbrust J. Enuresis and encopresis. Psychiatric Clinic of North America 1982; 5(2): 283-291.

PROBLEM #53: AN INFANT WITH FEVER AND NO LOCALIZING SIGNS

348. A 6 month old infant is seen in the emergency room for evaluation of fever. There are no localizing signs. The child's WBC is 17,000 cells/mm^3, and the ESR is 45 mm./hour. The probability of this child being bacteremic is approximately:

   a) 1%
   b) 5%
   c) 9%
   d) 15%
   e) 50%

349. The most common cause of occult bacteremia is:

   a) Neisseria meningitidis
   b) Hemophilus influenzae
   c) Streptococcus pneumoniae
   d) Salmonella
   e) Mycoplasma pneumoniae

350. Which of the following medications is NOT suitable as empiric therapy for the child at risk for occult bacteremia?

   a) trimethoprim-sulfamethoxazole
   b) amoxicillin
   c) cefaclor
   d) amoxicillin-potassium clavulanate
   e) erythromycin

CODE: (a:1, 2 and 3; b: 1 and 3; c: 2 and 4; d: 4 only; e: all of the above)

351. The child described in question #348 has a generalized seizure while the investigations are being performed. Which of the following is/are characteristic of febrile seizures in children?

   1) onset between 6 months and 5 years of age
   2) short duration (< 15 minutes)
   3) generalized tonic-clonic pattern
   4) no focal or lateralizing aspect

352. Which of the following is/are risk factors for occult bacteremia in children?

   1) age 6-24 months
   2) temperature greater than 39.4 °C
   3) white blood cell count greater than 15,000 mm^3
   4) ESR greater than 30 mm./hour

353. Which of the following investigations should routinely be done in children with fever and apparent focus of infection?

1) urinalysis
2) electrolytes
3) blood cultures
4) albumin/globulin ratio

ANSWERS

348. c) The probability of a child with a white blood cell count elevated above 15,000 mm³ and an ESR elevated above 30 mm./hour having occult bacteremia is 9/100. It appears that the positive predictive value of the elevated white blood cell count and elevated erythrocyte sedimentation rate are equivalent. Therefore, combining the two tests increases the sensitivity of the screening process.

439. c) The most common cause of occult bacteremia in children is Streptococcus pneumoniae (65%). Other common causative agents include Haemophilus influenzae type b (25%) and Neisseria meningitidis. Salmonella and Mycoplasma pneumoniae are uncommon causes of occult bacteremia.

350. e) Empiric antimicrobial therapy should be effective against the two most likely pathogens, Streptococcus pneumoniae and Haemophilus influenzae. Trimethoprim-sulfamethoxazole, amoxicillin, cefaclor, and amoxicillin-potassium clavulanate fulfill this criteria. Erythromycin does not cover H. influenza type b and thus should not be used as empiric therapy.

351. e) About 2% of children will have one or more febrile seizures by 5 years of age, and approximately 90% of these children will be free of seizures in later life. The seizures are usually tonic-clonic, generalized, and precipitated by fever. Classically, the following characteristics are associated with simple febrile seizures: (1) onset between 6 months and 5 years of age; (2) the convulsion usually occurs with a rise in temperature to above 39 degrees Celcius; (3) the seizures are short (15 minutes or less) and are generalized tonic-clonic with loss of consciousness during the event and post-ictal drowsiness; (4) there is no focal or lateralizing aspect to the seizures; (5) postictally, there is no neurologic deficit; (6) the interictal electroencephalogram is always normal; and (7) there may be recurrences (35% of children).

The following risk factors increase the probability that a child with febrile seizures will develop epilepsy later in adulthood: (1) history of seizures without fever in a parent or a sibling; (2) abnormal neurologic status prior to the first febrile seizure; (3) initial seizure with focal or lateralizing findings; and (4) seizure lasting longer than 15 minutes or a cluster of seizures in 24 hours. If a child has two or more risk factors he should be treated for at least two years with phenobarbitol.

352. e) Risk factors for occult bacteremia include: (1) age between 6 and 24 months, (2) temperature greater than 39.4°C, (3) white blood cell count greater than 15,000 mm³, (4) erythrocyte sedimentation rate greater than 30 mm./hour, (5) a normal chest X-ray, (6) a normal urinalysis and (7) a compromised immune system.

353. b) The laboratory investigations that should routinely be done in a child suspected of having occult bacteremia include: (1) CBC, (2) ESR, (3) urinalysis, (4) chest X-ray, (5) blood cultures and (6) urine cultures. Because of the subtle signs of meningitis in infancy, high-risk children under 12 months of age should probably have a lumbar puncture performed as well.

Measurement of serum electrolytes and albumin/globulin ratios do not increase the sensitivity of screening and therefore should not be done.

References

Gutierrez-Nunez J, Ibanez A, Stevens M, and David D. Fever Without a Focus. American Family Physician 1985; 32(1): 36, 138-144.

Crain E, Shelov P. Febrile Infants: Predictors of bacteremia. Journal of Pediatrics 1982; 101: 686-689.

PROBLEM #54: A 13 YEAR OLD GIRL WITH SHORT STATURE

354. A 13 year old girl presents with a height below the 5th percentile, a webbed neck, lack of breast bud development, a high-arched palate and a low set hairline. She most likely has:

    a) Noonan's syndrome
    b) Trisomy 21
    c) Turner's syndrome
    d) Fragile X syndrome
    e) constitutional delay of growth

355. The most common cause of short stature in children is:

    a) familial short stature
    b) chromosomal abnormality
    c) constitutional delay of growth
    d) hypothyroidism
    e) psychosocial dwarfism

356. Bone age can sometimes be used to differentiate certain causes of short stature in children. With respect to bone age, which of the following statements is true:

    a) bone age is normal in both familial short stature and constitutional delay of growth
    b) bone age is normal in familial short stature and delayed in constitutional delay of growth
    c) bone age is normal in constitutional delay of growth and normal in familial short stature
    d) bone age is delayed in both familial short stature and constitutional delay of growth
    e) bone age is variable in these two situations and cannot be used to differentiate them

357. Psychosocial dwarfism is a situation in which poor physical growth may be associated with an unfavorable psychosocial situation. With respect to psychosocial dwarfism, which of the following statements is FALSE?

    a) sleep and eating aberations occur in these children
    b) growth usually returns to normal when the stress is removed
    c) growth hormone levels are normal in these children
    d) behavioral problems are common

CODE: (a: 1, 2 and 3; b: 1 and 3; c: 2 and 4; d: 4 only; e: all of the above)

358. Isolated growth hormone deficiency is often suspected in children referred for evaluation of short stature. Which of the following statements regarding growth hormone deficiency is/are CORRECT?

1) the diagnosis of growth hormone deficiency rests on the basis of poor response to at least two stimuli
2) the bone age of a child with growth hormone deficiency will be delayed
3) somatomedin C determination is a good screening test for growth hormone deficiency
4) growth hormone replacement therapy has been associated with Creutzfeldt-Jakob disease

ANSWERS

354. c) The most common chromosomal abnormality associated with short stature in females is Turner's syndrome (45 XO or mosaicism). Noonan's syndrome may share some of the phenotypic features of Turner's syndrome but not the genotype. Trisomy 21 will usually be recognized long before the age of 13 years. The fragile X syndrome is a syndrome associated with mental retardation and macro-orchidism in males.

355. a) The most common cause of short stature is familial short stature. If one or both parents are short, the child has a greater chance of being short. Other causes are constitutional delay of growth, chromosomal abnormalities, intrauterine growth retardation, chronic diseases such as renal disease or inflammatory bowel disease, hypothyroidism, adrenal hyperplasia, growth hormone deficiency, bioinactive growth hormone, and psychosocial dwarfism.

356. b) Bone age determination is very useful in distinguishing between the two most common causes of short stature — familial short stature and constitutional delay of growth. In familial short stature the bone age is normal whereas in constitutional delay of growth it is delayed.

357. c) Psychosocial dwarfism is associated with behavioral disturbances, sleep and eating aberrations, and transient low levels of human growth hormone during periods of stress. These return to normal when the stress is removed or when the child is removed from the home.

358. e) The diagnosis of isolated growth hormone deficiency depends on poor response to at least two stimuli. These stimuli include the response to exercise and to sleep, arginine infusion, insulin tolerance. glucagon administration, and the oral administration of levodopa. Somatomedin C determination has recently become available and is a good screening test for growth hormone deficiency.

In growth hormone deficiency, bone age is delayed. This is corrected by the administration of growth hormone. However, recently two people treated with growth hormone derived from human pituitary glands have died of Creutzfeldt-Jacob disease. Thus, growth hormone replacement therapy has been temporarily suspended. Biosynthetic growth hormone, made from recombinant DNA is currently under investigation.

Reference

Kritzler R, Plotnick L. The short child — A matter of time or cause for concern. Postgraduate Medicine 1985; 78(4): 51-59.

PROBLEM #55: A 6 MONTH OLD CHILD WITH MULTIPLE BRUISES AND A FRACTURED HUMERUS

359. A 6 month old infant presents to the hospital emergency room with multiple bruises and a fractured right humerus. The mother states that the child sustained this injury while falling off a sofa. After examining the child, the next step is to:

    a) obtain an orthopedic consultation
    b) X-ray the fracture, support the arm, and send the mother and infant on their way
    c) investigate the child for possible osteogenesis imperfecta
    d) suggest that the mother purchase a walker instead of laying her child on a sofa
    e) discuss the details of the incident more fully with the mother and contact the hospital social worker

360. A 1 year old child is admitted to the hospital for investigation of failure to thrive. The child appears scared and clings to anyone who is present in his room. His mother states that he is a well-adjusted little boy and that this is most unusual behaviour for him. Physical examination and all laboratory investigations are within normal limits. The explanation for the child's behavior until proven otherwise is:

    a) the "white-coat syndrome"
    b) psychotic depression
    c) child abuse or neglect
    d) childhood schizophrenia
    e) acute paranoia of childhood

361. In the case of an abused child, the goal of treatment of the parents is not necessarily to terminate the relationship, but rather to terminate the abuse or neglect. What percentage of parents may be successfully treated so that they do not reabuse their children?

    a) 25%
    b) 35%
    c) 50%
    d) 60%
    e) 80%

CODE: (a:1, 2 and 3; b: 1 and 3; c: 2 and 4; d: 4 only; e: all of the above)

362. Which of the following is/are clues to the diagnosis of child abuse or neglect?

    1) discrepant history
    2) delay in seeking care
    3) family crisis
    4) higher socioeconomic class

363. An 8 month old child presents to the hospital emergency room with a large burn in the shape of an iron on his buttocks. The child's father states that the child dropped the iron on himself as he was reaching for his toys. As the casualty officer in charge, what should your next step(s) be?

    1) treat the burn and contact the hospital social worker
    2) call the police and have the father arrested
    3) try to obtain a more detailed history of the child's resent injury and his previous health
    4) use a confrontation approach and accuse the father of concealing information and abusing the child

364. Child abuse or neglect includes which of the following:

    1) physical abuse
    2) physical neglect
    3) sexual abuse
    4) emotional neglect

ANSWERS

359. e) In this case, the most striking element is the discrepant history. The explanation of how the injury occured does not fit the pattern or severity of the medical findings. This is a definite hint to child abuse or neglect. Other important clues to the diagnosis are (1) delay in seeking care, (2) a crisis in the family, (3) a trigger factor in the home environment, (4) unrealistic expectations of the child, (5) increasing severity of injuries assuming that this is not the first incident, (6) social and geographic isolation, and (7) a history of abuse of the parent in their family of origin.

   The treatment of the fracture itself, although important, is not the highest priority. An orthopedic consultation may be appropriate, depending on the severity of the fracture.

   It would be inappropriate to suggest the purchase of a walker at the best of times as this is associated with an increased incidence of falls and injuries.

   There are no associated findings to suggest the diagnosis of osteogenesis imperfecta.

360. c) The child discussed in the question is an abused or neglected child until proven otherwise. The combination of failure to thrive and clinging behavior is almost pathognomonic for child abuse. Once admitted to hospital, abused children often begin to gain weight well and develop more normal interactional behavior.

Psychotic depression, acute schizophrenia and acute paranoia are almost unheard of a 1 year old infant. The "white coat" syndrome, in which a child displays fear of anyone in a white coat, is not an adequate explanation for the combination of failure to thrive and clinging behavior.

361. e) Studies have shown that nearly 80% of abusive parents that have been treated do not reabuse their children. Treatment centres on education, training regarding the recognition of risk factors or situations, and ongoing support from a social or related health care worker.

362. a) Child abuse or neglect is increased in lower socio-economic groups. See the critique of question number 359 for a more detailed explanation of the clues to diagnosis.

363. b) The most appropriate step in the situation presented is to try and determine with as much accuracy as possible the circumstances surrounding the accident. If possible, the other parent should be interviewed as well. It is also appropriate to contact the hospital social worker who will go about reporting the case to the authorities.

It is not appropriate to have the father arrested with the amount of information that is currently available, nor is it wise to use a confrontational approach in dealing with the father. Accusations almost guarantee a poor outcome.

364. e) When the term "battered child syndrome" was originally described, it was used to refer to a child with multiple burises and multiple fractures at different stages of healing. This description is now infrequently seen. Instead, the term "physical abuse" is used for children who suffer bruises, welts, lacerations, fractures, burns, and head and abdominal injuries that are not accidental in nature.

As well, child abuse includes sexual abuse, physical neglect, medical neglect, emotional abuse and emotional neglect.

Reference

Krugman R. Child Abuse and Neglect. Primary Care 1984; 11(3): 527-534.

PROBLEM #56: A CHILD WITH A SKIN RASH

365. A 4-month-old infant presents with an excoriated diaper rash. It appears as a large erythematous area with discrete papules and some satellite lesions. Which of the following treatments may be helpful in this infant's condition?

   a) zinc oxide ointment
   b) a low potency topical steroid
   c) miconazole
   d) all of the above
   e) a and c

366. A 5-year old child presents with a skin rash on all four extremities. The extremities are dry and scaly, and areas of lichenification and hyperpigmentation are present. Some of the lesions are excoriated and weeping. Which of the following treatments may be useful in this condition?

   a) a low to medium potency topical steroid
   b) hydroxyzine (Atarax)
   c) erythromycin
   d) all of the above
   e) a and b

367. A 2-week old baby presents with a red, scaly, oily eruption occuring on the face and scalp. Which of the following treatments may be useful in the treatment of this condition?

   a) fluorinated topical corticosteroid
   b) a selenium containing shampoo
   c) mineral oil
   d) all of the above
   e) b and c

368. A 6-year old child presents with round, scaly scalp patches with hair loss. In addition, numerous annular plaques with red, papular, scaly borders and flat, hyperpigmented centers with a violet hue are seen. Which of the following treatments are indicated in this patient?

   a) a selenium containing shampoo
   b) high potency topical corticosteroids
   c) griseofulvin
   d) erythromycin
   e) a and c

369. A 6-year old child presents with an extensive gingivostomatitis with extensive perioral vesicles and pustules and intraoral vesicles and erosions. The fluid from a vesicle is scraped and demonstrates multinucleated giant cells on a Tzanck test. Which of the following are indicated in the therapy of this condition?

    a) burrow's solution (aluminum acetate) compresses
    b) intravenous acyclovir
    c) topical fluorinated corticosteroids
    d) all of the above
    e) a and b

CODE: (a:1, 2 and 3; b: 1 and 3; c: 2 and 4; d: 4 only; e: all of the above)

370. A 3-year old child develops a perioral skin rash consisting of honey-colored crusts. Which of the following statements regarding this skin rash is/are TRUE?

    1) staphylococci are the most likely cause of the rash
    2) wet compresses and topical antibiotics are usually sufficient for treatment
    3) the skin condition is most likely to become chronic
    4) a secondary bacteremia from this infection is unlikely.

ANSWERS

365. d) The infant described has a typical irritant diaper dermatitis with secondary candida infection. Discrete lesions occurring at a distance from the main rash called "satellite" lesions are most likely due to Candida infection. Irritant dermatitis is the most frequent type of dermatitis in childhood. In infants, irritation from urine, stool, and topical preparations may produce an acute or chronic diaper dermatitis.

    Initial management of diaper dermatitis includes frequent diaper changes and application of occlusive topical preparations (vasoline, zinc oxide ointment). Low or medium potency topical steroids are used for 7 to 10 days when the dermatitis is severe or persistent. In this case, because of the secondary Candida infection, an antifungal agent such as Ecostatin or Mycostatin cream should be added.

366. d) The child described in this question has atopic eczema. Patients with this condition usually respond to a twice daily application of low-to-medium potency corticosteroid, administration of an antihistamine such as hydroxyzine 5-10 mg. every 6 hours, and the liberal use of emollients such as Lubriderm or Nutraderm. In addition, when excoriation and weeping are present, the lesions are likely superinfected with bacteria and an antibiotic such as erythomycin should be added. Children with atopic dermatitis have a high incidence of associated allergies.

367. e) The child described in this question has seborrheic dermatitis. The etiology of this condition is unclear. Often the first manifestation is "cradle cap", a thick, tenacious, scaly eruption on the scalp. The oily lesions described in this child frequently follow. The condition usually improves spontaneously by six months of age.

Scalp lesions clear with daily use of antiseborrheic shampoos containing selenium, pyrithione zinc or salicylic acid. Scales may be loosened with mineral oil massage before shampooing. Generalized lesions respond within several weeks to application of low-to-medium potency topical steroids once or twice daily. Fluorinated topical corticosteroids should never be used on the face.

368. e) The child described in this question has tinea capitis. Scalp ringworm is particulary common in childhood and may become epidemic in schools and day-care centers. Topical antifungals are effective on glabrous skin, but in hair-bearing areas eradication of the fungus requires systemic griseofulvin in a dose of 10 mg./kg./day. Scalp lesions require six to eight weeks to clear. Selenium-containing shampoos are useful in the first few weeks of therapy to reduce the risk of shedding spores and spreading the fungus to siblings and classmates.

Antibiotics are not helpful in the treatment of this fungal infection unless a bacterial superinfection has developed.

369. a) The child described in this question has herpetic gingivostomatitis. The multinucleated giant cells seen on the Tzanck smear are virtually diagnostic of herpetic infection. In older children and adults, patterns of primary and recurrent herpes simplex respond well to symptomatic treatment with aluminum acetate compresses and analgesics. The lesions should be watched carefully for signs of infections, in which case a topical or oral antibiotic would also be indicated.

Intravenous acyclovir is indicated only in infants. Infants can rapidly develop a systemic infection, which has a 50% mortality rate.

As mentioned previously, fluorinated topical corticosteroids should never by used on the face.

370. c) The child descibed in this question has streptococcal impetigo. Impetigo caused by staphylococci tends to be a bullous impetigo, characterized by slowly enlarging bullous rings surrounding central umbilicated crusts.

In streptococcal impetigo, lesions usually clear with wet compresses and topical antibiotics (e.g. — bacitracin, polymyxin). This is an acute self-limiting condition which does not become chronic and a systemic bacteremia from it is unlikely.

Reference

Cohen B. Common Dermatoses of Childhood. American Family Physician 1985; 32(4): 186-203.

PROBLEM #57: AN ANXIOUS MOTHER WITH A YOUNG CHILD WHO "TOES IN"

371. A mother presents to the office with her 15-month old infant who is "toeing-in". The most common cause of "toeing-in" in infancy is:

    a) pes planus
    b) metatarsus adductus
    c) internal tibial torsion
    d) internal femoral torsion
    e) congenital dislocation of the hip

372. The treatment of choice for flexible metatarsus adductus is:

    a) serial casts
    b) a Denis-Brown splint
    c) reassurance and re-examination
    d) bilateral osteotomies
    e) special orthopedic shoes

373. Which of the following conditions usually require special orthotic footware to ensure correction?

    a) genu varum
    b) genu valgum
    c) flexible pes planus
    d) internal femoral torsion
    e) none of the above

CODE: (a:1, 2 and 3; b: 1 and 3; c: 2 and 4; d: 4 only; e: all of the above)

374. Which of the following statements regarding internal tibial torsion is/are CORRECT?

    1) it is usually noted in ages 8 months to 3 years
    2) it is due to intrauterine molding, maintained by the infant's sleeping posture
    3) it spontaneously resolves in 90% of cases
    4) in refractory cases tibial osteotomies may be required

375. Flat feet (pes planus) is a very common cause of concern of parents about their children. Which of the following statements regarding pes planus is/are CORRECT?

1) most children with flat feet have flexible flat feet
2) flexible flat feet can be differentiated from inflexible flat feet by their appearance on weight bearing
3) an X-ray can usually differentiate a flexible flat foot from an inflexible flat foot
4) most inflexible flat feet require operative correction

ANSWERS

371. b) The most common cause of "in-toeing" in children is metatarsus adductus. The characteristics of this deformity are (1) adduction of the tarsometatarsal joint, causing the individual to walk on the lateral side of the foot; (2) an increase in the height of the longitudinal arch; and (3) an increase in the space between the first and second toes.

The majority of pigeon toes from forefoot adduction will correct spontaneously by two or three years of age provided the child's foot is flexible. This flexibility is best demonstrated by stroking along the lateral border of the child's foot and ankle so as to stimulate the peroneal musculature. If the child is able to straighten out the forefoot adduction, the problem will usually correct spontaneously. Thus, further treatment is not required.

Intoeing can also be caused by internal tibial torsion and internal femoral torsion. They are less common causes of intoeing, and occur at a later age than metatarsus adductus.

Internal tibial torsion is noted from age 8 months to 3 years. It is due to intrauterine molding, maintained by the infant's sleeping posture, and spontaneously resolves in 90% of patients by the age of 4 years. Cases that do not resolve by age 4 may be corrected by shoes externally rotated on a Denis-Browne bar, worn at night.

Internal femoral torsion (femoral anteversion) becomes apparent at three to five years of age, when the legs have completed their medial rotation from the externally rotated and flexed neonatal position. Femoral anteversion tends not to resolve as quickly as flexible metatarsus adductus or internal tibial torsion. There will be some true correction until age seven or eight. The remainder of the in-toeing will be compensated for by the development of external tibial torsion during adolescence, when appearance becomes important to children and they make a voluntary effort to straighten their feet.

Pes planus and congenital dislocation of the hip do not cause intoeing in infants.

372. c) The treatment of choice for flexible metatarsus adductus is reassurance and periodic re-examination. Serial casts are only indicated if the child has an inflexible metatarus adductus (See critique of question #371 for differentiating features.).

    Denis-Browne splints may be useful in the treatment of internal tibial torsion.

    Bilateral osteotomies are not indicated in the treatment of flexible metatarsus adductus. Special orthopedic shoes have not been found to make any difference in the treatment of metatarsus adductus.

373. e) Special orthotic footwear has been suggested by manufacturers to be the answer for every normal variation in children's legs and feet. Studies have shown that they are not any more effective than nature in correcting the problem. True, children with genu varum (bow legs), genu valgum (knock knees), internal femoral torsion and flexible pes planus get better with orthotic footwear; but so do children who have these conditions and who wear ordinary footwear.

374. a) See the critique of question #371 for a more complete description of internal tibial torsion. Internal tibial torsion does not require tibial osteotomies, but rather reassurance or a simple device like the Denis-Browne splint for treatment.

375. b) Flat feet (pes planus) is an extremely common problem in pediatric practice. Approximately 98% of flat feet are flexible flat feet. In differentiating flexible flat feet from inflexible flat feet, the patient should be asked to stand on his toes. This will reconstitute the longitudinal arch and satisfy most parents that the feet really are not flat. X-ray examination can be used to discover the major causes of inflexible flat feet including congenital vertical talus, congenital tarsal coalition, and accessory navicular bones.

Reference

Wedge J. Assessing Children's Legs and Feet. Canadian Family Physician 1985; 31: 595-598.

PROBLEM #58: AN ANXIOUS MOTHER WITH A CHILD WHO IS DEVELOPMENTALLY DELAYED

Lack of achievement of certain developmental milestones may alert the family physician that a child is not developing normally and should be more completely investigated. Match the following developmental milestones with the approximate average age at which they occur. Each lettered time may be used once, more than once, or not at all.

376. Smiles on social contact   _____

377. Laughs out loud   _____

378. Lifts head and rolls over   _____

379. Sits up alone without support   _____

380. Creeps or crawls   _____

381. Utters repetitive consonant sounds (mama, dada)   _____

382. "Cruises" or walks holding on to furniture   _____

383. Walks alone, climbs up stairs   _____

384. Follows simple commands, names a familiar object   _____

385. Runs well, puts 3 words together   _____

     a) 1 month
     b) 2 months
     c) 4 months
     d) 6 months
     e) 9 months
     f) 12 months
     g) 15 months
     h) 18 months
     i) 24 months
     j) 30 months

386. The first primary tooth to erupt is the:

   a) lower cuspid
   b) upper central incisor
   c) lower central incisor
   d) upper cuspid
   e) lower lateral incisor

CODE: (a:1, 2 and 3; b: 1 and 3; c: 2 and 4; d: 4 only; e: all of the above)

387. Teething is a common cause of irritibility in infants. Which of the following is/are shown associated with teething?

   1) low-grade fever
   2) facial rashes
   3) mild diarrhea
   4) increased salivation

ANSWERS

376. b.
377. c.
378. d.
379. e.
380. e.
381. e.
382. f.
383. g.
384. g.
385. i.

Developmental pediatrics is an important part of family practice. Certain milestones have been suggested that should be assessed in every pediatric visit. The most common milestones have been illustrated in this matching question. Briefly, an infant should:

   1) smile on social contact at 2 months
   2) laugh out loud at 4 months
   3) lift his head and roll over at 6 months
   4) sit alone without support, creep or crawl and utter repetitive consonant sounds (mama, dada) at 9 months
   5) cruise or walk holding on to furniture at 12 months
   6) walk alone, crawl up stairs, and follow simple commands at 15 months
   7) run well and put 3 words together at 24 months

386. c) The primary dentition usually erupts in the following order: lower central incisor, lower lateral incisor, upper central incisor, upper lateral incisor, lower first molar, upper first molar, lower first cuspid, upper first cuspid, lower second molar, and upper second molar. The primary dentition begins to erupt at approximately 6 months of age.

387. d) As the teeth penetrate the gums, inflammation and sensitivity sometimes occur, a condition referred to as teething. The child may become irritable, and salivation may increase markedly. There is no definite evidence to support claims of accompanying temporary systemic disturbances, such as low-grade fever, facial rashes, and mild diarrhea.

Teething is best treated with mild analgesics such as acetaminophen, with or without mild antihistamine.

References

Behrman R, Vaughan V., editors Nelson Textbook of Pediatrics. 12th edition. W.B. Saunders Co., Philadelphia: 1983; pages 36-37, 876-877.

PROBLEM #59: AN ANXIOUS MOTHER WITH A 3 WEEK OLD INFANT AND MANY QUESTIONS CONCERNING FEEDING

388. A mother presents to the office with her 3 week old infant. She has many questions concerning infant feeding. She is currently breast feeding but is not sure she wishes to continue. You discuss with her the advantages of breast feeding. Which of the following statements comparing breast milk and cow's milk is FALSE?

   a) cow's milk may be responsible for diarrhea, intestinal bleeding and occult melena
   b) "spitting up", colic and atopic eczema are more common in formula fed babies
   c) human milk contains many bacterial viral antibodies, mainly of the IgA class
   d) breast fed infants do not require iron supplementation until 1 year of age
   e) breast milk is an adequate source of vitamin C

389. Which of the following vitamins may need to be supplemented in a breast fed baby?

   a) vitamin A
   b) vitamin C
   c) vitamin D
   d) b and c
   e) all of the above

390. Fluoride supplementation for formula-fed infants is usually not required if the fluoride concentration of the water in the community exceeds:

   a) 1.0 ppm
   b) 2.0 ppm
   c) 5.0 ppm
   d) 10.0 ppm
   e) 100.0 ppm

391. Breast milk in comparison to cow's milk has:

   a) a higher fat content
   b) a lower carbohydrate content
   c) a lower protein content
   d) a greater concentration of casein
   e) a greater number of calories/gram

392. Pablum and other solid foods do not usually have to be introduced into the infant's diet until:

    a) 1 month of age
    b) 2-3 months of age
    c) 4-6 months of age
    d) 9 months of age
    e) 12 months of age

393. A mother brings her 6 month old infant into the office. She states that he has been constipated since she switched him from breast to bottle 2 weeks ago. On careful questioning, you determine that the infant is having 1 hard bowel movement every 4 days. You should advise the mother to:

    a) go home and relax, the child will grow out of it
    b) to supplement with extra fluids, extra foods, and prune juice
    c) to use milk of magnesia at bedtime
    d) to add 2 tablespoons of bran to the pablum and feed it to him every 3 hours
    e) to give him a glycerine suppository at bedtime.

394. A mother brings her 6-week old infant into the office. She states that he has been spitting up all of his formula for the last 3 weeks and is obviously malnourished. You find that the infant weighs 11 lbs. 3 oz. His birth weight was 7 lbs. 6 oz. You should advise the mother to:

    a) go home and relax, the child will grow out of it
    b) increase the time spent burping the infant and put him on his abdomen for a nap immediately after feeding
    c) investigate the child for pyloric stenosis
    d) suggest the use of a GI tract motility modifier such as metoclopramide
    e) refer the child to a pediatrician

CODE: (a:1, 2 and 3; b: 1 and 3; c: 2 and 4; d: 4 only; e: all of the above)

395. A mother who is currently breast-feeding her 4-month old son presents to your office with a erythematous, swollen, tender area at the 11 o'clock position in the right breast. The swelling measures 4 cm. in diameter. Your initial impression is mastitis. You should advise her to:

    1) apply warm compresses to the area
    2) discontinue breast feeding
    3) begin antibiotic therapy with cloxacillin
    4) start the baby on prophylactic penicillin

ANSWERS

388. d) Breast milk has many advantages over cow's milk for the feeding of infants. These advantages include:

   a) it is easier to digest
   b) it has many bacterial and viral antibodies present in it, especially those of the IgA class
   c) it does not produce allergic manifestations such as diarrhea, GI tract bleeding and atopic dermatitis
   d) it has a lower incidence of regurgitation, constipation, colic, and other feeding problems
   e) it is the most important way to establish maternal-infant bonding

   Breast milk contains adequate supplies of all vitamins except for Vitamin D. Breast-fed babies should receive supplemental Vitamin D until they begin vitamin-fortified cereals or other foods. Vitamin C is not required for supplementation.

   Although breast milk contains some iron, and the iron that is present is well absorbed, the child probably should begin iron-fortified foods at 6 months of age to prevent an iron-deficiency anemia.

389. c) Vitamin D is the only vitamin that may be required for supplementation in a breast-fed baby. If a baby is not exposed to adequate sunlight or has dark skin, the quantity of Vitamin D may not be sufficient. It is recommended that the daily intake of Vitamin D be 400 IU/day. Whether or not all breast-fed babies should be supplemented with Vitamin D is still debated.

390. a) Fluoride supplementation of a formula-fed infant is not required if the fluoride concentration of the water supply exceeds 1.0 ppm. There is still some debate as to whether or not a breast-fed baby needs supplementation. The current opinion is that breast milk does not have a sufficient quantity of fluoride, even in a fluoridated community.

   Additional fluoride given to formula-fed babies in a community with a fluoridated water supply could result in fluorosis, which is mainly manifested by mottling of the teeth.

391. c) In comparison to cow's milk, breast milk has the following characteristics:

   a) a higher carbohydrate content — 7.0% to 4.5%. The main sugar, lactose, is the same in both.
   b) a lower protein content — 1.0% to 3.3%. As well, the predominant protein in breast milk is lactalbumin and lactoglobulin as compared to casein in cow's milk.
   c) a qualitative difference in fat but no difference in quantity — 3.5%
   d) the same caloric content — 20 kcal/oz.

392. c) Solid foods do not have to be introduced into an infant's diet until 4-6 months of age. Pablum is usually introduced at about 4 months of age. Other solid foods can wait until 6 months of age. The main concern in a child in which solid food is not introduced until later is the possibility of an iron deficiency anemia.

393. b) Constipation is a common problem in bottle-fed babies. It is practically unknown in breast-fed babies. Constipation in a formula-fed baby may be due to the insufficient amount of food or fluid. In other instances, it may result from diets too high in fat or protein or deficient in bulk. Simply increasing the amount of fluid or sugar in the formula may be corrective, especially if it occurs in the first few months of life. After this age, better results are obtained by adding or increasing the amounts of cereal, vegetables, or fruit. Prune juice (1/2-1 oz.) may also be helpful.

The use of milk of magnesia and glycerine suppositories as anything but a very temporary measure is inappropriate. The addition of 2 teaspoons of bran to the pablum, although theoretically sound as a measure of increasing the bulk in the infant's diet, would be somewhat unpalatable.

Telling the mother to go home and relax is not appropriate. In this case you have not given any constructive information to the mother, and your doctor-patient relationship is likely to be compromised.

394. b) Regurgitation or spitting up is a common problem in infants. The reason seems to lie in the immaturity of the gastroesophageal sphincter mechanism. Within limits, regurgitation is a natural occurence, especially during the first 6 months of life. It can be reduced to a negligible amount, however, by adequate eructation of swallowed air during and after eating, by gentle handling, by avoidance of emotional conflicts, and by placing the infant on the right side or abdomen for a nap immediately after eating. One should also ensure that the head is not lower than the rest of the body during the rest periods.

Unless the child (especially a male) demonstrates projectile vomiting and has a palpable mass in the pylorus, pyloric stenosis is not likely.

Metoclopramide and other GI tract motility modifiers have no place to play in the management of regurgitation in infants. The condition should be gently explained to the the mother in a calm, reassuring manner. She should be asked to try the simple measures outlined above. Inadequate explanation, along with advice to relax is inappropriate. Unless the mother is not happy with your advice, referral to a pediatrician is not indicated.

395. b) Mastitis is a common complaint in breast feeding mothers. Treatment should be begun with analgesics, warm compressess, and an anti-staphylococcal antibiotic such as cloxacillin. Breast feeding should be continued. It is very unlikely that the baby will develop an infection because of the infection in the mother, and thus prophylactic antibiotics in the infant are not recommended.

Reference

Behrman R, Vaughan V. Nelson Textbook of Pediatrics, 12th edition, W.B. Saunders Company, Philadelphia: 1983; pages 148-163.

PROBLEM #60: A 2 YEAR OLD BOY WITH DIARRHEA

396. A mother presents to the office with her 2 year old boy. The child has had diarrhea for the last 5 days. You recognize that the most common cause of diarrhea in the pediatric age group is a viral agent. The most common viral cause of diarrhea in the pediatric age group is:

a) Norwalk agent
b) rotavirus
c) coxsackie virus
d) echovirus
e) influenza Type A

397. The most common bacterial cause of diarrhea in the pediatric age group is:

a) Salmonella
b) Shigella
c) Campylobacter
d) E.Coli
e) enterococcus

398. The most common cause of antibiotic-associated diarrhea in the pediatric age group is:

a) ampicillin
b) clindamycin
c) erythromycin
d) penicillin
e) none of the above

CODE: (a: 1, 2 and 3; b: 1 and 3; c: 2 and 4; d: 4 only; e: all of the above)

399. The investigations that should be done on all children present with diarrhea include:

1) urine specific gravity
2) sigmoidoscopy
3) stool evaluation for blood and leukocytes
4) serum osmolarity

400. Which of the following oral fluids is/are suitable for rehydration of a dehydrated toddler with diarrhea?

1) apple juice
2) grape juice
3) decarbonated soda
4) Pedialyte

401. Which of the following pediatric infections often present with diarrhea?

    1) acute appendicitis
    2) otitis media
    3) urinary tract infections
    4) pneumonia

ANSWERS

396. b) The most common cause of gastroenteritis in the pediatric age group is rotavirus. The most severe rotaviral infections occur in young infants. Neonates may also have rotavirus and in some nurseries as many as 50% of babies are excreting it. Many are asymptomatic. Although there is now a rapid diagnostic test for rotavirus antigen in stool, (Rotazyme-Abbott) it is of little clinical value for the routine case because the results do not alter management. It may be helpful to evaluate complicated cases or to define isolation procedures in hopitals.

    The Norwalk agent is the most common cause of viral gastroenteritis in adults.

    Although enteroviruses (coxsackie virus and echovirus) may cause gastroenteritis, they more commonly produce a febrile respiratory syndrome that may be associated with a diffuse maculopapular rash.

    The clinical manifestations in influenza Type A infection in children are mainly respiratory, although gastrointestinal manifestations may be seen.

397. c) The most common bacterial cause of gastroenteritis in the pediatric age group is Campylobacter species. It has only been in the last few years that this organism has been recognized as a major cause of gastroenteritis. The manifestations of this illness include fever, cramps, vomiting, and loose stools that often contain mucus and blood. Untreated, it lasts a few days to several weeks. Specific antibiotic therapy with erythromycin usually eradicates the organism, but does not necessarily ameliorate the disease, which is usually self-limited.

    Other bacterial causes include Salmonella, Shigella, and Yersinia species. Pathogenic E.coli are a relatively infrequent cause of acute gastroenteritis in children.

398. a) The most common cause of antibiotic-associated diarrhea in children is ampicillin. This is currently a well recognized disease, presumably due to the presence of Clostridium difficile toxin. Most cases are mild and resolve with discontinuation of the drug. Bloody diarrhea or severe pseudomembranous colitis may occur. Diagnosis is best made by demonstrating the toxin in the stool. Treatment of severe cases usually consists of vancomycin hydrochloride or metronidizole.

399. b) The investigations that should be performed on all children with diarrhea include the urine specific gravity and stool analysis for blood and fecal leukocytes. If the urine specific gravity is below 1.015 you can be reassured that the hydration is adequate. Blood or fecal leukocytes in the stool suggests the presence of an inflammatory disease. Although rotavirus may produce heme-positive stools, gross blood is more suggestive of invasive bacteria or Entamoeba histolytica. Also, numerous leukocytes are not seen with viral or parasitic infections.

As well as an examination of the stool for blood and fecal leukocytes, the stool sample should be gram-stained and cultured.

Other investigations including a complete blood count, erythrocyte sedimentation rate, serum electrolytes, and serum osmolarity may be indicated in a toxic child, but are unlikely to change your management in mild infections.

Sigmoidoscopy, which is obviously a very traumatic procedure for a child unless done under anaesthesia, should not be part of a routine work-up.

400. d) The only solution listed that is acceptable for oral rehydration is Pedialyte. Pedialyte contains 45 mEq/litre of sodium, 20 mEq/litre of potassium, 35 mEq/litre of chloride, 30 mEq/litre of bicarbonate and 2.5 g/dl of glucose. The osmolarity of the solution is 390 mOsm/litre.

Apple juice, grape juice and decarbonated soda have no sodium and a very high osmolarity (700-1000 mOsm/L). A solution of this osmolarity will obviously aggravate an already inflammed gut.

401. e) Loose stools and vomiting may be seen in children who have nonenteric inflammatory diseases. In general, the younger the infant, the more likely this is to occur, perhaps due to the relative hypermotility and laxity of the gastroesophageal sphincter in the infant. The most common infections producing this syndrome are otitis media and urinary tract infection. In the case of urinary tract infection there is rarely a history suggesting dysuria or gross pyuria. The loose stools contain neither blood nor leukocytes because there is no true enteritis.

Acute appendicitis may present as a severe gastroenteritis. An inflamed appendix lying in the pelvis, near the distal colon, often causes colonic irritation and diarrhea. Fever, vomiting, toxicity, nonfocal abdominal tenderness without peritoneal signs, and an elevated leukocyte count complete the clinical picture.

Lower lobe pneumonia may present with abdominal symptoms as well. Demonstrating the consolidation on physical examination is challenging. Unexplained tachypnea should prompt radiographic evaluation in febrile children with enteric symptoms.

References

Paisley J. Acute Gastroenteritis Syndromes in Children. Primary Care 1984; 11(3): 513-526.
Rodriguez, W. Specific Diarrheal Disease. In: Current Therapy in Pediatric Infectious Disease. Nelson J, editor. B.C. Decker Inc., Philadelphia: 1986; pages 62-66.

PROBLEM #61: A 6 YEAR OLD CHILD WITH HYPERACTIVITY

CODE: (a:1, 2 and 3; b: 1 and 3; c: 2 and 4; d: 4 only; e: all of the above)

402. A mother presents to your office with her 6 year old son. As you enter the examining room he is in the process of destroying it. Which of the following is/are potential causes for overactivity and decreased attention span in this 6 year old boy?

    1) constitutional attention deficit
    2) emotionally based attention deficit
    3) neurologically based attention deficit
    4) attention deficit due to asthma and hay fever

403. Which of the following characteristics is/are found in children with constitutional attention deficit?

    1) traits traceable back to early infancy
    2) normal intelligence
    3) normal developmental history and school performance
    4) no neurologic abnormalities

404. Which of the following treatments is/are indicated for the child with emotionally based attention deficit?

    1) education and explanation to the parents
    2) methylphenidate (Ritalin) 10-40 mg./day
    3) exploration of psychological problems
    4) diazepam 2-6 mg./day

405. With regard to dietary manipulation of children with attention deficit syndrome, which of the following is/are TRUE?

    1) the Fiengold diet is often of considerable benefit
    2) megavitamin therapy is often successful
    3) increasing the dietrary fibre helps many children
    4) there does seem to be a subset of children who are adversely affected by large amounts of sugar

406. Attention deficit syndrome is often treated with stimulant medication such as methylphenidate (Ritalin). Which of the following types of attention deficit syndrome may this medication be indicated in?

    1) constitutional attention deficit
    2) emotionally based attention deficit
    3) neurologically based attention deficit
    4) attention deficit syndrome due to other illnesses

ANSWERS

402. e) The term "attention deficit disorder" has now replaced the terms "hyperactivity" and "minimal brain dysfunction" in the description of a child with overactivity and decreased attention span. Attention deficit disorder may be divided into several types:

   a) Constitutional attention deficit: the child is born with a distinct set of characteristics that can be collectively called temperament. The "temperament" can then be expressed as overactivity and decreased attention span.

   b) Emotionally based attention deficit: the child is expressing anxiety or depression as overactivity and decreased attention span.

   c) Neurologically based attention deficit: the child is overactive and has a decreased attention span because of some preexisting neurological condition such as perinatal asphyxia, prematurity, central nervous system infection, etc.

   d) Attention deficit disorder due to another medical condition: the child has overactivity and decreased attention span due to a chronic condition such as asthma, hay fever or a dermatologic condition producing pruritis.

   e) Medication-induced attention deficit: the child is overactive and has a decreased attention span due to medications such as aminophylline, sympathomimetics, antihistamines, steroids, phenobarbitol etc.

   f) Misdiagnosis: the child is diagnosed as hyperactive when in fact the adults in the child's environment have unrealistic expectations for the child's behavior.

403. e) The history is the most important instrument in establishing a diagnosis of attention deficit disorder. Children with "constitutional attention deficits" are those whose temperament profile is two standard deviations away from the mean in activity level, attention span, or persistence with tasks. The keys to the diagnosis in this group of children are that (1) the traits are traceable back to early infancy, (2) they have normal intelligence, (3) their developmental history and school performance are normal, and (4) they have no neurologic abnormalities. There is often a positive family history for these traits, as well.

404. b) Emotionally based attention deficit is often the first clue to a primary anxiety of depressive disorder. It is important to explore the child's behavior and his environment in light of this probability. Education of the parents, as well as exploration of the psychologic factors that may be involved are essential. Methylphenidate and other stimulant medications have not been shown to be beneficial in this subgroup of attention deficit disorder. Benzodiazepines are probably not indicated, even if the illness turns out to be a primary anxiety disorder. Rather, a manipulation of the child's routine and environment are the primary treatments. This could include additional rest periods, relaxation techniques such as soft music, quiet time, a warm bath, and deep breathing exercises.

405. d) The treatment of attention deficit disorder by dietary modification has been the subject of ongoing controversy. The Fiengold diet, which eliminates most food additives, is a costly and difficult diet to follow. It, along with mega-vitamin therapy and high fibre diets, have not been shown to have a significant impact on children with attention defict disorder. There does, however, appear to be a subset of children that are adversely affected by large amounts of sugar. Therefore, it may be reasonable to advise parents to avoid large boluses of sugar in their overactive child.

406. b) The only subgroups of attention deficit disorder in which methylphenidate and other stimulant medications have been found to be useful are constitu-tional attention deficit and neurologically based attention deficit. In those groups, therapy with methylphenidate (beginning at 5-10 mg. in the morning and repeated at noon) may be beneficial.

Emotionally based attention deficit should be treated by addressing the potential underlying anxiety or depression.

Attention deficit disorder due to other medical illness or medication can often be altered by treating the primary disease process more effectively, or discontinuing the offending medication.

Reference

Poole S. Hyperactivity. Primary Care 1984; 11(3): 431-442.

PROBLEM #62: A FULL-TERM INFANT WITH JAUNDICE

407. A full-term infant weighing 4000 grams develops jaundice on the 2nd day of life. The infant appears healthy and is breast feeding well. Vital signs are normal. The mother is group 0 positive and the infant is group A positive. The direct and indirect Coombs' tests are negative. The most likely cause of this baby's jaundice is:

    a) undiagnosed neonatal sepsis
    b) breast milk jaundice
    c) physiologic jaundice
    d) jaundice due to a minor antigen blood group incompatibility
    e) AB0 blood group incompatibility

408. A full-term infant weighing 3800 grams develops jaundice on the 4th day of life. He is being breast fed and is feeding well. Vital signs are normal. The mother is group 0 positive and the infant is group A positive. The direct and indirect Coombs' tests are negative. The most likely cause of this baby's jaundice is:

    a) undiagnosed neonatal sepsis
    b) breast milk jaundice
    c) physiologic jaundice
    d) jaundice due to a minor antigen blood group incompatibility
    e) AB0 blood group incompatibility

409. Jaundice in the newborn period develops in what percentage of full-term infants?

    a) 20%
    b) 40%
    c) 60%
    d) 80%
    e) 95%

410. A serum bilirubin in excess of what level is accepted as evidence of nonphysiologic jaundice in a full-term infant?

    a) 102.5 micromoles/litre (6 mg./dl)
    b) 205 micromoles/litre (12 mg./dl)
    c) 250 micromoles/litre (15 mg./dl)
    d) 307.5 micromoles/litre (18 mg./dl)
    e) 410 micromoles/litre (24 mg./dl)

411. A breast fed baby develops jaundice on the 4th day of life. At what level of serum bilirubin is it appropriate to initiate phototherapy?

   a) 102.5 micromoles/litre (6 mg./dl)
   b) 205 micromoles/litre (12 mg./dl)
   c) 250 micromoles/litre (15 mg./dl)
   d) 307.5 micromoles/litre (18 mg./dl)
   e) 345 micromoles/litre (20 mg./dl)

CODE: (a:1, 2 and 3; b: 1 and 3; c: 2 and 4; d: 4 only; e: all of the above)

412. Which of the following is/are complications of phototherapy in the treatment of newborn infants with jaundice?

   1) frequent loose stools
   2) a transient rash
   3) lethargy and abdominal distension
   4) hyperthermia and flushing

ANSWERS

407. c) The newborn infant most likely has physiologic jaundice. Physiologic jaundice usually begins on the 2nd or 3rd day of life. It is thought to be due to the accumulation in the skin of unconjugated, nonpolar, lipid-soluble bilirubin pigment (indirect reacting) formed from hemoglobin by the action of heme oxygenase, biliverdin reductase, and nonenzymatic reducing agents in the reticuloendothelial cells. It may also be due, in part, to the deposition of the pigment after it has been converted in the liver cell mircosome by the enzyme uridine diphosphoglucuronic acid glucuronyl transferase to the polar, water-soluble ester glucuronide of bilirubin (direct reacting).

   Physiologic jaundice usually does not exceed 205 micromoles/litre at its height, and usually clears in a full-term baby by 4-5 days.

   As the baby is feeding well and his vital signs are normal it is unlikely to be due to neonatal sepsis.

   Breast milk jaundice does not usually begin until at least the 4th day.

   Rh blood group incompatibility is ruled out because both mother and baby are Rh positive. AB0 blood group incompatibility and incompatibility due to other minor blood groups are unlikely with a negative direct and indirect Coombs' test.

408. b) Breast milk jaundice usually begins on the 4th day of life or later and may reach 520 micromoles/litre (30 mg./dl) or greater. Breast milk jaundice is thought to be due to the presence of certain inhibitors of the enzyme glucuronyl transferase in the breast milk. If the maximum concentration of bilirubin reached is less than 250 micromoles/litre no treatment is required. If

greater than 250 micromoles/litre but less than 345 micromoles/litre photo-therapy is indicated. If the maximum concentration reached is greater than 345 micromoles/litre the baby should be taken off the breast for 24-48 hours. This will usually result in a dramatic fall in the serum bilirubin.

The other choices in the question are incorrect for the same reasons given in question #407.

409. c) Jaundice is extremely common in newborn infants. Under usual nursery conditions jaundice is observed during the 1st week of life in approximately 60% of term infants and 80% of breast fed infants.

410. b) Physiologic jaundice rarely produces serum bilirubin levels in excess of 205 micromoles/litre (12 mg./dl). If the serum bilirubin level exceeds this level, other causes such as breast milk jaundice, jaundice due to various blood group incompatibilities and jaundice due to sepsis should be suspected.

411. c) Phototherapy should probably be initiated in the full-term infant at a level of 250 micromoles/litre (15 mg./dl). This applies to breast milk jaundice and jaundice due to blood group incompatibility problems. If it is begun at a level less than this, the potential complications (see critique of questin #412) probably outweigh the benefits. If it is not begun until the bilirubin has reached a higher level, the risk of kernicterus in increased.

412. e) The potential complications of phototherapy are:
   a) frequent and loose stools (an effect of light energy on Auerbach's plexus)
   b) transient rash
   c) lethargy and abdominal distension
   d) bronze baby syndrome — a gray brown discoloration of the skin in those infants with some degree of cholestasis
   e) hyperthermia and flushing
   f) potential dehydration — supplement of 25 mls./kg./24 hrs. water is suggested.

References

Behrman R, Vaughan V III, Editors. Nelson Textbook of Pediatrics 12th edition. W.B. Saunders Co., Philadelphia: 1983; pages 378-381.
Sankaran K. Hyperbilirubinemia. University of Saskatchewan, CME News 1985; 15(7): 1-3.

PROBLEM #63: A 3 YEAR OLD CHILD WITH PHARYNGITIS

413. A 3-year old child who has had rhinitis and pharyngitis for 3 days develops a barking cough and stridor. He is brought into the hospital emergency room where he is given humidified oxygen and improves. The most likely diagnosis of this child's condition is:

a) acute laryngotracheitis
b) acute spasmodic croup
c) acute epiglottitis
d) spontaneous pneumothorax
e) acute viral pneumonia

414. The agent most frequently implicated as the cause of the condition described in question #413 is:

a) respiratory syncytial virus
b) adenovirus
c) rhinovirus
d) parainfluenza virus

415. The test of choice for the diagnosis of streptococcal pharyngitis is:

a) antibody coated latex particles
b) throat culture
c) total neutrophil count
d) acute and convalescent sera using immunodiffusion techniques
e) C-reactive protein

416. The diagnosis of streptococcal pharyngitis is often difficult by clincial examination alone. Which of the following clinical features is sensitive in distinguishing a streptococcal pharyngitis from a viral pharyngitis?

a) the presence of exudate on the tonsils
b) the presence of cervical lymphadenopathy
c) the presence of a temperature greater than 39°C
d) none of the above
e) all of the above

417. The viral agent most frequently responsible for the common cold is:

a) adenovirus
b) rhinovirus
c) echovirus
d) coxsackie virus
e) influenza A virus

418. The viral agent most frequently responsible for acute bronchiolitis in children is:

    a) adenovirus
    b) rhinovirus
    c) parainfluenza virus
    d) respiratory syncytial virus
    e) influenza A virus

ANSWERS

413. a) The child described in the question most likely has acute laryngotracheitis. This is one of three croup syndromes which includes acute spasmodic croup and acute epiglottitis.

    Acute laryngotracheitis is most often caused by a parainfluenza virus. Symptoms include the history of an upper respiratory tract infection and the development of a severe "barking" nocturnal cough with increasing stridor and hoarseness. Treatment is symptomatic with oxygenation and humidity. Inhalation of racemic epinephrine as 0.5 mls. in 4 mls. of saline is controversial but may be of benefit.

    Acute epiglottitis is the most serious form of croup, as complete airway obstruction may develop. The infection is caused by Haemophilus influenzae type b and responds to appropriate antibiotic therapy with ampicillin or chloramphenicol.

    Acute spasmodic croup is a variation of the croup syndrome in which there appears to be a host-specific characteristic. Symptoms of stridor and a barking cough develop in the evening in a child who was previously well with no other respiratory symptoms. Recent evidence suggests that his problem may have an atopic etiology. Treatment with beta-mimetic bronchodilators or steroids may be helpful.

    Spontaneous pneumothorax would not usually present with any infective signs or symptoms. Acute viral pneumonia would likely present with symptoms and signs of lower airway involvement, rather than a barking cough.

414. d) The causative agent of acute laryngotracheitis is parainfluenza virus. See the critique of question #413 for a description of the syndrome.

415. b) Although the diagnosis of streptococcal pharyngitis has been revolutionized by rapid tests utilizing antibody coated latex particles, the gold standard of diagnosis is still the throat culture. Serious questions have arisen regarding the sensitivity of some of the newer rapid antibody tests. There seems to be a critical number of colonies below which the antibody tests lose their sensitivity. Also, some cases of streptococcal pharyngitis are due to streptococci other than Lancefield Group A. These streptococci are not detected using the rapid antigen detection kits.

416. d) The differentiation of streptococcal pharyngitis from viral pharyngitis on clinical grounds alone is impossible. Both streptococcal and viral pharyngitis may present with high fever, the presence of exudates on the tonsils and the presence of cervical lymphadenopathy. The only distinction tends to be the presence of other symptoms of respiratory tract infection, such as rhinitis and congestion, in the case of viral pharyngitis.

417. b) The most common cause of the common cold is rhinovirus. Other viruses that have been implicated are adenovirus, echovirus, coxsackie virus, and influenza and parainfluenza virus. Nasal discomfort, congestion, sneezing, and rhinorrhea are the chief complaints. Treatment is symptomatic and antibiotics should not be prescribed either to prevent bacterial complications or to treat the cold itself.

418. d) Acute bronchiolitis is most often caused by the respiratory syncytial virus. The syndome is characterized by tachypnea, wheezing and fever. The differential diagnosis includes asthma and pneumonia. Most children with bronchiolitis can be managed as outpatients with oxygenation and hydration. A trial of systemic or nebulized beta-receptor agoinst bronchodilators is often helpful.

References

Gerber M. Latex aggultination test for rapid identification of group A streptococci directly from throat swabs. Journal of Pediatrics 1984; 105: 702-705.

Nicholson D, Bower A. Pulmonary medicine. Textbook of Family Practice 3rd edition. Rakel R, editor. W.B. Saunders Co., Philadelphia: 1984:, pages 371-374.

Stillerman M. Streptococcal Tonsillopharyngitis and Scarlet Fever. Current Therapy in Pediatric Infectious Disease. Nelson J, editor. B.C. Decker Inc., Philadelphia: 1986, pages 23-26.

Kellogg J, Manzella J. Detection of Group A Streptococci in Laboratory or Physician's Office. JAMA 1986; 255(19): 263802642.

PROBLEM #64: A 5 YEAR OLD GIRL WITH RECURRENT ABDOMINAL PAIN

419. A 5 year old girl presents to the office with her mother. Her mother states that she has had recurrent abdominal pain for the last 18 months. Which of the following symptoms is MOST COMMON in recurrent abdominal pain in children?

a) diarrhea
b) constipation
c) school phobia
d) depression
e) anxiety

420. Which of the following statements about recurrent abdominal pain in children is FALSE?

a) a child with no organic disease found can be assumed to have an emotional problem
b) 10-15% of school children at some time experience recurrent abdominal pain
c) children with recurrent abdominal pain often have parents with the same symptom
d) school problems are often a triggering factor
e) parents of children with recurrent abdominal pain often seek numerous medical opinions

CODE: (a:1, 2 and 3; b: 1 and 3; c: 2 and 4; d: 4 only; e: all of the above)

421. Which of the following may be involved in the etiology of recurrent abdominal pain in children?

1) a somatic predisposition, dysfunction or disorder
2) life style and habit
3) temperament and learned response patterns
4) milieux and critical events

422. Which of the following laboratory investigations is/are MANDATORY in children with recurrent abdominal pain?

1) complete blood count
2) erthyrocyte sedimentation rate
3) urinalysis
4) a plain supine X-ray of the abdomen

423. Which of the following MAY BE indicated in the treatment of a child with recurrent abdominal pain?

    1) long term laxative therapy
    2) dietary modification
    3) modification of the child's daily routine
    4) yearly GI and barium enema

419. b) All of the symptoms listed can be part of the recurrent abdominal pain syndrome in childhood. However, the most common sympton is constipation. This fits into the "life style and habit" category. Children are often in a hurry to proceed with the events of the day and don't even have time to have a proper bowel movement. In addition, dietary habits such as a lack of fiber may play a contributing role.

420. a) Recurrent abdominal pain is common in the school age population. Various studies have estimated that 10-15% of children will at one time or another manifest recurrent abdominal pain.

    Recurrent abdominal pain seems to be more common in families with recurrent abdominal complaints. It does not appear to be correlated with previous symptoms in the parents as children, but rather the present or recent situation.

    School problems or school phobias are one of the most common factors contributing to recurrent abdominal pain. It fits into the multifactorial model previously discussed under "milieux and critical events".

    Parents of children with recurrent abdominal pain often seek numerous medical opinions for their children. As physicians, it is our duty of offer a second (or third) opinion if the parents ask for it. By so doing, we will be seen as caring and concerned about the problem.

    A child should never be assumed to have emotional problems simply because the traditional organic evaluation has failed to yield an identifiable disease. Rather, the multifactorial model should be kept in mind, and repeated visits and counselling aimed at changing the factors involved in the child's total health undertaken.

421. e) The etiology of recurrent abdominal pain in children can best be thought of as multifactorial with contributions from (1) somatic predisposition, dysfunction or disorder such as constipation, peptic ulcer or any other cause of acute abdominal pain; (2) life style and habit, including the child's daily schedule, routine, and dietary habits; (3) milieu and critical events including stressess at home, in the neighborhood and at school and (4) temperament and learned response patterns in early life.

422. e) All children with recurrent abdominal pain should have a complete blood count, an erythrocyte sedimentation rate, a urinalysis and a plain X-ray of the abdomen. The single most common positive finding will be retained stool on

KUB. A urinary tract infection, especially in a young girl is a common cause of recurrent abdominal pain. This will be discovered by the finding of WBC's or bacteria in the urine. A urine culture would then be appropriate. The erythrocyte sedimentation rate is a nonspecific screening test for inflammatory conditions. A hemoglobin will often detect occult anemia which would indicate ongoing blood loss from the GI tract.

Further targeted investigations should be in response to findings suggestive of a particular disease process or one or more of the following "red flags".

1) a history of weight loss and/or reduced appetite
2) alteration of function or symptom progression related to a specific organ system
3) abnormalities of the complete blood count
4) occult or frank bleeding from any orifice
5) abnormal urinalysis and/or culture
6) compelling family history of a particular disorder (eg. ulcer disease)
7) constitutional symptoms of chronic illness such as recurrent fever, ill-appearance, growth failure, swollen joints, and lack of energy

423. a) Treatment of recurrent abdominal pain is directed to the multifactorial model. If a specific somatic dysfunction such as constipation is present, long term laxative therapy is often helpful. In this regard, life-style and habit can be altered by including time in the daily routine for proper bowel movements and changing the diet to include more fiber (if constipated).

Stressess occurring in the child's life, such as problems at school and home can be explored and work done towards their resolution.

Temperament and learned response patterns can also be altered by providing supportive counselling regarding their effects on the etiology of the pain. Encouraging the child and parent to return to the office at regular intervals is often the most helpful treatment.

Reference

Levine M, Rappaport L. Recurrent Abdominal Pain in School Children. Pediatric Clinics of North America 1984; 31(5): 969-991.

PROBLEM #65: A CHILD WITH FEVER AND A SKIN RASH

The 6 numbered descriptions of exanthems are followed by six childhood exanthems. Match the appropriate exanthem to the numbered description. Each exanthem may be used once, more than once or not at all.

Answer

424. Koplik's spots   _____

425. circumoral pallor   _____

426. "blueberry muffin" baby   _____

427. bullous eruption   _____

428. "slapped cheek" appearance   _____

429. characteristic sequence of fever, defervescence, and
     rash   _____

    a. rubeola
    b. rubella
    c. roseola
    d. Filatov-Dukes disease
    e. scarlet fever
    f. erythema infectiosum

ANSWERS

424. a) Although the incidence of measles has been reduced very substantially by the introduction of a measles vaccine, it still affects 1,500 children/year in the United States.

    Measles has an incubation period of eight to fourteen days. Early signs and symptoms include fever, malaise, and the three C's (cough, coryza, and conjunctivitis). After the fever reaches a peak on about the fifth day, at the height of the eruption, the characteristic enanthem, Koplik's spots, appear on the buccal mocosa.

    By the third or fourth day the characteristic exanthem begins to appear-discrete, dusky-red maculopapules. The rash starts on the forehead, behind the ears, and on the neck and the upper torso. Over the next few days, the initial skin lesions coalesce and become confluent, and new lesions appear on the extremities. The rash then fades over the next 3-4 days.

    Treatment is symptomatic. Complications include otitis media, primary viral or secondary bacterial pneumonia, and encephalitis.

425. e) Scarlet fever develops after an incubation period of one to seven days, with the abrupt onset of fever, chills, headache, and sore throat. Abdominal pain and vomiting may also be prominent.

The exanthem which appears quickly, consists of 1-to 2-mm fine, punctate, erythematous lesions that give the skin a rough, sandpapery texture. The rash appears on the trunk, becomes generalized within 24 hours, and has a characteristic distribution. It is most intense in the skinfolds, such as the axillae and groin, and spares the face. However, the face becomes flushed, except for the area around the mouth, which remains pale. The generalized rash is commonly followed by desquamation.

Examination of the pharynx reveals exudative tonsillitis, often with petechiae on the soft palate. The lingual papillae become red and swollen. Early in the course of the illness the tongue has a whitish coating; with the protruding papillae it resembles a white strawberry. Later, when the coating has disappeared, it resembles a red strawberry. The treatment of choice for scarlet fever is oral penicillin.

426. b) A "blueberry muffin" baby is the name applied to an infant that has developed thrombocytopenic purpura as a manifestation of the congenital rubella syndrome. During the first weeks of life these babies also develop hepatitis, hepatosplenomegaly, bone lesions and hemolytic anemia.

Rubella in older children is usally a mild disease. After an incubation period of 14-21 days, a prodrome of malaise, low-grade fever, and lymphadenopathy may develop, especially in the postauricular and suboccipital areas. Coryza, cough and sore throat may occur, but they usually are not prominent. The rash, which may be the sole complaint, generally begins on the face as a discrete, pink, maculopapular eruption. Over the next one to two days, the lesions spread to the chest, abdomen, and extremities. The rash pattern is not specific for rubella, and may be seen in many other viral exanthems. Treatment is symptomatic.

427. d) Filatov-Dukes disease is synonomous with staphylococcal scalded skin syndrome. In this syndrome, the patient is colonized by a strain of Staphylococcus aureus that produces an exfoliative exotoxin. The toxin causes an erythematous rash with separation of the epidermis at the level of the stratum granulosum.

Several features distinguish Filatov-Dukes disease from scarlet fever: lack of prodromal symptoms, a benign or only mildly erythematous pharynx, the absence of strawberry tongue and palatal petechiae and the failure to isolate group A Beta-hemolytic streptococci from the throat.

Treatment involves an antistaphylococcal drug such as cloxacillin or methacillin.

428. f) Erythema infectiosum is an acute, probably viral, illness with a very distinctive rash. It occurs most commonly in temperate climates during the winter and spring. Cases may be sporadic or clustered. During some community epidemics, the incidence among school-aged children has approached 25%.

The onset is abrupt, usually without prodromal symptoms, and follows a four-to 14 day incubation period. The characteristic rash generally progresses through three stages. In the first stage, the cheeks become fiery red and the child has a "slapped cheek" appearance.

In one to four days, a discrete maculopapular, erythematous rash appears on the proximal extremities and spreads to the trunk and buttocks. It becomes confluent, forming a reticular or lacy pattern.

In the third stage, the rash waxes and wanes for up to three weeks. During that time its intensity changes markedly, and it may even disappear only to recur with exposure to light or heat. The rash is frequently pruritic, is most prominent on extensor surfaces, and may involve the hands and feet.

Arthritis, the most frequent complication, is less common in children than in affected adults, about half of whom develop it. Treatment is symptomatic.

429. c) Roseola infantum is a syndrome probably associated with many viral infections. It is characterized by the acute onset of fever with few associated signs or symptoms. The fever lasts three to five days and ranges from 38.9-40.6 degrees Celcius.

The exanthem usually coincides with defervescence, but may occur hours to two days after the fever has subsided. It consists of discrete, erythematous, 2-to-5 mm macules or maculopapules, which blanch to pressure. It most often appears on the neck and proximal trunk.

On physical examination, the patient may have inflamed tonsils; a red pharynx; or small ulcerative lesions on the uvula, soft palate, or tonsils.

Roseloa is diagnosed when the characteristic sequence of fever, defervescence, and rash is recognized. It may be associated with enterovirus, adenovirus, and parainfluenza virus infections. Treatment is symptomatic.

Reference

Hayden G, Powell K. Rash and fever: Six childhood infections. Diagnosis 1985; 2(2): 95-107.

PROBLEM #66: A CHILD WITH AN EARACHE

430. A 5 year old child presents with otalgia, fever, and irritability. On examination a bulging tympanic membrane is seen, with pneumatoscopic evidence of effusion. According to standard nomenclature, the child has:

    a) acute otitis media
    b) acute suppurative otitis media
    c) purulent otitis media
    d) otitis media with effusion — acute
    e) acute serous otitis media

431. Otitis media is a frequent condition in childhood. What percentage of children, by the age of 2 years have at least three documented episodes of acute otitis media?

    a) 10%
    b) 20%
    c) 33%
    d) 50%
    e) 66%

432. The most common causative organisms in acute otitis media in order of frequency are:

    a) pneumococcus, Hemophilus influenzae, group A streptococci
    b) pneumococcus, Hemophilus influenzae, staphylococci
    c) pneumococcus, Hemophilus influenzae, Branhamella catarrhalis
    d) Hemophilus influenzae, pneumococcus, group A streptococcus
    e) Hemophilus influenzae, pneumococcus, Branhamella catarrhalis

433. The drug of choice for acute otitis media is:

    a) penicillin
    b) erythromycin
    c) erythromycin-sulfisoxazole
    d) amoxicillin
    e) cefaclor

434. The drug used in the treatment of otitis media that has the most serious side effects is:

    a) amoxicillin-potassium clavulanate
    b) erythromycin-sulfisoxazole
    c) trimethoprim-sulfamethoxazole
    d) cefaclor
    e) amoxicillin

Questions 435-436 are TRUE and FALSE questions. If the statement is TRUE, mark "a". If the statement is FALSE, mark "b".

435. Decongestants shorten the duration of middle ear effusion in otitis media.

436. Decongestants reduce the inccidence of otitis media when given to children with upper respiratory infections.

CODE: (a:1, 2 and 3; b: 1 and 3; c: 2 and 4; d: 4 only; e: all of the above)

437. Which of the following statements regarding persistent middle ear effusion is/are correct:

    1) young children tend to have effusions more frequently than older children patients with frequent respiratory infections and/or acute otitis are at
    2) increased risk of persistent middle ear effusion patients with an allergic history or atopic disease are more often affected
    3) with persistent middle ear effusion tobacco used in the home is associated with a significantly increased risk of
    4) chronic middle ear effusion

438. Drugs of choice for phrophylaxis in recurrent otitis media is/are:

    1) amoxicillin
    2) trimethoprim-sulfamethoxazole
    3) sulfamethoxazole
    4) erythromycin-sulfamethoxazole

ANSWERS

430. a) To reduce confusion due to the use of different terms, a standard nomenclature for otitis media has recently been suggested:

    1. *Otitis media without effusion:* This entity was often called myringitis in the past. It is defined as inflammation of the mucous membranes of the middle ear and drum, without evidence of fluid in the middle ear on pneumatic otoscopy.
    2. *Acute otitis media:* This refers to the clinical syndrome of otalgia, fever and irritability (either singly or in combination) in association with a full or bulging tympanic membrane, with pneumatoscopic evidence of effusion. This condition corresponds to what various authors have termed "acute suppurative otitis media" or "purulent otitis media".
    3. *Otitis media with effusion:* This differs from acute otitis in that signs and symptoms of acute infection or inflammation are absent. Otitis media with effusion is further classified according to its duration: Acute —

present for less than three weeks; subacute — present for three weeks to three months; and chronic — present for more than 3 months. Otitis media with effusion includes the condition often called "secretory", "non-suppurative", or "serous" otitis media; as well as that known as "glue ear".

431. c) By the age of two years, nearly one out of three children have already experienced at least three documented episodes of acute otitis. These children typically have repeated bouts of acute otitis until age 5 or 6 when the frequency begins to decline. The most likely explanation for the marked differences is that children with recurrent otitis have eustachian tube dysfunction related to delayed innervation of the tensor veli palatini muscle.

432. c) The bacteriology of acute otitis shows the following frequency: pneumococcus, 35%; Hemophilus influenzae, 20-25%; Branhamella catarrhalis, 10-15%; Group A streptococci, 8-10%; and Staphylococcus aureus, 1-2%.

433. d) Amoxicillin remains the drug of choice for acute otitis media. It is usually administered in a dose of 25 mg./kg./day in divided doses. The drug is highly effective in pneumococcal infections, and it performs remarkably well against H. influenzae even though 20-25% of these organisms may prove resistent on sensitivity testing.

Penicillin V produces good results in pneumococcal infections but is relatively ineffective against Hemophilus species.

Erythromycin does not penetrate well into the middle ear and thus should never be used alone. However, when erythromycin is combined with a sulfonamide such as sulfisoxazole, a highly synergistic effect is produced against Hemophilus. On the other hand, there are some data to suggest that the concurrent administration of erythromycin and a sulfonamide has an antagonist effect in acting against pneumococci.

Cefaclor is active against all bacterial causes of otitis. Cure rates for pneumococcal and Hemophilus otitis are similar to those produced by amoxicillin. Cefaclor, however, has two disadvantages: it is expensive and repeated courses are occasionally associated with the appearance of a serum-sickness like illness.

434. c) Of all the drugs used in the treatment of otitis, trimethoprim-sulfamethoxazole is the one most likely to produce severe reactions, which include generalized vasculitis manifested as Stevens-Johnson syndrome or Lyell's syndrome. Hepatitis, various hematologic changes and acute deterioration of renal function have also been reported. If trimethoprim-sulfamethoxazole is used in a child, the parents should be told to stop therapy immediately if fever recurs or if a rash appears; these events may represent the earliest signs of a vasculitis.

435. b)

436. b) Controlled studies have shown that decongestants fail to reduce the incidence of otitis when they are given to children with upper respiratory infections, including simple head colds. Similary, decongestants do not benefit patients with acute otitis media; they do not prevent or shorten the duration of middle ear effusion. In fact, studies have shown that decogestants may prolong the duration of middle ear effusions in children with a strong allergic history.

437. e) Several risk factors for persistent middle ear effusion have recently been identified. Younger children tend to have effusions more frequently than older children; patients with frequent respiratory infections and/or acute otitis are at increased risk, and patients with an allergic history or atopic disease are more often affected. Tobacco use in the home is also associated with a significantly increased risk of chronic middle ear effusion.

    Since hearing loss associated with persistent middle ear effusion almost always disappears with the clearing of the effusion, a nonaggressive approach seems reasonable. No therapy is required in a child with unilateral effusion; a child with bilateral effusion should be observed for at least 3 months. By that time, most problems will have resolved spontaneously. A persistent effusion at that time can be treated with a tympanostomy and the insertion of ventilatory tubes.

438. b) Amoxicillin and sulfamethoxazole are the preferred agents for prophylaxis in patients who have recurrent otitis media. Trimethoprim-sulfamethoxazole is not a good choice because of its relative toxicity. Erythromycin-sulfamethoxazole is not a good choice because of its combination antagonistic effect in acting against pneumococcus.

Reference

Eichenwald H. Developments in Diagnosing and Treating Otitis Media. American Family Physician 1985; 31(3): 35, 155-163.

PROBLEM #67: AN ADOLESCENT GIRL WITH KNEE PAIN

439. A 15-year old girl comes to your office complaining of pain in the area of the knee associated with running, jumping and kicking. Discomfort is often aggravated by ascending and descending stairs. Which of the following entities would be the most common cause of these symptoms?

   a) chondromalacia patellae
   b) patellofemoral arthralgia
   c) Osgood-Schlatter disease
   d) medial meniscal tear
   e) partial collateral ligament disruption

440. Which of the following statements concerning overuse syndrome of the knee is INCORRECT?

   a) chondromalacia patallae is the most common overuse syndrome of the knee encountered in clinical practice
   b) chondromalacia patallae is a pathological diagnosis
   c) chondromalacia patallae is best managed by intensive physiotherapy
   d) non-steroidal anti-inflammatory drugs are often useful in the management of overuse syndromes of the knee
   e) patients with patellofemoral arthralgia need not curtail their activities once the acute condition settles down

441. Osgood-Schlatter's disease is a:
   a) suprapatellar tendinitis
   b) a tendinitis of the origin of the infrapatellar tendon
   c) a tendinitis of the insertion of the infrapatellar tendon
   d) a prepatellar bursitis
   e) a pes anserine bursitis

442. A 17-year old boy develops a sudden pain in the region of the lateral femoral condyle while running the 100-yard dash. He begins to walk towards the finish line. As he does so, the pain decreases. As he starts to run again, the pain returns. What is the most likely diagnosis?

   a) Osgood-Schlatter disease
   b) prepatellar bursitis
   c) fat pad impingement syndrome
   d) iliotibial band bursitis
   e) pes anserine bursitis

CODE: (a:1, 2 and 3; b: 1 and 3; c: 2 and 4; d: 4 only; e: all of the above)

443. Which of the following statements about meniscal tears of the knee is/are CORRECT?

    1) medial meniscal tears are 5-7 times more common than lateral meniscal tears
    2) the medial meniscus is usually torn by a twisting injury with the knee partially flexed
    3) medial meniscal tears are the most common cause of knee joint pain
    4) the diagnosis of meniscal tears is usually confirmed by McMurray's test

ANSWERS

439. b) The most common overuse syndrome of the knee is patellofemoral arthralgia. It is more common than true chondromalacia of the patella, fat pad impingement syndrome, and other overuse syndromes including patellar tendonitis, Osgood-Schlatter disease, prepatellar bursitis, iliotibial band bursitis, pes anserine bursitis and retinaculitis.

Patellofemoral arthralgia results from a combination of abnormal patellar pressures and abnormal patellar excursion. The most common presenting symptom is pain in or around the knee, associated with running, jumping, kicking, kneeling or crouching. Discomfort is commonly aggravated by ascending and descending stairs; a sensation of instability or crepitus may be noted. On examination, the only positive findings may be tenderness to palpation around or over the patella and its tendons, or to compression of the patella against the femoral condyles. There are no signs of internal derangement, there is no effusion, no lost range of motion or ligamentous instability. There may be some mild quadriceps wasting and occasionally, some retropatellar crepitus, but usually the examiner is unable to detect major abnormality. True patellofemoral crepitus will be elicited when the knee is extended against resistance from a flexed position, and should be confirmed with the knee in full extension, with the patella pressed down and moved gently sideways, medially and laterally. If crepitus is elicited in this position, the patella itself is involved and chondromalacia patalla is present.

440. a) Patellofemoral arthralgia is the most common overuse syndrome of the knee. Chondromalacia patallae can be thought of as a type of patellofemoral overload syndrome in which patients actually have true degenerative wear. The etiology is not well understood. Trauma may or may not be involved. During adolescence, and particularly during the growth spurt, the patella's articular cartilage appears to proliferate, without the orderly regulation of growth that normally prevails. As a result, the ground substance breaks down, and the collagenous fibrils of the articular cartilage become disrupted, instead of forming normal arcades. Thus, chondromalacia patellae is really a pathological diagnosis.

Both patellofemoral arthralgia and chondromalacia patellae are best managed by intensive physiotherapy. Isometric quadriceps setting and straight leg raising, followed by progressive, resisted exercises over the final five to ten degrees of knee extension are emphasized.

Non-steroidal anti-inflammatory agents are very beneficial in the treatment of all knee overuse syndromes.

In contrast to chondromalacia patalla, patients with patellofemoral arthralgia must be reassured that continuing the activity is safe and will not lead to degeneration. Patients with chondromalacia will probably have to significantly alter their activity programs to prevent further degeneration.

441. c) Osgood-Schlatter's disease is a tendinitis of the insertion of the infrapatellar tendon into the proximal tibial epiphysis. Pressures on the sensitive growth area evoke a local discomfort which can be disabling. Ice, stretching exercises, and an infrapatellar strap may control pain and allow patients to resume sports activites. A localized ossicle of ununited epiphysis may be identifed on plain X-rays, and excision required.

Suprapatellar tendinitis, tendinitis of the origin of the infrapatellar tendon, prepatellar bursitis and pes anserine bursitis are all common overuse syndromes of the knee that are sometimes confused with Osgood-Schlatter's disease.

442. d) The patient described in this question has iliotibial band bursitis. This is a troublesome inflammation of the bursa underlying the distal portion of the iliotibial tract on the lateral aspect of the knee. It results from the friction of the repetitive knee flexion and extension, associated with impact loading of the knee, as in jogging. It often strikes suddenly, with a sharp pain over the lateral femoral condyle. It becomes so painful that the athlete is forced to discontinue the activity. On walking, the knee seems to improve spontaneously, but the pain returns when attempts are made to run again.

Ice friction treatments, ultrasound, stretching and strengthening exercises and oral anti-inflammatory medication are often necessary to alleviate the condition. Occasionally local steroid injection into the bursa may be indicated.

443. e) Medial meniscus tears are the most common cause of knee joint pain. The medial meniscus, which is five to seven times more susceptible than the lateral meniscus to tearing, is torn by a twisting injury with the knee partially flexed. The meniscus in this position is forced toward the center of the joint and becomes caught between the femur and the tibia. It is then torn longitudinally by shearing forces when the joint is suddenly extended.

The diagnosis of medial meniscal tears is usually confirmed clinically by the McMurray test. In this test, the patient lies supine with the hip and the knee flexed acutely and maximally. The posterior medial joint line is palpated with one hand and then the foot and the leg are externally rotated as far as possible with the other hand. The externally rotated and flexed knee is then slowly extended. As the torn meniscus is caught between the femur and the tibia, a click is felt which the patient describes as painful.

Confirmation of the diagnosis by arthroscopy offers the advantage of removal of the torn meniscus at the same time.

Reference

Welsh R. Patellofemoral Arthralgia, Overuse Syndromes of the Knee and Chondromalacia Patella. Canadian Family Physician 1985; 31: 573-576.

Psychiatry

PROBLEM #68: A 35 YEAR OLD FEMALE WITH AGORAPHOBIA

444. A 35 year old female presents to the office with a 6 month history of an intense fear of being alone and recurrent panic attacks. You suspect agoraphobia. Which of the following is NOT a characteristic of agoraphobia?

a) a loss of contact with reality, including hallucinations and delusions
b) an intense fear of being in public places
c) acute bursts of terrifying levels of anxiety (panic attacks)
d) fear of panic attack or other calamity, leading to chronic anxiety and restriction of activities
e) avoidance of supermarkets, shopping malls, church services, meetings, or other places where help is unavailable or escape is difficult

445. Recent epidemiologic studies have shown that a large number of North Americans suffer or have suffered from agoraphobia in the past. This number is currently thought to be:

a) 20% of the population
b) 30% of the population
c) 10% of the population
d) 5% of the population
e) 1% of the population

446. The two roles for the use of medication in the treatment of agoraphobia are the prevention of panic attacks and the management of anticipatory anxiety. Which of the following medications has been shown to fulfill both of these roles?

a) imipramine
b) alprazolam

c) phenelzine
d) diazepam
e) chlorpromazine

CODE: (a:1, 2 and 3; b: 1 and 3; c: 2 and 4; d: 4 only; e: all of the above)

447. Which of the following is/are included in the goals of treatment for agoraphobia?

1) patient education: informing the patient that panic attacks are harmless
2) appropriate medication including antidepressants and sedatives
3) programmed practice of feared activities
4) relaxation techniques

448. Tricyclic antidepressants are often used in the treatment of agoraphobia because they may:

1) relax the patient and significantly decrease anticipatory anxiety
2) prevent panic attacks
3) effectively treat the delusions that accompany agoraphobia
4) effectively treat a secondary depression that may accompany agoraphobia

ANSWERS

444. a) Agoraphobia is characterized by the following clinical features: (1) intense fear of being alone or in a public place; (2) acute bursts of terrifying levels of anxiety (panic attacks); (3) fear of panic attacks or other calamity, leading to chronic anxiety and restriction of activities, often to the point of becoming housebound; and, (4) avoidance of supermarkets, shopping malls, church services, meetings, parties, elevators, tunnels, bridges, buses, subways and other places where help is unavailable or escape is difficult. Agoraphobia is not characterized by hallucinations, delusions, or any other loss of contact with reality.

445. d) Recent epidemiologic studies have indicated that about 5% of North Americans have suffered from agoraphobia at some time in their lives. About three times as many women as men are effected.

446. b) Alprazolam, a relatively new benzodiazepine, has recently been shown to both prevent panic attacks and treat the anticipatory anxiety accompany agoraphobia. It is usually administered in a dose of 0.25-0.5 mg. t.i.d.
        The antidepressants, including both tricyclics and MAO inhibitors, have been shown to be successful in the prevention of panic attacks. Imipramine (tricyclic) is usually administered in a dose of 75-150 mg./day. Phenelzine

(MAO inhibitor) is usually administered in a dose of 15 mg. t.i.d.

The benzodiazepines such as diazepam or lorazepam have been shown to be useful in diminishing anticipatory anxiety.

The phenothiazines, such as Largactil, have no place in the treatment of agoraphobia.

447. e) The components of treatment in agoraphobia include the following: (1) Patient education: informing the patient that panic attacks are harmless, that agoraphobia develops as a result of fear of the panic attacks, and that activities surrendered to the anxiety disorder must be gradually regained. (2) Appropriate medication, including the antidepressants and benzodiazepines. (3) Programmed practice of feared activities, beginning with the least anxiety provoking and working toward more intensely feared situations. (4) Relaxation techniques, to diminish anticipatory anxiety and interrupt panic attacks and (5) The exploration of psychodynamic factors.

448. c) Tricyclic antidepressants have been shown to prevent panic attacks that occur in agoraphobia. They are also useful in the treatment of a secondary depression that may accompany agoraphobia. However, they do not diminish anticipatory anxiety. Delusions are not part of the clinical picture of agoraphobia, and in any case, are not effectively treated by antidepressants.

Reference

Horn H. Agoraphobia. American Family Physician 1985; 32(1): 35, 165-173.

PROBLEM #69: A 25 YEAR OLD FEMALE WITH MULTIPLE BRUISES

449. A 25 year old female presents to the emergency room with multiple bruises. You suspect battered wife syndrome. The estimated incidence of battered wife syndrome in Canada is:

   a) 1/100
   b) 1/50
   c) 1/25
   d) 1/10
   e) 1/2

450. All of the following are characteristics of the battered wife syndrome EXCEPT:

   a) the association of violence with alcohol intake in the batterer
   b) violent behavior in the family of origin in both victim and batterer
   c) high risk of suicide attempt or gesture in the victim
   d) high incidence of neurotropic drug use in the victim
   e) a syndrome associated with lower socioeconomic class

451. The main goal of psychotherapy in battered wife syndrome is:

   a) to try to establish a framework by which the couple can work out their problems
   b) to try to establish a cause for the violence
   c) to overcome fear and reverse the concept of "learned helplessness" in the victim
   d) to try to find some common ground whereby the victim and batterer can begin a new relationship
   e) to convince the victim that to stay in the present relationship is an exercise in futility

CODE: (a:1, 2 and 3; b: 1 and 3; c: 2 and 4; d: 4 only; e: all of the above)

452. A woman with battered wife syndrome often presents with:

   1) chronic pelvic pain
   2) dyspareunia
   3) chronic back pain
   4) chronic abdominal pain

453. The purpose of an interval or transition house is to:

    1) provide an environment in which the woman and her children can feel safe
    2) provide an atmosphere where supportive counselling of both victim and batterer can take place
    3) provide education for the woman about the battered wife syndrome
    4) facilitate the wife in seeking a divorce from her husband

ANSWERS

449. d) The estimated incidence of battered wife syndrome in Canada is 1/10. There is some suggestion that the incidence has been increasing in recent years due to the economic recession and unemployment.

450. e) Alcohol intake been associated with battered wife syndrome in all of the relevant studies. The association has ranged from 60% to 93%. In some cases the batterer uses alcohol to disavow his behavior and convince others that he was not responsible for his actions at the time of the assault.

    A family of origin in which violence occured is common in both victims and batterers. It seems that victims sometimes subconciously seek to enter into another battering relationship. This supports the theory of "assortive mating".

    In one series, 71% of victims were taking neurotropic drugs. As well, 46% of these women has sought a psychiatric opinion and 42% had made a suicide attempt or gesture.

    Although battered wife syndrome may occur more commonly in the lower socioeconomic class because of chronic unemployment, it is not per se associated with the lower socioeconomic class. It occurs in ALL classes of society.

451. c) The main goal of psychotherapy in battered wife syndrome is to overcome fear and reverse the concept of "learned helplessness" in the victim. This is accomplished by encouraging an increase in the victim's self-confidence and the development of a new self-concept, from "victim" and "failure" to a competent, autonomous person.

452. e) Victims of battered wife syndrome often present with somatic or conversion symptoms or psychophysiologic reactions. Their most frequent complaints are headache, insomnia, a choking sensation, hyperventilation, chronic pelvic pain, dysparenunia, chronic back pain, chronic abdominal pain, chest pain, anxiety, depression and suicidal behavior.

453. b) The primary purpose of an interval or transition house is to provide a safe environment for the woman and her children. The combination of continuing threats and violence by the husband and the absence of provisions for safety are universally identified as deterrants to actions. In addition, once this barrier of fear is removed, productive education about the syndrome and supportive counselling can take place. The batterer has no place in an interval or transition house, and "couples" counselling has had limited success. The purpose of psychotherapy is not to steer the woman in the direction of divorce, but rather to develop a new self-concept in which she is capable of making her own decisions.

Reference

Swanson R. Battered wife syndrome. Canadian Medical Association Journal 1984; 130: 709-712.

PROBLEM #70: A 35 YEAR OLD FEMALE WHO HAS JUST LOST HER HUSBAND

454. A 35-year old wife and mother of two calls you six days after suffering the loss of her husband in an automobile accident. She has been unable to sleep for the past six days and asks you for some medication to help her sleep and cope during the initial few weeks. You would now:

    a) tell the patient that tranquillizing medication will postpone the grief work and she should try to make it on her own
    b) prescribe a tricyclic antidepressant to help her sleep and combat acute anxiety in the first few weeks
    c) prescribe a minor tranquillizer to help her sleep and combat acute anxiety in the first few weeks
    d) prescribe an antipsychotic to help her sleep and combat acute anxiety in the first few weeks
    e) schedule immediate counselling sessions to try and nip the problem in the bud

455. Four weeks later the patient described in question #454 returns to your office. She describes seeing her husband walking through her room at night. When she speaks to him he answers her and tells her that he will be coming back soon. At this time you should:

    a) refer the patient to a psychiatrist for treatment of a pathological grief reaction
    b) reassure the patient that such visions are a normal component of a grief reaction
    c) prescribe an antipsychotic medication to eliminate the visions
    d) tell the patient to "snap out of it" and get on with her life
    e) prescribe a tricyclic antidepressant to treat an underlying masked depression

456. A mother who has spent the last 6 weeks at the bedside of her infant son who is being maintained on life-support systems in the neonatal intensive care nursery heaves a sigh of relief when the infant finally dies. She shows no visible emotion or sadness and leaves the unit quickly. Her lack of emotion at this time is probably due to:

    a) significant anticipatory grieving
    b) a pathological grief reaction
    c) lack of concern
    d) an underlying depressive illness
    e) none of the above

CODE: (a:1, 2 and 3; b: 1 and 3; c: 2 and 4; d: 4 only; e: all of the above)

457. Which of the following is/are normal physical sensations associated with acute grief reactions?

    1) a hollowness in the stomach
    2) a tightness in the chest
    3) an oversensitivity to noise
    4) a sense of depersonalization

458. Which of the following is/are basic principles to follow in helping someone through an acute grief reaction?

    1) to help the survivor actualize the loss
    2) to help the survivor identify and express feelings
    3) to assist the survivor in living without the deceased
    4) to facilitate emotional withdrawal from the deceased

ANSWERS

454. c) There has been much discussion about the use of medication in the management of acute, normal grief. The consensus of opinion is that, if possible, it is better to avoid it. However, in this case, the patient has not slept for six nights and her anxiety level is extremely high. Therefore, the prescription of a minor tranquillizer like diapezam to take up to three times a day and at bedtime is appropriate. This dosage will not postpone the grief reaction, but rather will make the functioning of this particular patient a little better in the first few weeks.

    The use of antidepressants and antipsychotic medications is not indicated in the treatment of acute, normal grief.

    Counseling sessions will not "nip this problem in the bud". This is a problem that must be worked through.

455. b) Hallucinations of both the visual type and the auditory type are a frequent experience of the bereaved. They are usually transient experiences, often occurring within a few weeks following the loss, and generally do not portend a more difficult or complicated mourning experience.

    The prescription of antidepressant or antipsychotic medication in this situation is not appropriate as we are not dealing with a pathological process. A referral to a psychiatrist for treatment of a pathological grief reaction is likewise inappropriate as we are dealing with a normal part of grieving. A suggestion to the patient that she "snap out of it" shows a lack of empathy and understanding for the whole grief process.

456. a) The term "anticipatory grieving" refers to grieving that occurs prior to the actual loss. It represents the absence of overt manifestations of grief at the actual time of death in survivors who have already experienced the phases of normal grief and who have freed themselves from their emotional ties with the deceased.

   In the case described the mother has probably done most of the grieving for her infant son in the six weeks spent in the neonatal unit. It is important to recognize this type of grieving as it may leave the impression that the survivor really does not care.

457. e) Physical sensations are common following the death of a loved one. Patients may describe feelings of (1) hollowness in the stomach; (2) a tightness in the throat; (3) a tightness in the chest; (4) an oversensitivity to noise; (5) a sense of depersonalization; (6) acute shortness of breath; (7) weakness in the muscles; (8) lack of energy; and (9) a dry mouth and many others.

458. e) Grief counseling is based on a number of principles. They are:

   1) help the survivor actualize the loss
   2) help the survivor identify and express feelings
   3) assist the survivor in living without the deceased
   4) facilitate emotional withdrawal from the deceased
   5) provide time to grieve
   6) interpret "normal" behavior for the survivor
   7) allow for individual differences in the survivor
   8) provide continuing support
   9) examine defenses and coping styles
   10) identify pathology and refer to a specialized grief counselor if necessary

Reference

Worden J. Grief Counseling and Grief Therapy. New York: Springer, 1984, pages 1-146.

PROBLEM #71: A 45 YEAR OLD MALE WITH A SLEEP DISTURBANCE

459. A 45-year old man presents to the office with a 6-month history of insomnia. He states that he has difficulty falling asleep and usually awakens in the middle of the night. He then paces the floor for an hour before he is tired enough to go back to bed. The physical examination is normal. Your next step should be to:

   a) reassure the patient that we all have problems sleeping at one time or another and not to worry about it
   b) refer the patient to a sleep laboratory for a polysomnogram
   c) prescribe triazolam 0.5 mg. h.s. and review the patient in 1 month
   d) prescribe hot milk before the patient goes to bed
   e) take a more detailed history

460. A 50-year old male comes in for his annual physical examination. He weighs 240 lbs and complains of excessive sleepiness during the day. His blood pressure is 200/110 mm. Hg. On further questioning you obtain a history of excessive snoring that seems to be bothering his wife. The most likely cause of this man's sleep disturbance is:

   a) narcolepsy
   b) sleep-apnea syndrome
   c) generalized poor physical condition
   d) an underlying psychiatric problem
   e) idiopathic insomnia

461. A 35-year old male presents to your office with a chief complaint of "weak muscles" especially after laughing. On further questioning you discover that the patient has excessive daytime sleepiness and "wierd imaginings" just before going to sleep at night. The patient appears anxious and tense. Your tentative diagnosis is:

   a) narcolepsy
   b) hysterical conversion reaction
   c) psychosomatic symptoms secondary to chronic anxiety
   d) hypochondriasis
   e) serious psychiatric disturbance NYD

CODE: (a:1, 2 and 3; b: 1 and 3; c: 2 and 4; d: 4 only; e: all of the above)

462. Which of the following medications may be associated with disordered sleep?

   1) propranolol
   2) antihistamines
   3) cimetidine
   4) amitriptyline

463. Which of the following statements regarding the use of hypnotic medication is/are TRUE?

   1) hypnotics generally lengthen total sleep time by 1 hour or more
   2) hypnotics generally shorten sleep latency by 1/2 hour or more
   3) hypnotics with short half-lives generally do not cause significant side effects and can be used for extended periods of time
   4) hypnotics have an adverse effect on REM sleep

ANSWERS

459. e) Insomnia accounts for 1/3 of patients who come to a sleep-disorders clinic. It has many causes including (1) psychiatric disorders of affect or personality; (2) psychophysiologic sleep disorders which involve only the onset of sleep and occur in patients with anxiety; (3) illicit drug or alcohol dependency; (4) abuse of hypnotic medication; (5) medications including major and minor tranquillizers, tricyclic antidepressants, antihistamines, antihypertensive agents such as methyldopa and propranolol, and cimetidine; and (6) caffeine and nicotine.

   Thus, a careful history with careful attention to clues to the above conditions is essential. In addition, precise information about the onset and timing of symptoms is important. Most insomnia problems can be sorted out by the family physician without referral to a sleep laboratory for polysomnography.

   Reassurance that everyone has insomnia from time to time is inappropriate as no attempt has been made to come up with a diagnosis.

   Hot milk is usually not effective in helping patients go to sleep.

   The prescription of hypnotics such as triazolam is generally not indicated. A recent Institute of Medicine study of hypnotic medication use in the United States concluded that "prolonged" use of hypnotic medication is never indicated, and 'automatic' prescriptions are inappropriate.

460. b) This patient has the classical symptoms of sleep-apnea syndrome. Sleep-apnea syndrome is the most common of the "hypersomnias", which account for about 50% of sleep disorders. The other major disorder in this category is narcolepsy.

   Sleep-apnea syndrome is characterized by temporary cessation of breathing lasting longer than 10 seconds. In most cases, there is upper airway obstruction. Since relief of the obstruction and resumption of breathing depend on CNS arousal, patients may waken briefly hundreds of times each night.

   Sleep-apnea syndrome should be suspected in massively obese individuals who snore and exhibit excessive daytime sleepiness. Hypertension, peripheral edema, excessive movements, hypnagogic hallucinations, autonomic behavior, excessive sweating, nocturnal enuresis, impotence, morning headache, personality changes, and impaired intellect are also common.

The only widely available and useful non-surgical approach to obstructive sleep-apnea is weight loss. Surgical treatments include uvulopalatopharyngoplasty and tracheostomy. Hypnotic medication of any kind is ABSOLUTELY CONTRAINDICATED in patients with obstructive sleep apnea.

461. a) The patient described in this question has the classical symptoms of narcolepsy. This patient describes a sudden weakness or loss of muscle control associated with strong emotional expression. This symptom is known as cataplexy and is virtually pathognomonic of narcolepsy. Other symptoms include excessive daytime sleepiness, hypnagogic hallucinations, sleep paralysis and automatic behavior.

The diagnosis of narcolepsy can be confirmed by polysomnography, in which the characteristic finding is sleep-onset rapid eye movement sleep (SOREM).

Treatment consists of stimulant medication such as methylphenidate hydrochloride and dextroamphetamine for sleepiness and tricyclic antidepressants for associated symptoms.

462. e) Many medications are associated with disordered sleep. Propranolol is notorious for producing hallucinations. Antihistamines and antidepressants may produce hypersomnia or insomnia. Cimetidine interferes with sleep by altering the metabolism of hypnotics such as the benzodiazepines.

Other medications commonly implicated in sleep disorders are the major and minor tranquillizers and the antihypertensive agent alpha methyldopa. It is important to be aware, however, that virtually any medication can be associated with a sleep disorder in a particular patient.

463. d) Most patients with sleep disorders have been prescribed hypnotic-sedative drugs by their physicians. The prescription for the medication often becomes "automatic" over the months and subsequent years. Patients find themselves unable to discontinue the pills, and frequently, also complain of daytime symptoms resulting from their use.

Hypnotics shorten the latency to sleep onset by only a few minutes and lengthen the total sleep-time by only a few minutes. Unfortunately, within a few weeks to a few months, these beneficial effects disappear. Because of this, HYPNOTIC MEDICATION CANNOT BE VIEWED AS A SOLUTION TO THE PROBLEM OF CHRONIC SLEEPLESSNESS.

Patients taking sleeping pills frequently suffer withdrawal symptoms during efforts to stop the medication. Symptoms include agitation, gastrointestinal upset, headache, muscle stiffness and pain, palpitations, diaphoresis, and nightmares. These are wrongly interpreted as primary symptoms rather than withdrawal symptoms by both the patient and the physician. The patient, therefore, restarts the medication despite lack of beneficial effect at night and "hangover" symptoms during the day. Eventually, hypnotic medication can fragment sleep by altering REM sleep and produce the same elements of insomnia for which it was originally prescribed. This results in the ironic situation in which a patient will become dependant on a medication that is producing the symptom for which the medication was originally prescribed.

References

Sassin J. Disorders of Sleep and Wakefulness. Primary Care 1984; 11(4): 573-581.
Dement W. Disordered Sleep — Why? Diagnosis 1985; 2(2): 32-43.

PROBLEM #72: A 50 YEAR OLD FEMALE WITH CHRONIC ANXIETY

464. A 50 year old female with chronic anxiety presents to the office for counseling. Which of the following is the MOST COMMON reason for a patient to present for psychotherapy?

   a) demoralization
   b) anger
   c) depression
   d) anxiety
   e) shame

465. Which of the following statements regarding medical psychotherapy is FALSE?

   a) medical psychotherapy is used for patients in crisis
   b) in medical psychotherapy there is intense interaction between the patient and the therapist
   c) to be effective, medical psychotherapy must provide a rationale that can be believed by both patient and therapist
   d) medical psychotherapy requires specialized training to be performed properly
   e) physicians can frequently use medical psychotherapy to help a patient cope with a chronic illness

CODE: (a:1, 2 and 3; b: 1 and 3; c: 2 and 4; d: 4 only; e: all of the above)

466. Which of the following statements BEST describes the psychotherapy performed by family physicians?

   1) it provides support for the patient
   2) it attempts to provide introspective exploration
   3) it provides reassurance for the patient
   4) it usually requires frequent, long sessions to be successful

467. Which of the following aspects of medical psychotherapy are important in CRISIS counseling?

   1) a careful history
   2) an exploration of the previous methods of problem solving that the patient has found useful
   3) suggestions of strategies for dealing with the current problem
   4) implementation of the regime discussed before the next visit

468. Which of the following statements regarding medical psychotherapy in the treatment of chronic conditions is/are TRUE?

    1) goal setting is extremely important
    2) the aim of the therapist differs greatly depending on the patient
    3) the opportunity for ventilation usually provides the patient with substantial relief
    4) the therapist should assume the patient is totally helpless; this often enhances medical psychotherapy

ANSWERS

464. a) Demoralization is the most common problem that brings people to psychotherapy. This state of mind, which occurs in individuals unable to cope with problems in their lives, is associated with a host of painful feelings, such as anxiety, guilt, shame, depression and a sense of diminished self-worth. At times, demoralization presents in the guise of somatic complaints or preoccupations. Such symptoms interact with demoralization in a destructive, dynamic equilibrium: they increase the degree of demoralization, which in turn increases the severity of the symptoms.

465. d) Medical psychotherapy is used in patients with crisis (onset of physical illness, loss of a job, threatened loss of a spouse) or in a chronic state of difficulty (persistent physical illness, severe mental illness).

    Medical psychotherapy involves an intense interaction between those defined as patient and therapist. This relationship, which promotes emotional arousal and discharge, exists within a healing setting that is deemed safe by the patient.

    To be effective, medical psychotherapy must provide a rationale that can be believed by both the patient and the therapist. From such rationales arise specific psychotherapeutic procedures that serve as guidelines for restoration of morale. These techniques strengthen the therapeutic relationship, inspire hope, provide opportunities for cognitive and experiential learning, and offer experiences of success to help patients gain a sense of mastery.

    It is clear that knowledgeable physicians use psychotherapy when they help a patient cope with illness. This may include helping him to grieve over his loss of health or helping him to understand that his physical symptomatology represents the expression of grief for a loved one who has died. It follows, then, that family physicians provide psychotherapy when they simply provide support and reassurance for patients in all sorts of trouble. Therefore, medical psychotherapy does not require extensive training to be performed properly. It requires a physician who cares and is sensitive to the needs of patients.

446. b) The family physician's role in psychotherapy is best described as providing reassurance and support. By so doing, he helps the patient strengthen his own usual psychologic mechanisms. This role parallels the early mother-child

relationships, and tends to alleviate fears about separation that demoralize the patient. Paradoxically, when this therapeutic bond exists in the medical setting, the patient's adult resources can be marshalled toward the task of problem solving.

Although psychotherapy can include introspective exploration of the psychic causes for the patient's demoralization, this is usually left to someone with more formal training in psychotherapy.

Psychotherapy does not have to involve lengthy, frequent sessions to be effective. A few minutes is often all that it takes to make a considerable difference in the patient's persception of a problem. In many cases the family physician is performing psychotherapy without even being aware that he is doing it.

467. e) When in crisis, an individual is faced with a set of problems that defy resolution through the usual patterns. Frustrated in his attempts to apply an old formula to a new stress, the person frequently experiences rising tension. Varying degrees of anxiety, depression, and disequilibrium create a new, dysphoric emotional state that persists until problem-solving approaches are implemented.

As in any other medical situation, the first step in crisis counseling is taking a good history. This is particularly important in identifying the individual's potential to harm himself or others. While obtaining the history, the physician should investigate the patient's perception of his crisis situation. States of anxiety, depression and tension need to be connected to precipitating events in an effort to reeducate the individual as to the etiology of the crisis. Only then can the physician and the patient begin the necessary treatment.

The next step in crisis resolution is a thorough exploration of previous methods of problem solving that the patient has found useful. The patient can be encouraged to use these methods to decrease tension during the current situation, or he can be given alternative suggestions that can be carried out either by the patient himself or by his support network.

Before the next scheduled visit, the patient implements the regimen discussed. Its effectiveness is then evaluated by both the patient and the physician. Should the regimen fail to reduce the patient's mounting tension and demoralization, alternative approaches are explored. Thoughtful collaborative planning with patients in crisis can rapidly restore those individuals to an acceptable emotional equilibrium.

468. a) In many instances, the physician intuitively provides medical pyschotherapy for patients suffering from chronic mental disorders or chronic physical disorders with concomitant emotional difficulties.

In this situation, goal setting is extremely important. Goals need to be realistic in a chronic illness that may last for many years or the rest of the patient's life. Lacking such realism, the physician will often experience demoralization himself.

Medical psychotherapy should aim to promote the best psychologic function for a given patient. Obviously, this differs greatly with the situation of the patient. For example, the best psychologic function of a chronic schizophrenic is far different from that of a patient who has just gone through an acute grief reaction.

As pointed out previously, reassurance and support are the major techniques of the family physician. The patient's particular strengths are pointed out, and doubts and misconceptions about his illness are removed. To be effective, reassurance must be realistic; groundless reassurance is detrimental.

Explanation is another technique of medical psychotherapy that is useful in chronic conditions. Explanation should be provided in straightforward, everyday language. Explanations are not just designed to promote self-understanding; they also enhance a patient's ability to cope by clarifying the problems that he must face.

Psychotherapy also offers the patient an opportunity for ventilation. Although ventilation in itself is not curative, the relief it provides often helps the patient accept other techniques used.

Medical psychotherapy encompassess more than intervention with the target patient. Initiating changes in the patient's environment can also be helpful. This may involve family members, employers, and social workers.

The patient must never be regarded as helpless in this whole process; this can lead to sustained debility. Rather, the physician practicing supportive psychotherapy attempts to maximize the patient's autonomous functional assets. This results in more effective psychotherapy with the ongoing support of the patient.

Reference

Goldberg R, and Green S. Medical Psychotherapy. American Family Physician 1985; 31(1): 173-178.

PROBLEM #73: A 45 YEAR OLD MALE WITH AN ENLARGED LIVER

469. A 45 year old executive comes into your office for his yearly physical examination. He is found to have a liver span of 20 cm. When questioned about alcohol intake he states that he often consumes 10-12 ounces of hard liquor when spending an afternoon with a client. He denies work or family problems associated with his consumption of alcohol. He has not increased his consumption lately and he has not noticed any lessening of the effect that the alcohol has on him. He denies withdrawal symptoms. With this history, your initial impression of his drinking problem would be:

a) excessive social drinking
b) alcohol abuse
c) alcoholism
d) heavy drinking
e) potential alcohol abuse

470. The same individual described in question #470 returns in 6 months complaining of a tremor in his hands if he does not consume at least two or three drinks in the morning. All other aspects of his life are unchanged. With this history your diagnosis would now be:

a) excessive social drinking
b) alcohol abuse
c) alcoholism
d) withdrawal symptoms associated with alcohol abuse
e) potential alcohol abuse

471. Alcoholics have a mortality rate that is approximately:

a) the same as nonalcoholics
b) one and one half times that of nonalcoholics
c) twice that of nonalcoholics
d) two and one-half times that of nonalcoholics
e) five times that of nonalcoholics

472. The treatment of choice for alcohol withdrawal symptoms is:

a) phenobarbitol
b) amitriptyline
c) chlordiazepoxide
d) chlorpromazine
e) phenytoin

CODE: (a:1, 2 and 3; b: 1 and 3; c: 2 and 4; d: 4 only; e: all of the above)

473. Which of the following conditions may result from the excessive ingestion of alcohol?

    1) acute hepatitis
    2) acute and chronic gastritis
    3) skeletal and cardiac myopathy
    4) esophageal and gastric carcinoma

474. Disulfiram:

    1) interferes with the metabolism of alcohol
    2) may cause an acute hypertensive reaction when used with alcohol
    3) may cause nausea, vomiting, malaise, flushing and dizziness when used with alcohol
    4) should be reserved for a few carefully selected alcoholics

475. Which of the following conditions is/are more common in alcoholics than in nonalcoholics?

    1) cigarette smoking
    2) obesity
    3) diabetes
    4) hypertension

ANSWERS

469. b) This patient can best be described as an alcohol abuser. An alcohol abuser has pathologic alcohol use and/or has impaired social or occupational functioning as a result of alcohol. Pathologic alcohol use is manifested by one or more of the following criteria:

    1) need for daily use of alcohol for adequate functioning
    2) inability to cut down drinking or to stop drinking
    3) repeated efforts to control or reduce excess drinking by periods of temporary abstinence
    4) binges (periods of intoxication lasting at least 2 days)
    5) occasional consumption of 10 ounces of spirits or its equivalent in wine or beer
    6) blackouts (amnesia for events occurring while intoxicated)
    7) continual drinking despite known medical contraindications
    8) drinking of nonbeverage alcohol

Evidence of impaired social or occupational functioning includes:

1) violence while intoxicated
2) absence from work or loss of job because of drinking
3) legal difficulties such as arrests for intoxicated behavior or traffic accidents while intoxicated
4) arguments or difficulties with family or friends because of excessive alcohol use

If a patient is to be labelled as an "alcoholic" then he must display either tolerance or withdrawal. Tolerance is the need for markedly increased amounts of alcohol to achieve the desired effect, or markedly diminished effect with regular use of the same amount of alcohol. Withdrawal is the development of a coarse tremor of the hands, tongue, and eyelids; and nausea, vomiting, malaise, weakness, autonomic hyperactivity (tachycardia, sweating, elevated blood pressure), anxiety, depressed mood, irratibility or orthostatic hypotension within several hours after cessation of or reduction in heavy, prolonged drinking. The patient described in question #469 fulfills the criteria for alcohol abuse but not for alcoholism.

470. c) When the patient returns for his next visit he has developed withdrawal symptoms. By definition, he is now an alcoholic. (see critique of question #469).

471. d) Alcoholics have a mortality rate 2.5 times greater than nonalcoholics. Common causes of death include cirrhosis, motor vehicle accidents, drowning, falls, homicide and suicide. Alcoholics are at risk of developing disorders of almost any organ of the body. These include:

1) neuropsychiatric syndromes including intoxication and idiosyncratic intoxication, withdrawal and withdrawal delirum, hallucinosis, amneic syndrome (Wernicke-Korsakoff), dementia, polydrug abuse, exacerbation of pre-existing mental illness and cerebellar degeneration.
2) hepatic disorders including acute and chronic gastritis, peptic ulcer, esophageal and gastric cancer and pancreatitis
3) digestive disorders including acute and chronic gastritis, peptic ulcer, esophageal and gastric cancer and pancreatitis
4) hematological effects including bone marrow suppression and anemia
5) nutritional deficiencies including polyneuropathy, beriberi, pellagra and amblyopia
6) other conditions such as skeletal and cardiac myopathy, hypertriglyceridemia, hypoglycemia, increased frequency of infections, and an increased predisposition to hypertension, obesity, diabetes and heavy cigarette smoking

472. c) In most instances, the symptoms of alcohol withdrawal are relatively mild and without specific complications. Treatment involves placing the patient in a quiet, alcohol free environment and administering moderate doses of a minor tranquillizer such as chlordiazepoxide 25 mg. every 4 hours or diazepam 5-10 mg. every 4 hours. Patients with more severe withdrawal symptoms including delerium tremens may need up to 400 mg. of chlordiazepoxide/day. Seizures are treated with intravenous diazepam or phenytoin. Although phenobarbitol and chlorpromazine could be used for the treatment of withdrawal symptoms they are not first-line agents. Phenytoin is used only if seizures occur. Amitriptyline is not recommended for the treatment of withdrawal symptoms.

473. e) See critique of question #471.

474. b) Because even the best intentioned alcoholics may succumb to the temptation to resume drinking, they should be encouraged to take the deterrent drug disulfiram 250 mg./day. This drug interferes with the metabolism of alcohol, resulting in acetaldehyde accumulation with the rapid onset of nausea, malaise, flushing, and dizziness. Severe hypotensive reactions may occur if the patient drinks heavily. Hypertensive reaction do not occur when disulfiram and alcohol are combined.

475. e) Cigarette smoking, obesity, diabetes and hypertension are much more common in alcoholics than in nonalcoholics. Some studies have shown that alcoholism is a very common cause of hypertension.

Reference

Favazza A. Alcoholism. American Family Physician 1983; 27(2): 274-278.

PROBLEM #74: A 31 YEAR OLD FEMALE WITH FATIGUE

476. A 31 year old female presents with a 6 month history of fatigue. She also states that for the past 3 months she has had difficulty falling asleep. You feel that she may have an underlying depression. Which of the following symptoms is MOST CHARACTERISTIC of a depressive illness?

a) fatigue
b) weight loss
c) headache
d) anhedonia
e) memory loss

477. A complete psychiatric history is most important in evaluating depressed patients. In taking a history from a patient with depression, which of the following questions is the MOST IMPORTANT to ask?

a) family history of psychiatric problems
b) personal history of previous episodes of depression
c) suicidal ideation
d) presence or absence of hallucinations
e) presence or absence of delusions

478. Of the following antidepressants, which of the following has the LEAST anticholinergic activity?

a) desipramine
b) amitriptyline
c) imipramine
d) amoxapine
e) maprotiline

479. With most tricyclic antidepressants, clinical response may not appear until adequate dosage has been used for:

a) 2-4 days
b) 5-7 days
c) 7-14 days
d) 14-28 days
e) 2-4 months

480. When a favorable response to a particular antidepressant has occurred during the acute phase of treatment, therapy with that drug should be continued for a period of:

a) 1-2 months
b) 3-4 months
c) 5-6 months
d) 6-12 months
e) 18-24 months

CODE: (a:1, 2 and 3; b: 1 and 3; c: 2 and 4; d: 4 only; e: all of the above)

481. Which of the following statements regarding tricyclic antidepressants is/are CORRECT?

1) all tricyclic antidepressants are equally efficacious
2) the most common limiting side effects of tricyclic antidepressants are anticholinergic side effects
3) doxepin has a lower cardiotoxicity than amitriptyline
4) if therapy with one tricyclic antidepressant is unsuccessful, it is unlikely that another one will be of benefit

ANSWERS

476. d) All of the symptoms listed can be presenting symptoms of a depressive disorder but anhedonia, or the inability to experience pleasure is an almost universal characteristic of depression. When questioned about their mood, many patients complain not of feeling sad or depressed, but rather of being unable to feel any kind of emotion.

Depression usually presents as a combination of physical, emotional and cognitive manifestations. One of the most frequent symptoms is insomnia. Insomnia may be either initial insomnia (inability to get to sleep), middle insomnia (waking in the middle of the night and experiencing difficulty getting back to sleep) or late insomnia (waking early in the morning and being unable to return to sleep). Other symptoms include headache, blurred vision, dry mouth, hyperventilation, a sense of constriction in the chest, tachycardia, back pain, abdominal and pelvic pains, anorexia, weight loss, digestive upsets, nausea, vomiting, constipation, diarrhea, alterations in menstrual function, urinary frequency and decreased libido. Emotional symptoms other than anhedonia include anxiety, irritability, feelings of unworthiness and hopelessness, incompetency and inadequacy, feelings of guilt and self-doubt, and suicidal ideation. Cognitive manifestations include inability to concentrate, recent memory loss and indecision.

477. c) The most important question in the psychiatric history of a patient with depression is the question of feelings or thoughts of self-harm or suicide. Patients should be questioned directly and openly about their feelings in this area. If the patient admits to thoughts of suicide he should be questioned about his plan, previous attempts and a family history of suicide. At that point the physician should attempt to classify him as low or high risk. Any patient thought to be at high risk of suicide should be admitted. Family history of other psychiatric problems, previous episodes of depression in the patient, and the presence or absence of hallucinations or delusions are all part of a complete psychiatric history but not as important as the immediate risk of suicide.

478. a) The degree to which an antidepressant causes sedation and produces anticholinergic and cardiovascular side effects is an important consideration. There is a great difference among tricyclic antidepressants in anticholinergic activity. Anticholinergic activity is manifested by dry mouth, blurred vision, constipation and urinary retention. Tricyclic antidepressants with high anti-cholingeric activity include amitriptyline and imipramine. Amoxapine and maprotiline are intermediate in anticholinergic activity. Desipramine has the least anticholingeric effect of any tricyclic, and trazadone, a triazolopyridine derivative, has almost no anticholingeric activity.

479. d) Tricyclic antidepressants, along with psychoptherapy are the treatment of choice for patients with depressive illnesses. Most tricyclic antidepressants require 14-28 days to exert their antidepressant effect. A possible exception is amoxapine. Some studies have shown that this agent is fully effective by 14 days.

480. d) When favourable response to a particular antidepressant agent has occurred during the acute phase of treatment, therapy with that drug should be continued for an additional six to twelve months. The correct dose for long-term therapy varies from patient to patient but averages 100-150 mg./day. When individual dosage is established the entire daily dose can be given at night to reduce anticholingeric and antihistaminic side effects. Failure to continue the drug for at least 6 months often results in relapse.

481. a) All tricyclic antidepressants are equally efficacious on a milligram to milligram basis but differ considerably in their side effect profile. The most common side effects are the anticholinergic ones and include dry mouth, blurred vision, constipation and urinary retention. Thus, an agent with few anticholingeric side effects is often preferrable, unless insomnia is a major symptom. As well, patients with chronic diseases such as glaucoma and prostatic hypertrophy are better treated with agents that are low in the anticholingeric spectrum. The antidepressant should be tailored to the symp-toms of the patient. If you wish to stimulate a patient who is lethargic you

should use an agent such as desipramine. If, on the other hand, you wish to treat a patient whose major symptom is anxiety you should choose an agent such as trimipramine or doxepin.

These agents also differ in their cardiotoxic potential. Orthostatic hypotension, sinus tachycardia, arrthymias and disturbances of atrioventricular and intraventricular conduction appear to be dose related and more common with amitriptyline and imipramine than with doxepin or maprotiline.

In individualizing tricyclic antidepressant therapy it is important to remember that individuals show great variation in their response to these drugs. Dosage may have to be increased to 300 mg./day in some individuals to obtain a therapeutic response. On the other hand, elderly patients often require considerably less, averaging 50-75 mg./day. If one agent has been taken to full therapeutic dose and no response has been obtained, it is useful to try another tricyclic agent. Alternatives to this include switching to either an MAO inhibitor or lithium as second-line therapy.

Reference

Ayd F, Taylor B. The depressed office patient. American Family Physician 1983; 28(1): 155-161.

PROBLEM #75: AN 18 YEAR OLD MALE REQUESTING MEPERIDINE AND PENTAZOCINE FOR CHRONIC BACK PAIN

482. An 18 year old male presents to your office requesting meperidine and pentazocine for back pain. He was in a motor vehicle accident two years ago and has had back pain since the mishap. You suspect narcotic analgesic abuse. Which of the following signs is MOST CHARACTERISTIC of intoxication with narcotic analgesics?

a) pupillary constriction
b) mydriasis
c) increased alertness and hyperactivity
d) hyperventilation
e) diarrhea

483. Treatment of opiate withdrawal syndrome is best accomplished by substitution therapy with:

a) codeine
b) naloxone
c) methadone
d) clonidine
e) pentazocine

484. Intoxication with PCP (phenylcylidine) includes all of the following symptoms EXCEPT:

a) vertigo
b) nausea and vomiting
c) flushing
d) hypotension
e) diaphoresis

485. A 23 year old male presents to your office and tells you that he wants to "quit doing downers". He is currently taking 80 mg. of diazepam/day. You should manage this patient's withdrawal from diazepam by:

a) stopping the diazepam "cold turkey"
b) stopping the diazepam over 72 hours
c) gradually decreasing the diazepam over 6 months
d) substituting phenobarbitol for diazepam and reducing the dose of diazepam by no more than 10%/day
e) substituting oxazepam for diazepam and gradually decreasing the dose over a one week time interval

486. According to recent surveys, the drug preferred and most frequently abused by American teenagers is:

   a) amphetamines
   b) heroin
   c) alcohol
   d) marijuana
   e) phencyclidine (PCP, angel dust)

CODE: (a:1, 2 and 3; b: 1 and 3; c: 2 and 4; d: 4 only; e: all of the above)

487. The definition of substance abuse requires the presence of which of the following conditions?

   1) a pattern of pathologic abuse
   2) duration of at least one month
   3) impairment in social or occupational functioning
   4) suicidal ideation upon withdrawal of the agent

ANSWERS

482. a) The patient presenting is almost certainly abusing opiates. The most characteristic finding with opiate intoxication is pupillary constriction. Other signs of mild intoxication include drowsiness, slurred speech, impaired attention and memory, and constipation. Mydriasis, increased alertness, hyperactivity, hyperventilation and diarrhea are associated with opoid withdrawal rather than opiate intoxication.

483. c) Treatment of the opiate withdrawal syndrome is best accomplished by substitution therapy with methadone, which is preferred because of several pharmocokinetic advantages: it can be administered orally and produces minimal euphoria by this route; it has a long duration of action needing to be administered no more than twice daily; its effects tend to persist with constant dosage; and it will suppress withdrawal at a relatively moderate dose. If symptoms of withdrawal occur after stopping methadone the drug of choice is clonidine for 1-2 weeks; it is hypothesized that this drug blocks a noradrenergic mechanism that mediates opiate withdrawal.

   Codeine and pentazocine are both narcotic agonists (with pentazocine also being an antagonist) and therefore are not appropriate for treatment. Naloxone is the agent that will acutely reverse narcotic overdose but it is not useful for treatment of withdrawal syndrome.

484. d) Intoxication with PCP (phenylclidine) may induce hypertension, vertigo, vertical nystagmus (this is almost diagnostic), nausea and vomiting, decreased

sensory acuity, hyperreflexia, paraesthesias, constricted pupils, decreased pupillary light reflexes and ptosis. Hypotension is usually not a feature of acute PCP intoxication.

485. d) The sedative-hypnotic withdrawal syndrome involves generalized hyperarousal of the central nervous system, with insomnia, anxiety, tremor, vulnerability to convulsions, and sometimes delirium or other organic brain syndromes. Abrupt withdrawal of these drugs is much more dangerous than abrupt withdrawal of opiates.

Substitution therapy with phenobarbitol or pentobarbitol is usually the most convenient approach for detoxification of a patient with possible physical dependence on sedative-hypnotics. The appropriate starting dose of pentobarbitol is first empirically determined by administration of a 200 mg. test dose which is then repeated every hour until symptoms of withdrawal have disappeared and mild sedation is noted. The total dose should then be administered in several portions for each of the next 2 days, followed by gradual reduction at a rate of no more than 10%/day. Withdrawal can usually be accomplished within 7-10 days. Stopping the diazepam "cold turkey" or decreasing the diazepam over too short (such as 72 hours) or too long (such as six months) is not appropriate. Oxazepam is not an appropriate substitution as it produces just as much dependence as diazepam.

486. c) In every recent survey, alcohol was the drug most frequently used and most frequently preferred by teenagers. It is the first mind-altering drug tried by a large majority, and young people who do not use alcohol tend not to use any intoxicating drug. It is estimated that there are 1.3 million problem drinkers and 750,000 hard-core alcoholics between the ages of 12 and 17 in the United States today.

487. a) Substance abuse denotes the pathologic use, repeatedly over a period of time, of any substance that affects the central nervous system in such a manner that the behavior interferes with the person's normal social or occupational functioning. As defined in DSM-III, diagnoses in this category require the presence of all three of the following:

1) A pattern of pathologic use manifested by features such as: (a) intoxication throughout the day; (b) inability to reduce or terminate the use of the substance; (c) repeated unsuccessful attempts to control use by temporary abstinence or self-imposed restriction; (d) continued use of the substance in spite of knowledge that a serious health problem is being exascerbated; (e) inability to function adequately without daily use of the substance, or (f) episodes of some complication, such as blackouts or overdosage.
2) Duration of at least one month for the pattern of pathologic use.
3) Impairment in social or occupational functioning due to substance use, manifested by features such as: (a) disruption of social relationships with

a) family or friends; (b) failure to meet important obligations; (c) irresponsible or impulsive behavior; (d) inappropriate expression of sexual or aggressive feelings; (e) criminal or antisocial behavior, such as assault or fighting, driving an automobile while intoxicated, or stealing to obtain money for purchase of the substance; (f) excessive absence from school or work; or (f) poor occupational or academic performance due to intoxication.

Suicidal ideation upon withdrawal of the substance is not recognized as a diagnostic criteria, but this behavior would certainly suggest dependence.

Reference

Gregory I, Smeltzer D, editors. Psychiatry-Essentials of Clinical Practice. Little, Brown and Company, Boston: 1983; pages 218-244.

PROBLEM #76: AN 18 YEAR OLD FEMALE WITH A RAPID WEIGHT LOSS

488. An 18 year old female presents to the office with a 40 lb. weight loss in the last six months. You suspect anorexia nervosa. Anorexia nervosa occurs most commonly in:

    a) females
    b) lower socioeconomic groups
    c) males
    d) Chinese
    e) children under the age of 12

489. Anorexia nervosa is characterized by all of the following EXCEPT:

    a) self-imposed dietary limitations
    b) intense fear of gaining weight
    c) normal menses
    d) disturbed body image
    e) profound weight loss

490. Which of the following is LEAST characteristic of anorexia nervosa?

    a) lowered vital signs when the weight is low
    b) denial of illness
    c) history of obesity
    d) decreased physical activity
    e) episodes of bulimia, followed by vomiting

491. Anorexia nervosa may have a mortality rate of up to:

    a) 3%
    b) 22%
    c) 26%
    d) 30%
    e) 50%

492. Bulimia is characterized by sudden, compulsive ingestion of large amounts of food in a very short time. What percentage of obese patients show behavior characteristic of bulimia?

    a) less than 5%
    b) 10%
    c) 15%
    d) 20%
    e) 25%

493. The most consistent indicator of a good outcome is anorexia nervosa is:

   a) early onset of illness
   b) late onset of illness
   c) gradual weight loss
   d) obesity prior to anorexia nervosa
   e) absence of compulsive behavior other than that related to food and losing weight

494. Initial treatment of anorexia nervosa should center on:

   a) behavior conditioning
   b) family psychotherapy
   c) group psychotherapy
   d) restoring the patient's nutritional state to normal
   e) treating an underlying depression with E.C.T.

ANSWERS

488. a) Anorexia nervosa occurs predominantly in females. Various studies report that a range of 4-6% are males. The risk for a sister of an anorectic patient developing anorexia is about 6.6%, which greatly exceeds the normal expected risk. Often mothers or fathers have had an explicit history of significantly low adolescent weight or weight phobia. At the present time, the evidence available does not permit any conclusions as to the role of heredity in the development of this disorder. Recent prevalence studies have shown anorexia nervosa to be a common disorder in the 12-30 year age group, and in the higher socioeconomic classes.

489. c) Anorexia nervosa is a disorder characterized by self-imposed dietary limitations, behavior directed toward losing weight, peculiar patterns of handling food, weight loss of at least 25% of original body weight, intense fear of gaining weight, disturbance of body image, and in women, amenorrhea. It is one of the few psychiatric illnesses that may have a course that is unremitting until death.

490. d) Anorexia nervosa involves great variation in nutritional intake, and may include episodes of overeating (bulimia), vomiting (which may be self-induced), pica, and a "premorbid" history of obesity. There is denial of illness, of disability, of painful affect, and of unacceptable motivation (eg. — aggressive or sexual). Physical activity is often increased except when there is extreme cachexia.

491. b) The course of anorexia nervosa may result in (1) spontaneous recovery without treatment; (2) recovery after a variety of treatments; (3) a fluctuating course of weight gains followed by relapses; or (4) a gradually deteriorating course resulting in death due to complications of starvation. The short term response of patients to almost all hospital programs is good. Studies have shown a range of mortality of from 5-21.5%.

492. a) Bulimia, which is found in fewer than 5% of obese patients, is one of the rare exceptions to the pattern of impaired satiety. It is characterized by the sudden, compulsive ingestion of very large amounts of food in a very short time, usually with subsequent agitation and self-condemnation. It appears to represent a reaction to stress. In contrast to the night eating syndrome, these bouts of overeating are not periodic, and they are far more often linked to specific precipitating circumstances. Binge eaters can sometimes lose large amounts of weight by adhering to rapid and unrealistic diets, but such efforts are almost always interrupted by a resumption of eating binges.

493. a) The most consistent indicator of a good prognosis in anorexia nervosa is early onset of disease. The most consistent indicator of poor outcome is late onset of disease. Such factors as childhood neuroticism, parental conflict, bulimia, vomiting, laxative abuse and various behavioral manifestations such as obsessive compulsive, hysterical, depressive, psychosomatic, neurotic and denial of symptoms have been related to poor outcome in most studies.

The expected outcome may vary from complete recovery with normal weight maintenance and usually effective functioning to an inability to maintain weight with a gradual starvation course and an inability to function because of extreme weakness and a severe interfering preoccupation with losing weight. The mortality rate has been reported to be as high as 21.5%.

494. d) The immediate aim of treatment in anorexia nervosa is to restore the patient's nutritional state to normal. This is necessary because of complications of emaciation, dehydration and electrolyte imbalance, which may lead to death. Usually, a hospitalized treatment program that provides considerable environmental structure is necessary for the weight restoration stage of treatment. Later, behavior conditioning and family therapy offer the greatest promise for long-term success. Group psychotherapy may be helpful in some patients and treatment of underlying major depression is obviously necessary.

References

Kaplan H, Sadock B, editors. Modern Synopsis of Comprehensive Textbook of Psychiatry III. Williams and Wilkins Co., Baltimore: 1981; pages 607-612.

Kaplan H, Sadock B; editors. Study Guide and Self-Examination Review for Modern Synopsis of Comprehensive Textbook of Psychiatry III. Williams and Wilkins Co., Baltimore: 1983; pages 211-222.

Gregory I, Smeltzer D; editors. Psychiatry. Little, Brown and Company, Boston: 1983; pages 194-211.

PROBLEM #77: A 40 YEAR OLD FEMALE WITH CHRONIC ABDOMINAL PAIN

495. A 40 year old woman walks into your office holding her abdomen. She comes to you seeking advice for an abdominal pain she has had for 10 years. She has had 5 operations in the last 2 years to try and correct this pain. These include vagotomy and pyloroplasty, cholecystectomy, appendectomy and hysterectomy. You are the 24th doctor she has consulted. On further questioning you discover that her husband is 30 years older than her and is very possessive. He never lets her go out by herself and she feels like a prisoner. The most likely diagnosis is:

   a) obsessive-compulsive disorder
   b) somatization disorder
   c) conversion disorder
   d) psychogenic pain disorder
   e) hypochondriasis

496. A 45 year old woman presents to your office in an anxious, tearful state. She states that she has chronic upper abdominal pain and is certain she has cancer of the stomach and nobody will believe her. She has attended 16 different physicians in the past year and has had a GI series performed six times; a barium enema performed three times, an ultrasound of her abdomen performed four times and a CT scan performed twice. She is coming to you as a last resort before going to an herbal clinic in Mexico. Based on the history, the most likely diagnosis is:

   a) obsessive-compulsive disorder
   b) somatization disorder
   c) conversion disorder
   d) psychogenic pain disorder
   e) hypochondriasis

497. A 43 year old woman presents to the emergency department with paralysis of both lower limbs and paraesthesias in both upper limbs beginning two hours ago. When first seen she is lying on a stretcher and is unable to move either lower extremity. A neurologist is consulted and states that the presentation does not fit any known neurological disease. On further questioning you discover that the patient is being regularly beaten by her husband. Her last beating occurred two hours before her symptoms began. The most likely diagnosis is:

   a) obsessive-compulsive disorder
   b) somatization disorder
   c) conversion disorder
   d) psychogenic paralysis
   e) hypochondriasis

498. A 35 year old female presents to your office for the first time. She has seen 20 other physicians in the past 3 years. She presents with the following list of symptoms: headache, dizziness, vomiting spells, chest pain, hyperventilation, back pain, upper abdominal pain, pelvic pain, numbness and tingling in all four extremities, pruritis and a sensation of fullness in the head. She has had six operations including three back operations for presumed spinal stenosis, cholecystectomy, appendectomy and 3 exploratory laparotomies. She denies being depressed and says that she enjoys life and meeting new people (especially new doctors). The most likely diagnosis is:

a) obsessive-compulsive disorder
b) somatization disorder
c) conversion disorder
d) psychogenic pain syndrome
e) hypochondriasis

499. A few months ago after his mother died of abdominal cancer, a 46 year old man with no previous psychiatric problems became preoccupied with the belief that he too had cancer. He complains of marked anergia, malaise, anorexia and a "bloating feeling" in the abdomen. An intensive workup reveals no evidence of organic pathology, but he insists he has cancer and constantly talks about it. He then begins to lose weight and experiences difficulty staying asleep at night for longer than 3 to 4 hours. He loses interest in most of his previous activities and becomes unable to experience pleasure even momentarily. The correct diagnosis is:

a) adjustment disorder with depressed mood
b) hypochondriasis
c) major depression
d) obsessive compulsive disorder
e) somatization disorder

500. Each of the following may be a form of conversion disorder EXCEPT:

a) dystonias and dyskinesias
b) gait disturbance
c) gun barrel vision
d) pseudodementia
e) stocking and glove anesthesia

501. The treatment of choice for neurotic disorders is generally considered to be:

a) benzodiazepines
b) long term intensive individual psychotherapy
c) group psychotherapy
d) short term supportive psychotherapy
e) tricyclic antidepressants

CODE: (a:1, 2 and 3; b: 1 and 3; c: 2 and 4; d: 4 only; e: all of the above)

502. Neurotic disorders are diagnosed more frequently:

    1) among persons of high socioeconomic status than among persons of low socioeconomic status
    2) among psychiatric outpatients than among inpatients
    3) among patients with higher education than among those with lower education
    d) among men than among women

503. Neurotic disorders as a group are:

    1) distressing to the person and regarded as unacceptable and alien (ego-dystonic)
    2) are associated with no major impairment of reality testing (such as hallucinations and delusions)
    3) are not limited to temporary reactions to external stress
    4) are associated with no demonstratable organic etiology

ANSWERS

495. d) The characteristic finding in psychogenic pain disorder is severe and prolonged pain, which is often but not necesarily inconsistent with the anatomic distribution of the nervous system, and for which no organic pathology or pathophysiologic mechanism can be found after thorough evaluation. There must be evidence of either primary gain (such as initiation or exacerbation of the pain immediately following environmental stimuli related to a psychological conflict or need) or secondary gain (when the pain results in avoidance of some unpleasant activity or increased support from the environment).

    In early stages these disorders are usually responsive to non-reinforcement (after adequate medical evaluation), along with appropriate psychotherapies or environmental manipulation. However, they may be greatly aggravated and prolonged by inappropriate medical or surgical procedures. This patient's somatic pain and disability have resulted in obvious secondary gains through escape from the intolerable aspects of her married life. The other options in the question will be discussed in subsequent questions.

496. e) Hypochondriasis is characterized by preoccupation with bodily functions and with fears of presumed diseases of various organs. These fears are not delusional in intensity, but persist in spite of reassurance concerning normal findings from physical examination and laboratory investigations.

497. c) Conversion disorder involves the psychogenic loss or disturbance of sensory, motor or other physical functions in a manner suggestive of neurologic or other somatic disease, but without any acutual finding of the latter. There must be some evidence that psychological factors (confilcts or unfulfilled needs) are involved in producing the symptoms, but the latter must not be under voluntary control by the patient. The main forms of conversion include:

   1) altered sensations such as anesthesia or paresthesia, partial or complete blindness, or deafness
   2) atoxia or paralysis, including inability to stand or walk and loss of voice with inability to whisper
   3) involuntary movements or dystonias, and pseudoepileptic convulsions.

   The onset of conversion symptoms is sudden and dramatic. the symptoms appear neurologic, but careful examination and tests are likely to reveal obvious discrepancies between the dysfunction and actual anatomic distributions of motor and sensory nerves (eg. anesthesia with a stocking and glove distribution). There may be gross disability about which the patient shows no apparent anxiety or concern (la belle indifference).

498. b) Somatization disorder includes a complicated history, extending over a period of years, and a pattern of seeking medical attention for a large variety of physical symptoms that are often described in a vague, dramatic, or exaggeratered manner. In spite of continued failure to find a physiologic basis for their symptoms, these patients believe they have been sickly for a good part of their lives. Often their histories include episodes of conversion disorder or of dissociative symptoms such as psychogenic amnesia or multiple personality. Otherwise, the main symptoms involve complaints of physical pain, such as abdominal pain, vomiting spells, back pain, joint pain, pain in the extremities or frequent headaches. Women are likely to complain of dysmenorrhea or excessive menstrual bleeding. There is often pain or lack of pleasure during intercourse. The somatic complaints are apt to lead the person to consult many different doctors, to be admitted to hospitals, and to be subjected to polysurgery.
   The only other disorder not discussed up to now is obsessive compulsive disorder. This is characterized by recurrent and persistent obsessions (unwanted ideas, thought, images, or impulses) or compulsions (repetitive and seemingly purposeful actions performed according to certain rules) or in a stereotyped manner, that are not fully rational.

499. c) The only correct diagnosis is major depression. Loss of interest in previous activities and the inability to experience pleasure strongly suggest a diagnosis of depression. Also characteristic of depression are anergia, malaise, anorexia, loss of weight, and early morning awakening. Delusions of having cancer or other serious somatic illness are depressive in nature, although delusional thinking is found in only the most severe depressions. Obsessive

thoughts, hypochondriasis, and other neurotic symptoms often occur in major depression and are not separately diagnosed unless they are also present when the person is not depressed.

500. d) The only symptom listed that is not a form of conversion disorder is pseudodementia. Pseudodementia refers to a depressive illness in which the person appears to have dementia.

501. b) The treatment of choice for neurotic disorders is long-term intensive psychotherapy. Neurotic disorders, which have often been going on for many years usually cannot be quickly reversed. Although benzodiazepines may be used for a short time, long-term use is not recommended because of addictive potential. Antidepressant medication is not indicated unless major depression is the primary problem. Short-term psychotherapy and group psychotherapy have not been shown to be as effective as long-term intensive psychotherapy.

502. a) Neurotic disorders are more common in women than in men (or at least they present more frequently), and tend to be associated with patients that are both better educated and in a higher socioeconomic class. They occur much more frequently in outpatients than in inpatients.

503. e) Neurotic disorders are groups of symptoms having all of the following characteristics: (1) they are distressing to the person and regarded as unacceptable and alien (ego-dystonic); (2) there is no major impairment of reality testing (such as hallucinations or delusions), and behavior does not actively violate important social norms (although it may be socially or occupationally disabling); (3) the symptoms tend to be relatively enduring or recurrent unless effective treatment is obtained; (4) the symptoms are not limited to temporary reactions to external stress; and (5) there is not demonstratable organic etiology involved.

Reference

Gregory I, Smeltzer D; editors. Psychiatry. Little, Brown and Company, Boston: 1983; pages 285-300.

PROBLEM #78: A 65 YEAR OLD HYPERTENSIVE MALE WITH IMPOTENCE

504. A 65 year old male with hypertension, congestive cardiac failure and peptic ulcer disease presents to your office for his regular blood pressure check. Although his blood pressure is now under control, he complains of an inability to maintain an erection. He is currently taking the medications listed below. Which of the medications listed is the LEAST LIKELY to be the cause of this man's impotence?

a) alpha-methyldopa
b) propranolol
c) digoxin
d) hydrochlorothiazide
e) cimetidine

505. Regarding the patient described in question #504, which of the following medications is the MOST LIKELY cause of his impotence?

a) alpha-methyldopa
b) propranolol
c) digoxin
d) hydrochlorothiazide
e) cimetidine

506. Impotence due to organic causes seems to be somewhat less common than impotence due to psychologic factors. Which of the following conditions is the most common organic cause of impotence?

a) prostatism
b) hyperthyroidism
c) Parkinson's disease
d) diabetes mellitus
e) atherosclerosis of the abdominal aorta

507. The single most important aspect in the evaluation of impotence is:

a) the history
b) the physical examination
c) nocturnal penile tumescence measurement
d) ratio of penile/brachial blood pressure
e) serum testosterone measurement

CODE: (a:1, 2 and 3; b: 1 and 3; c: 2 and 4; d: 4 only; e: all of the above)

508. Which of the following is/are important in the treatment of psychogenic impotence?
    1) reducing performance anxiety by prohibiting intercourse
    2) anxiety reduction by identification and verbalization
    3) introduction of the process of sensate focus
    4) instruction in interpersonal communication skills

509. which of the following is/are important in the treatment of premature ejaculation
    1) reducing performance anxiety by prohibiting intercourse
    2) anxiety reduction by identification and verbalization
    3) introduction of the process of sensate focus
    4' teaching of the penile squeeze technique

ANSWERS

504. c) Drugs are probably the most common recognized cause of impotence. Antihypertensives, sedatives, antipsychotics and cimetidine are the most common offenders. Digoxin is rarely a cause of impotence.

505. a) Antihypertensives are the most common class of pharmaceutical agents associated with impotence. Although thiazide diuretics, propranolol and other beta-blockers, and clonidine are often associated with impotence, alpha-methyldopa is the antihypertensive agent most frequently associated with this condition.

506. d) Diabetes mellitus is the most organic cause of impotence. It is now reasonably certain that the impotence of diabetes mellitus is caused principally by diabetic neuropathy; a process of microscopic damage to nerve tissue that occurs throughout the body of the diabetic. Although the exact cause of this neuropathy is not known, current experimental evidence suggests that it is the result of an abnormal accumulation of chemical substances called polyols in nerve fibers. This accumulation produces segmental demyelination and defective myelin synthesis. The accumulation of these substances appears to be a direct result of hyperglycemia. In some diabetic men microvascular or macrovascular changes resulting from diabetes may be important causes of impotence.

Impotence secondary to hyperthyroidism, Parkinson's disease and atherosclerosis of the abdominal aorta as well as many other diseases is less common than impotence secondary to diabetes. Because of the association between impotence and diabetes mellitus, all patients with impotence probably should have a 3-hour glucose tolerance test.

507. a) The single most important aspect in the evaluation of impotence is the history. If a man achieves erections under certain conditions but not others, the likelihood is high that the impotence is psychogenic. Thus, the impotent man who experiences erections with masturbation, during homosexual activity, during extramarital sex, and in response to reading or looking at erotic materials is unlikely to have a physical or metabolic explanation for his difficulties. For the same reason, the common history of the man who has no difficulty in achieving a firm erection, only to lose it promptly upon attempting vaginal insertion is strong evidence for a psychogenic cause. Similarly, the presence of a firm erection at the time of awakening indicates that the capacity for normal erectile response is present physiologically.

The physical examination is very important but more useful information is obtained from the history.

Measurement of nocturnal penile tumescence, the ratio of penile/brachial blood pressure and the serum testosterone are investigations that have an important role to play in the overall evaluation of impotence.

508. e) Most cases of impotence are characterized by fear of performance, a debilitating set of sexual anxieties that arise when the male is unable to obtain or maintain a normal erection and begins pressuring himself to improve his functioning. Sometimes the partner contributes to such anxieties either purposely (by making derogatory remarks, for example) or indirectly (by pretending that nothing is wrong or by attempting to be supportive) and thus compounding the difficulties.

The first step in reducing performance anxieties at the outset of therapy is the prohibition of any direct sexual activity. The couple is told that after a therapeutic plan has been formulated, the therapists will make specific suggestions for reestablishing sexual activity to facilitate learning. The second step in anxiety reduction is the process of identification and verbalization. Bringing the man's anxieties into the open, assuring him that such concerns are quite common, acquainting the wife or partner with the problems that the impotent man has been facing, and offering hope that such problems can be overcome allows a dialogue to develop that may materially reduce the intensity of pressures to perform and simultaneously facilitate the establishment of the therapeutic rapport.

The third, and probably the most important step in anxiety reduction involves the introduction of the principles of sensate focus. Early in therapy, the couple is instructed to participate in semistructured touching opportunities that will permit them to focus on their sensory awareness without any need to perform sexually. In fact, at the initial levels of sensate focus touching the genitals or female breasts are "off limits". As time goes on the levels of sensate focus are gradually increased. Lastly, instruction in interpersonal communication with the ability to tell your partner how you are feeling is constantly stressed.

509. e) The initial treatment of premature ejaculation is the same as that of impotence. In addition, the very helpful "squeeze" technique, in which the female partner puts her thumb on the frenulum of the penis and places her first and second fingers just above and below the coronal ridge on the opposite side of the penis is taught.

References

Sacks S. Evaluation of Impotence. Postgraduate Medicine 1983; 74(4): 182-197.
Braunstein G. Endocrine causes of impotence. Postgraduate Medicine 1983; 74(4): 207-217.
Golden J. Psychiatric aspects of male sexual dysfunction. Postgraduate Medicine 1983; 74(4): 221-229.
Kudish H. Treatment of impotence. Postgraduate Medicine 1983; 74(4): 233-240.
Kolodny R, Masters W, and Johnson V. Textbook of Sexual Medicine. Boston: 1979; Little Brown and Company, pages 507-532,

PROBLEM #79: A 75 YEAR OLD MALE ALCOHOLIC WITH "NO WILL TO CARRY ON LIVING"

510. A 75 year old alcoholic male presents to the office in a tearful, depressed state. He states that he no longer has anything to live for. You are concerned about possible suicide. Which of the following variables has the best correlation with suicide risk?

   a) prior psychiatric inpatient hospitalization
   b) loss of physical health
   c) age
   d) male sex
   e) alcoholism

511. In a patient who presents to the emergency department and is actively suicidal and a severe alcoholic the best treatment is:

   a) immediate psyciatric hospitalization
   b) exacting a promise not to kill himself
   c) daily psychotherapy sessions
   d) daily group psychotherapy sessions
   e) large doses of antipsychotics

512. A large percentage of persons who eventually commit suicide have had medical attention within what period of time before taking their own lives:

   a) one week
   b) one month
   c) three months
   d) six months
   e) one year

513. The ratio of male to female successful suicides is:

   a) 1 to 3
   b) 4 to 1
   c) 3 to 1
   d) 7 to 2
   e) 1 to 2

514. Among persons who successfully commit suicide, the two most frequent psychiatric diagnoses are major depression and:

a) alcoholism
b) borderline personality disorder
c) dementia
d) schizophrenia
e) somatization disorder

CODE: (a:1, 2 and 3; b: 1 and 3; c: 2 and 4; d: 4 only; e: all of the above)

515. Which of the following groups have age-adjusted suicide rates that are markedly higher than the age-adjusted rates for the entire United States population?

1) adults who have never married
2) physicians and medical students
3) persons whose socioeconomic status is declining
4) persons living in inner city slums

516. Increased risk of successful suicide attempts is associated with being:

1) male
2) divorced
3) depressed
4) age under 45

ANSWERS

510. c) One study showed that the most predictive items associated with high suicide risk are, in descending order of risk: advancing age, presence of alcoholism, rage, high lethality of prior suicidal behavior, male sex, not accepting help at the time of evaluation, long episode of current suicidal behavior, no prior psychiatric inpatient experience, recent loss or separation, somatic depression and loss of physical health.

Another study showed age; male sex; divorced, widowed, or separated marital status; living alone and choice of a highly lethal attempt as the major risk factors.

511. a) Any patient who is suspected of being suicidal should be directly asked if he feels so bad that he would like to end it all. A straightforward clinical ploy is to ask any patient considered suicidal whether he will agree to call when he reaches a point beyond which he is uncertain of controlling his suicidal impulses. If a patient can commit himself to such an agreement, he is reaffirming his belief that he has sufficient strength to cry out for help. If a patient who is considered seriously suicidal cannot make this committment, or if you have any doubt about his intensions, then immediate hospitalization is indicated.

512. d) Prior medical care appears to be a negatively correlated risk factor of suicide; 42% of suicides have had medical attention within six months of death. Seventy percent of victims are affected by one or more active, and for the most part chronic, illnesses at the time of death. Among suicide attempts studied, more than one third of the persons were actively ill at the time of the attempt, and more than 90% of the attempts were influenced by the illness. In both groups, psychosomatic illnesses constituted the majority of diagnoses.

513. Men commit suicide more than three times as often as women do, a rate that is stable over all ages. Women, on the other hand are three times as likely to attempt suicide than are men.

514. a) Major depression and alcoholism are the two diagnostic categories associated with exceptionally high rates of suicide. Patients with borderline personality disorder, schizophrenia or somatization certainly attempt and commit suicide, but the correlation is not nearly as great as it is with major depression and alcoholism.

515. a) Age-adjusted suicide rates are markedly higher in adults who were never married (as well as those separated or divorced or who have lost a spouse and are living alone); physicians and medical students (with suicide being the most common cause of death in physicians under the age of 40); and persons whose economic status is declining. Persons in inner-city slums do not have significantly higher age-adjusted suicide rates.

516. a) See critique of question #510.

References

Kaplan H, Sadock B; editors. Modern Synopsis of Comprehesive Textbook of Psychiatry III. Williams and Wilkins Co., Baltimore: 1981; pages 704-710.

Kaplan H, Sadock B; editors. Study Guide and Self-Examination Review for Modern Synopsis of Comprehensive Textbook of Psychiatry III. Williams and Wilkins Co., Baltimore: 1983; pages 241-249.

Gregory I, Smeltzer D; editors. Psychiatry. Little, Brown and Company, Boston: 1983; pages 700-702.

PROBLEM #80: A 35 YEAR OLD FEMALE WITH SEXUAL DYSFUNCTION

517. A 35 year old female presents to the office with a 6-month history of painful sexual intercourse. From the history you suspect vaginismus. Which of the following statements regarding vaginismus is FALSE?

    a) most women with vaginismus also have difficulty with sexual arousal

    b) there is a strong association between vaginismus and an intense childhood and adolescent exposure to religious orthodoxy

    c) there is a strong association between vaginismus and a traumatic sexual experience

    d) vaginismus is a condition of involuntary spasm or constriction of the musculature surrounding the vaginal outlet

    e) vaginismus may begin with a poorly healed episiotomy following childbirth

518. Regarding the diagnosis and treatment of vaginismus, which of the following statements is FALSE?

    a) throughout the diagnostic examination the woman must feel that she is in control, and may terminate the examination at any time

    b) the diagnosis of vaginismus can often be made without inserting a speculum

    c) the sexual partner should be involved in all aspects of the treatment process

    d) the insertion of vaginal dilators is not a recognized part of the treatment protocol

    e) sensate focus techniques are an important part of the treatment protocol

519. The percentage of sexually active women who have never experienced coital orgasm is:

    a) <1%

    b) 1-4%

    c) 5-10%

    d) 11-20%

    e) >20%

CODE: (a:1, 2 and 3; b: 1 and 3; c: 2 and 4; d: 4 only; e: all of the above)

520. Which of the following methods is/are useful in the treatment of female orgasmic dysfunction?

    1) sexual anatomy and physiology education

    2) sensate focus exercises

    3) treatment of underlying anxiety and depression

    4) long term use of a vibrator

521. Which of the following medications have been implicated in the etiology of inhibited sexual desire?

 1) alpha-methyldopa
 2) clonidine
 3) propranolol
 4) diphenylhydantoin

ANSWERS

517. a) Vaginismus is a condition of involuntary spasm or constriction of the musculature surrounding the vaginal outlet and the outer third of the vagina. The most dramatic instances of vaginismus often present as unconsummated marriages, since penile insertion into the vagina may not be possible due to spasm, resistance and attendant pain. The woman with vaginismus may be quite fearful of sexual activity, thus limiting her overall sexual response. Women with vaginismus have little difficulty with sexual arousal. Vaginal lubrication occurs normally, noncoital sexual activity may be pleasurable and satisfying, and orgasmic responsiveness is often intact. Women with vaginismus usually have normal libido and are distressed by their inability to participate pleasurably in coitus.

Vaginismus may arise from a natural protective reflex to pain originating from any lesion of the external genitalia or vaginal introitus. The percentage of cases of vaginismus that are initially attributable to organic pathology of this type is not certain; one difficulty is that repeated episodes of such pain may produce a conditioned response so that even if the original lesion heals spontaneously or is eliminated by proper medical therapy, the vaginismus may remain. Thus, a woman who initially experiences vaginismus in association with a poorly healed episiotomy may continue to be dysfunctional after perineal and vaginal tissue have healed normally. More commonly, however, no organic process can be implicated as the cause of the vaginismus. In these cases, a variety of psychosocial factors may be operative. There appears to be a conditioning to sex fostered by intense adolescent exposure to religious orthodoxy and the later occurrence of vaginismus. It should be emphasized that the development of vaginismus (or any sexual dysfunction) from this background has little to do with the specific theological content of relgious upbringing; rather, the major difficulty seems to stem from the rigid, often punitive thinking that regards sex as dirty, sinful and shameful.

Vaginismus may also stem from a traumatic sexual experience. Although this etiology is seen most typically in the case of women who were raped during childhood and adolescence, the occurrence of rape at any age may precipitate a subsequent pattern of secondary vaginismus, even when previous sexual function had been well established. Vaginismus is also common following an incestuous relationship in childhood.

518. d) The evaluation and treatment of vaginismus begins with a carefully performed physical examination in which the patient is always in full control. She may elect to have the examination terminated at any time. The pelvic examination begins by simple inspection of the external genitalia. Often at this point it is possible to detect spasm about the vagina and rigidity in the muscles along the interior of the thighs or along the perineum. After examination and palpation of the external genitalia, the next step is the insertion of a single examining finger into the vaginal outlet. If no significant discomfort is present, the examining finger is very gradually inserted into the vagina to a depth of 1-2 inches. The diagnosis of vaginismus can be made if involuntary spasm or constriction of the musculature surrounding the outer portion of the vagina is detected. If the diagnosis is made, it is not usually necessary to go to a more detailed pelvic examination at this time. The use of vaginal dilators in gradually increasing sizes has proved very helpful in the treatment of vaginismus. Starting with the smallest size and gradually increasing it, the woman is allowed to insert these herself, so that she begins to become more confident and more relaxed. By the time the largest plastic dilator can be inserted, the couple can make the transition to coitus. It is very important to invlolve the partner in all aspects of treatment. He should ideally be present during the entire evaluation and treatment process. Along with education about the anatomy and physiology of the female, The couple learns the concept of sensate focus exercises, which play a major part in the therapy of any sexual dysfunction problem.

519. c) Primary orgasmic dysfunction (primary anorgasmia) is defined as the condition of a woman who never has attained orgasm under any circumstances. Situational orgasmic dysfunction applies to women who have achieved orgasm on one or more occasions, but only under certain conditions. Women who are orgasmic by some means but are nonorgasmic during intercourse are described in subcategory of situational orgamic dysfunction known as coital orgasmic inadequacy (coital anorgasmia). Secondary orgasmic dysfunction describes women who were regularly orgasmic at one time but no longer are. The percentage of married women who have never experienced coital orgasm is variably quoted as 5-10%. Up to 17% of women seen in a general gynecologic parctice have difficulty in reaching orgasm with a partner.

520. a) Education for the patient and her partner regarding sexual anatomy and physiology is essential in the treatment of orgasmic dysfunction. As in vaginismus, sensate focus exercises play an important role. If an underlying anxiety state or a depression is present, it too must be treated. Although a vibrator may be initially helpful in providing a woman with an opportunity to experience orgasm as a frame of reference, the ongoing use of a vibrator in sex therapy is problematic for several reasons. First, the intensity of physical stimulation delivered by the vibrator cannot be duplicated by the man. Second, the use of the vibrator may alarm the woman if she preceives it as

unnatural. Third, the use of the vibrator may have a distancing effect on the couple; either or both partners may view it as reducing intimacy. Finally, repeated use of a vibrator over time may result in a degree of either psychological or physical dependence on the vibrator as the only possible source or orgasmic release.

521. e) Although inhibited sexual desire may have many causes, drugs and medication are one of the most common. The drugs and medications implicated include alcohol, alpha-methyldopa, antihistamines, barbiturates, clofibrate, clonidine, diphenylhydantoin, cannibis, monoamine oxidase inhibitors, phenothiazines, propranolol, reserpine and spironolactone.

Reference

Masters W, Johnson V, Kolodny R. Textbook of Sexual Medicine. Little, Brown and Company, Boston, 1979: pages 533-574.

General Surgery and Surgical Specialties

PROBLEM #81: A 45 YEAR OLD MALE WITH AN OSTOMY

522. A 45 year old male and his wife present to the office to discuss an ostomy which he has just undergone. Which of the following is the most common ostomy and indication for ostomy performed in North America?

   a) ileostomy-colorectal cancer
   b) ileostomy-inflammatory bowel disease
   c) colostomy-colorectal cancer
   d) colostomy-inflammatory bowel disease
   e) ileal conduit-bladder cancer

523. In a male undergoing an abdomino-perineal resection for colorectal cancer and a subsequent colostomy, the probability of impotence is:

   a) 10%
   b) 20%
   c) 30-50%
   d) 70-80%
   e) 100%

524. In a female undergoing an abdomino-perineal resection for colorectal cancer and a subsequent colostomy, which of the following statements is TRUE regarding subsequent sexual functioning?

   a) libido may be decreased
   b) vaginal lubrication may be decreased
   c) frequency of orgasm may be decreased
   d) all of the above are true
   e) none of the above are true

CODE: (a:1, 2 and 3; b: 1 and 3; c: 2 and 4; d: 4 only; e: all of the above)

525. With regard to the management of the patient with an ostomy, which of the following statements is/are TRUE?

1) adequate medical information in the pre-operative phase is essential
2) the post-operative care should include the enterostomal therapist
3) ostomy groups in the community play a major role in the patient's adjustment to his condition
4) psychological support for the spouse is not usually required

526. Which of the following is/are common problems in ostomy patients?

1) irrigation of the stoma, changing bags, and leakage
2) fears of sexual undesirability
3) strain in the work situation imposed by stoma care
4) depression

ANSWERS

522. c) The incidence of different ostomies among the population of Canada and the United States is as follows:
Colostomy for colorectal cancer — 51%
Ileostomy for inflammatory bowel disease — 35%
Urostomy (ileal conduit) for bladder cancer — 12%

523. c) In a male undergoing abdomino-perineal resection for colorectal cancer the probability of subsequent impotence is 30-50%. As well, there is a 50-75% chance of infertility following the same operation.
For ileostomy the incidence of subsequent sexual dysfunction is somewhat less and depends upon the age of the patient; for patients under age 35, the probability of impotence is 15%, over the age of 45 it is 53%.
Altered sexual function can be explained by damage to the pelvic sympathetic nerves L-1, L-2, and L-3 which are responsible for ejaculation and the pelvic parasympathetic nerves S-2, S-3, and S-4 which are responsible for erection.

524. d) In a woman undergoing abdomino-perineal resection for colorectal cancer, subsequent sexual dysfunction may include decreased libido, decreased vaginal lubrication, and decreased incidence of orgasm.

525. a) Management of a patient with an ostomy can be divided into 3 phases.
The first phase is the pre-operative phase in which adequate explanation of the actual medical situation, the needed surgical procedure, and possible (especially sexual) sequelae are discussed. The spouse or "significant other"

should be included in these discussions. During this phase also, a visit by a veteran patient or ostomy/enterostomal therapist is essential.

The second phase is the immediate post-operative phase. During this phase the postoperative care is directed by the ostomy therapist or experienced surgical nurse. Self-care must be learned before discharge. Again, inclusion of "significant other" is important.

The last or long-term adjustment phase is facilitated by clinic visits in which questions about the emotional state and sexual function of the patient should be addressed. During this phase, the coping of the spouse or significant other should be explored, as this individual is often having more problems coping than the patient himself. Involvement in a community-based ostomy group is encouraged.

526. e) The common problems encountered by ostomy patients can be divided into three categories.

The physical problems include the practical problems of handling the stoma and bowel/urinary function: irrigation, changing bags, finding the adequate appliance and leakage.

The emotional problems include impaired self-esteem and psychological dysfunction with depression and anxiety, anxiety in social situations, and fear of sexual undesirability.

The interpersonal problems include impaired sexual function or fears about sexual function; strain on key relationships (partner, family, friends); strain in the work situation imposed by stoma care and concerns about odors; and social isolation resulting from sense of stigma, low self-esteem, and withdrawal due to depression and anxiety.

Reference

Hurny C, Holland J. CA-A Cancer Journal for Clinicians 1985; 35(3) 170-181.

PROBLEM #82: A 35 YEAR OLD FEMALE WITH A BREAST LUMP

527. A 35 year old female presents with a 3 month history of a right breast lump, which seems to be larger and more tender in the week immediately before the menstrual period. On examination, a tender 3 cm rubbery mass with distinct borders is palpated in the right upper quadrant. The most likely diagnosis is:

    a) fibrocystic disease
    b) fibroadenoma
    c) carcinoma of the breast
    d) mastitis
    e) normal breast lump

528. The diagnostic procedure of choice for the patient described in question #527 is:

    a) ultrasound
    b) mammography
    c) excisional biopsy
    d) needle aspiration
    e) thermography

529. A 30 year old female presents with a 3 month history of a left-sided breast lump, which does not seem to vary in response to the menstrual cycle and is non-tender. On examination, a 2 cm hard, non-tender, mobile lump is palpated in the left upper quadrant. The most likely diagnosis is:

    a) fibrocystic disease
    b) fibroadenoma
    c) carcinoma of the breast
    d) mastitis
    e) normal breast lump

530. The diagnostic procedure of choice for the patient described in question #529 is:

    a) ultrasound
    b) mammography
    c) excisional biopsy
    d) needle aspiration
    e) thermography

531. The single most important factor in the prognosis of carcinoma of the breast is:

    a) size of the primary tumor
    b) length of time since the lump was first noticed
    c) age of onset
    d) family history of breast cancer
    e) presence or absence of positive axillary lymph nodes

532. A 40 year old female presents with a 3 cm mass in the right breast that is suspicious of carcinoma. She wishes to discuss alternatives to modified radical mastectomy. In discussing lumpectomy you should state that:

    a) it's not an effective operation and you don't want to discuss it further
    b) lumpectomy will probably result in a recurrence before modified radical mastectomy will
    c) the cure rate with lumpectomy is significantly lower than with modified radical mastectomy
    d) a combination of lumpectomy, axillary node dissection and external beam radiation appears to be an acceptable alternative to mastectomy in the treatment of primary breast cancer in selected patients
    e) modified radical mastectomy has been consistently shown to be the treatment of choice for primary breast cancer and you recommend that she go ahead with this operation

Questions 533-537 are TRUE and FALSE questions related to breast cancer risk factors. If the statement is TRUE mark "a"; if it is FALSE mark "b".

533. In a woman with a maternal family history of premenopausal breast cancer, the risk is 3X that of the general population of developing breast cancer.

534. A woman with a late menarche has a risk that is 2X that of the general population of developing breast cancer.

535. A nulliparous woman has a risk 4X that of the general population of developing breast cancer.

536. A woman with benign fibrocystic breast disease has a risk 4X that of the general population of developing breast cancer.

537. A woman who has an early natural menopause has a risk 2X that of the general population of developing breast cancer.

ANSWERS

527. a) Fibrocystic disease presents as a mass with a distinct border, rubbery consistency, with no fixation to underlying tissues and a growth pattern that is stable over time. In addition it fluctuates in size and tenderness in response to the menstrual cycle; being larger and more tender prior to menstruation. Fibroadenoma and carcinoma of the breast usually present as hard, non-tender masses that do not fluctuate in response to the menstrual cycle. Fibroadenomas are usually mobile and carcinomas of the breast are often fixed to fascia or muscle. Mastitis usually presents as a warm, erythematous, tender, swollen area in the breast of a woman who is breast feeding.

528. d) Needle aspiration is the diagnostic procedure of choice for a patient with suspected fibrocystic disease. The fluid is usually clear. A Papanicolaou smear can then be done on the fluid to look for malignant cells. Ultrasound, mammography and thermography are all useful in the diagnosis of breast lumps but are not necessary if fluid is obtained and the lump disappears. Excisional biopsy is usually not necessary.

529. b) A fibroadenoma usually presents as a distinct, hard, non-tender, mobile mass that rarely fluctuates in size in response to the menstrual cycle. It's growth pattern is stable over time. It is also known as a "breast mouse" due to its tendency to escape from palpation.

530. c) Because of its hard consistency and it's lack of fluid obtained on aspiration, a fibroadenoma can usually be diagnosed most accurately by excisional biopsy.

531. e) The most important single factor in the prognosis of carcinoma of the breast is the presence or absence of axillary lymph nodes. Patients with 1-3 axillary lymph nodes have a 5-year relapse rate of 50%, and those with 4 or more axillary nodes present have a 5-year relapse rate of 79%.

    The size of the primary tumor has considerable significance if axillary nodes are positive. The length of time since the lump first appeared correlates with both the stage of the disease and the size of the primary tumor. The age of onset and the presence of a positive family history do not ultimately correlate with the prognosis of an established breast cancer.

532. d) Currently, attention is focused on alternatives to full mastectomy in the primary treatment of breast cancer. From 1927 to 1982 at least 5,314 patients were treated with "lumpectomy" and/or radiation therapy. In 23 of 25 studies with follow-up of up to 30 years, survival rates with these forms of therapy were similar to survival rates with variations of radical mastectomy. It appears that a combination of lumpectomy, axillary lymph node dissection, and

external beam radiation are acceptable alternatives to mastectomy in primary breast cancer in patients with a primary tumor no greater than 4 cm. in diameter. Regardless of the mode of primary therapy, there is no significant difference in survival because local/regional therapy fails to eliminate distant metastases.

533. —a;   534. —b;   535. —a;   536. —a;   537. —b.

Breast cancer risk factors include:
1) maternal family member with premenopausal breast cancer: risk three times that of the general population
2) maternal family member with postmenopausal breast cancer: risk one-and-one-half times that of the general population
3) maternal family member with bilateral breast cancer at diagnosis: risk five and one-half times that of the general population
4) maternal family member with premenopausal and bilateral breast cancer at diagnosis: risk nine times that of the general population
5) early menarche or late natural menopause: risk more than twice that of the general population
6) nulliparous woman: risk four times that of the general population
7) woman older than 30 at her first pregnancy: risk five times that of the general population
8) woman with benign breast disease: risk four times that of the general population
9) North American and North European women: risk five times that of Asian and African women, and two and one-half times that of South American and South European women
10) ionizing radiation reaching more than 100 rads: risk significantly increased
11) hypothyroidism: believed to increase risk slightly
12) obesity (only in post-menopausal women): risk statistically increased
13) estrogen therapy in women: risk slightly but inconsistently increased (no increased risk is seen with use of combination-type oral contraceptives)

Reference

Hatfield H, Guthrie T. Breast Cancer Concepts: American Family Physician 1984; 30(2): 195-200.

PROBLEM #83: A 75 YEAR OLD MALE WITH RECTAL BLEEDING

538. A 75 year old male presents to the office with a 3-month history of bright red rectal bleeding. The rectal bleedings appears to be confined to the toilet tissue. The most common cause of rectal bleeding in adults is:

a) colorectal cancer
b) diverticulitis
c) hemorrhoids
d) ulcerative colitis
e) angiodysplasia

539. Which of the following colorectal polyps is MOST CLOSELY associated with colorectal carcinoma?

a) hyperplastic polyp
b) juvenile polyp
c) tubular polyp (tubular adenoma)
d) villous polyp (villous adenoma)
e) mixed polyp (tubulovillous adenoma)

CODE: (a:1, 2 and 3; b: 1 and 3; c: 2 and 4; d: 4 only; e: all of the above)

540. Which of the following is/are known risk factors for colorectal cancer?

1) age greater than 40 years
2) ulcerative colitis
3) family history of multiple adenomatous polyposis
4) genital or breast cancer in females

541. The treatment of hemorrhoids includes:

1) high fiber diet
2) psyllium hydrophilic mucilloid
3) stool softeners
4) zinc sulfate hydrocortisone acetate

542. Which of the following statements about C.E.A. (carcinoembryonic antigen) is/are CORRECT?

1) CEA may be elevated in tumors of the gastrointestinal tract
2) CEA is a glycoprotein that has little role in cancer screening or diagnosis
3) elevation of a previously normal CEA implies recurrent disease and is the most sensitive non-invasive indicator of tumor recurrence when performed regularly every 3 to 4 months
4) CEA is elevated in cigarette smokers

543. Which of the following screening tests have been recommended by the American Cancer Society after age 40 for the detection of colorectal carcinoma?

1) stools for occult blood annually
2) air contrast barium enema every 2 years
3) sigmoidoscopy every 2 years
4) colonoscopy every 2 years

ANSWERS

538. c) The most common cause of rectal bleeding is hemorrhoids. Hemorrhoids are dilated veins of either the internal or external hemorrhoidal plexus. In the United States, over 50% of patients over the age of 50 have hemorrhoids. Bleeding is the predominant manifestation of hemorrhoids. It is not dark as one might expect from venous bleeding; rather it is bright red and arterial in appearance. Bleeding usually occurs only with defecation and is noticed on the toilet tissue or coating the stools. It may color the toilet water red or drip from the anus following defecation.

Even though hemorrhoids have been identified as a possible source of rectal bleeding, sigmoidoscopic examination is mandatory to prove that bleeding is not from neoplasm or inflammatory bowel disease. In addition, an air-contrast barium enema should be done on any one over the age of 40 years who presents with rectal bleeding (an alternative to this is colonoscopy).

Colorectal cancer, diverticulitis, ulcerative colitis and angiodysplasia are all causes of rectal bleeding. However, they are uncommon compared to hemorrhoids.

539. d) Most colorectal carcinomas are thought to originate within polyps. There are several subtypes of colonic polyps, each with a different potential for malignant change. Hyperplastic polyps constitute 25% of all colonic polyps and 90% of polyps less than 3 mm. in diameter. They are found in areas of mucosal irritation and have no malignant potential. Juvenile polyps are harmatomas that are large and commonly found in the rectum. They have no malignant potential. Colonic adenomas are definately premalignant lesions, and the size of the polyp correlates with the liklihood of malignancy. Polyps of less than 1 cm. in diameter have a 1% chance of malignancy. A 10% malignant rate is found in polyps of 1-2 cm., whereas polyps greater than 2 cm. have nearly a 50% incidence of carcinoma. There are three types of colonic adenomas: adenomatous polyps (tubular adenomas); villous polyps (villous adenomas); and mixed polyps (tubulovillous adenomas). Tubular polyps make up 75% of adenomas less than 1 cm; while 60% of adenomas greater than 2 cm. are villous.

Polyps precede the onset of invasive cancer by an average of 5 years, and it is hypothesized that some time must elapse before malignant change occurs. Because it is impossible to tell one histologic type from another either radiographically or colonoscopically, all colon polyps should be removed if possible.

540. e) Risk factors for colorectal cancer include age greater than 40 years; associated disease such as ulcerative colitis or multiple adenomatous polyposis syndrome; a past history of colorectal adenomas, colorectal cancer or genital or breast cancer in females; and a family history of multiple adenomatous polyposis syndromes, colorectal cancer or colorectal polyps.

541. e) The treatment of hemorrhoids is aimed primarily at avoiding straining at stool. High fiber diets, psyllium hydrophilic mucilloid, stool softeners such as docusate sodium and agents such as zinc sulfate hydrocortisone cream or suppositories are useful, practical treatments for hemorrhoids. Sitz baths 2-3 times/day may help to reduce irritation and inflammation. Most patients will respond to this minimal therapy.

  Bothersome internal hemorrhoids can be removed by rubber-band ligation. The rubber banding of external hemorrhoids is very painful and not recommended; instead surgical removal is indicated.

542. e) CEA is a glycoprotein with a molecular weight of approximately 200,000. It is present in fetuses and was initially believed to be present postnatally only in colonic carcinomas. Further study has proved CEA to be associated with tumors of the gastrointestinal tract, pancreas, ovary, lung and breast, as well as in cigarette smokers and patients with chronic inflammatory diseases such as ulcerative colitis. CEA, then, is a non-specific substance that has little role in cancer screening or diagnosis. CEA does not appear to be useful in patients with known malignancy. Patients with colorectal cancer and perhaps those with bronchial carcinoma who also have low CEA values appear to have a better prognosis than patients with CEA levels greater than 10 mg./mL. An elevated CEA level should fall to normal 6 weeks following cancer surgery. If it does not, it indicates residual disease and is the most sensitive non-invasive indicator of tumor recurrence when performed every 3 to 4 months.

543. b) Colorectal cancer is the second leading cause of cancer death. Therefore, certain recommendations for screening the population over age 40 years have been developed. These include annual stools for occult blood and sigmoidoscopy every two years. Some authors have argued against these recommendations in that they have not yet been shown to be effective in decreasing the death rate from colorectal cancer. Also, they argue that the number of false positives obtained from fecal occult blood screening will tax the resources of radiologists and endoscopists necessary to perform subsequent air-contrast barium enema and colonoscopy studies. These latter two test are used as evaluation tools rather than as screening tools.

Reference

Boydstun J, Barker J, Lawhorne L. Gastrointestinal Disorders. Textbook of Family Practice 3rd edition; Rakel R, editor. W.B. Saunders Co., Philadelphia: 1984; pages 1015-1017.

PROBLEM #84: A 22 YEAR OLD FEMALE WITH ABDOMINAL PAIN

544. A 22 year old female presents with an acute onset of right upper quadrant pain. This is accompanied by nausea, vomiting, and a low-grade fever. Examination reveals maximal tenderness in the right upper quadrant of the abdomen, along with voluntary guarding. The most likely diagnosis is:

a) biliary colic
b) acute cholecystitis
c) ascending cholangitis
d) perforated peptic ulcer
e) acute pancreatitis

545. The treatment of choice for the patient described in question #544 is:

a) nasogastric suction, parenteral fluids, analgesics, IV antibiotics, and elective cholecystectomy in 3-6 months
b) nasogastric suction, parenteral fluids, analgesics, IV antibiotics, and urgent cholecystectomy
c) nasogastric suction, parenteral fluids, analgesics, IV antibiotics, and cholecystectomy as soon as the inflammation has been controlled
d) nasogastric suction, parenteral fluids, analgesics, IV antibiotics, and repair of perforated ulcer
e) none of the above

546. Which of the following statements about biliary colic is FALSE?

a) oral cholecystography is the diagnostic procedure of choice
b) biliary colic has cholelithiasis as its cause
c) biliary colic may be produced by ingestion of the oral contraceptive pill
d) biliary colic implies supersaturation of bile with cholesterol
e) cholesterol gallstones are responsible for most cases of biliary colic

547. The patient described in question #544 makes an uneventful recovery. She is readmitted to hospital 6 months later with acute periumbilical pain, followed by nausea and vomiting with movement of the pain into the right lower quadrant. On examination she has a fever of 39 degrees Celcius, and is acutely tender in the right lower quadrant. She does not appear jaundiced. Which of the following is the most likely diagnosis?

a) ascending cholangitis with referred pain to the right lower quadrant
b) twisted right ovarian cyst
c) bowel obstruction secondary to adhesion formation from the previous surgery
d) acute appendicitis
e) perforated ulcer

CODE: (a:1, 2 and 3; b: 1 and 3; c: 2 and 4; d: 4 only; e: all of the above)

548. Which of the following laboratory parameters is/are commonly elevated in a patient with acute cholecystitis?

1) serum bilirubin
2) serum alkaline phosphatase
3) white blood cell count
4) serum amylase

ANSWERS

544. b) The patient described in the question has a typical history of acute cholecystitis. There is an acute onset of right upper quadrant pain associated with systemic symptoms including nausea, vomiting, and fever. Examination usually reveals a tender right upper quadrant with voluntary guarding. Acute cholecystitis can be thought of as an extension of biliary colic, with the latter term applied to recurrent right upper quadrant pain associated with blockage of the cystic duct or the ampullary end of the gallbladder by a stone, but not associated with actual gallbladder inflammation (manifested by systemic signs). The symptoms associated with biliary colic often follow the ingestion of a meal rich in fat or containing foods that cause the patient digestive difficulty.

   Ascending cholangitis usually presents a much more toxic picture, with right upper quadrant pain accompanied by high fever, chills, jaundice and other systemic symptoms.

   Perforated peptic ulcer, acute pancreatitis, strangulating small bowel obstruction, pneumonia, myocardial infarction, congestive cardiac failure and pulmonary embolism are also causes of right upper quadrant pain but are distinctly less common than acute cholecystitis.

545. c) The treatment of choice for acute cholecystitis is nasogastric suction, parenteral fluids, analgesics, IV antibiotics, and cholecystectomy as soon as the acute inflammation has subsided. Cholecystectomy does not have to be performed on an urgent basis but likewise should not wait for 3-6 months.

   The antibiotic of choice in the treatment of acute cholecystitis is probably cefamandole 1 gram q6h.

546. a) Biliary colic implies pre-exisiting cholelithiasis. Cholelithiasis results from a supersaturation of bile with the excess cholesterol being deposited in the gallbladder and leading to the formation of cholesterol gallstones, the most common type. Young women taking the oral contraceptive pill are at increased risk for biliary colic, as estrogen increases the saturation of bile with cholesterol and subsequent gallstone formation. The diagnostic procedure of choice for biliary colic is abdominal ultrasound. If an abdominal ultrasound is negative, oral cholecystography is indicated as a second test.

547. d) The most common cause of the surgical abdomen is acute appendicitis. The patient presents with the "classical history" of periumbilical pain followed by nausea, vomiting, and movement of the pain into the right lower quadrant. The other possibilities listed in the question could present as right lower quadrant abdominal pain but would be much less common than acute appendicitis.

548. e) Patients with acute cholecystitis often have the white blood cell count, the serum bilirubin, the serum alkaline phosphatase and the serum amylase elevated. The elevation of amylase is a result of a secondary pancreatitis from blockage to bile flow. This is sometimes difficult to distinguish from a primary pancreatitis.

Reference

Mason G.R. Cholelithiasis and Cholecystitis. Conn's Current Therapy. Rakel R, editor. W.B. Saunders Co., Philadelphia: 1984, pages 353-356.

Boydstein J, Barker J and Lawhorne L. Gastrointestinal Disorders. Textbook of Family Practice 3rd edition. Rakel R, editor. W.B. Saunders Co., Philadelphia: 1984; pages 1031-1032.

PROBLEM #85: A 55 YEAR OLD MALE WITH PNEUMONIA

549. A 55 year old male who has C.O.P.D. and smokes 2 1/2 packs of cigarettes/day presents to your office with fever, chills, and hemopytsis. A CXR is performed and shows a left upper lobe pneumonia. Sputum cultures show a heavy growth of Hemophilus. The treatment of choice in this patient at this time is:

   a) ampicillin
   b) penicillin
   c) gentamicin
   d) carbenicillin
   e) cloxacillin

550. The patient described in question #549 continues to experience intermittant fever, chills, purulent sputum and hemoptysis for the next 3 months. He finally returns to see you. A CXR done at that time reveals no change from the previous examination — he appears to have a persistent left upper lobe pneumonia. The most likely explanation for the non-resolution of the left upper lobe pneumonia is:

   a) patient non-complicance with the treatment regime
   b) wrong antibiotic
   c) comprimised immune status secondary to C.O.P.D.
   d) endobronchial obstruction in the left upper lobe
   e) needle biopsy of the left upper lobe

551. The diagnostic procedure of choice for the patient described above is:

   a) tomograms of the left upper lobe
   b) CT scan of the left upper lobe
   c) monthly Chest X-rays for 6 months
   d) fiberoptic bronchoscopy
   e) needle biopsy of the left upper lobe

552. At this time, the most likely diagnosis in the patient described above is:

   a) fungal pneumonia
   b) tuberculosis
   c) bronchogenic carcinoma
   d) metastatic carcinoma from an unidentified primary site
   e) C.O.P.D. with chronic bacterial pneumonia

553. At this time, the treatment of choice for the patient described above is:

    a) hospitalization and IV gentamicin, clindamycin, and ampicillin
    b) isoniazid, rifampin and streptomycin
    c) surgery
    d) radiotherapy
    e) chemotherapy

554. The most common cause of cancer death in women is:

    a) breast cancer
    b) lung cancer
    c) colorectal cancer
    d) ovarian cancer
    e) endometrial cancer

ANSWERS

549. a) The treatment of choice in this patient is ampicillin. Hemophilus influenzae is a Gram-negative organism that is commonly cultured from patients with C.O.P.D. It responds well to both ampicillin and trimethoprim-sulfamethoxazole. It tends to be relatively resistant to penicillin. Gentamicin and carbenicillin are not first line agents for the treatment of uncomplicated pneumonia.

550. d) The most likely explanation for the non-resolution of the left upper lobe pneumonia is endobronchial obstruction in that region. This is most likely due to a neoplasm. Although patient non-compliance with the treatment regimen, incorrect antibiotic choice, compromised immune status and superinfection can all lead to non-resolution of a pneumonia that are unlikely to be the cause of a pneumonia that does not change over 3 months.

551. d) The diagnostic procedure of choice for this patient is fiberoptic bronchoscopy. This will locate an obstructing endobronchial lesion and will allow for its biopsy. Tomograms of the left upper lobe and CT scan of the left upper lobe and left hilum may provide useful information but they will not provide a definite diagnosis; fiberoptic bronchoscopy and biopsy will. Monthly chest X-rays for 6 months will simply delay diagnosis. Needle biopsy of the left upper lobe may well miss an obstructing lesion.

552. c) The most likely diagnosis in this patient is bronchogenic carcinoma. Fungal pneumonia, although a possibility, would be less likely since a bacterial source was already established. Although the tuberculin test should be done early in the evaluation, it is much less likely that TB is the cause of the persistent pneumonia. Metastatic carcinoma usually does not produce an obstructive pneumonia. A bacterial pneumonia (even with C.O.P.D.) should clear relatively rapidly.

553. c) The treatment of choice for bronogenic carcinoma (if it is resectable) is surgery. If the lesion is resectable a pneumonectomy, a lobectomy or a segmentectomy should be carried out. Although antibacterial treatment is initially indicated in this patient, the most important aspect of treatment is to remove the endobronchial obstruction as quickly as possible. Radiotherapy and chemotherapy have not been found to be of therapeutic benefit in most cases of bronchogenic carcinoma.

554. a) The most common cause of cancer deaths in women is still breast cancer. However, lung cancer is close behind and will soon overtake breast cancer as the number one cause of cancer deaths in women.

Reference

Matthews J, Blanton H. Lung Cancer. Primary Care 1985; 12(2): 267-281.

PROBLEM #86: A 35 YEAR OLD MALE WITH EAR PAIN

555. A 35 year old male presents to the office with a 2-day history of acute ear pain. On examination, you determine that the patient has acute otitis externa. The organism most frequently associated with otitis externa is:

a) Pseudomonas aeruginosa
b) Streptococcus pneumoniae
c) Mycoplasma pneumoniae
d) Haemophilus influenzae
e) Actinomyces

556. The most frequent direct cause of otitis externa is:

a) taking frequent baths or showers and allowing water to collect in the external ear
b) an infection secondary to otitis media
c) interference with the self-cleaning mechanism of the ear canal
d) an external ear canal blocked by cerumen
e) an infection spread from the paranasal sinuses

557. Otitis externa is most commonly encountered in:

a) military recruits
b) farmers
c) rock musicians
d) swimmers
e) deep sea fishermen

CODE: (a:1, 2 and 3; b: 1 and 3; c: 2 and 4; d: 4 only; e: all of the above)

558. The treatment of otitis externa involves

1) thoroughly cleansing of the ear with suction or a solution of merthiolate
2) the application of an antibacterial, antifungal otic solution containing a corticosteroid
3) the insertion of a wick in closure of the external canal is emminent
4) normal saline irrigation four times/day

559. Malignant otitis externa is most commonly seen in:

1) young children with repeated episodes of suppurative otitis media
2) patients with diabetes mellitus
3) competitive swimmers
4) patients on immunosuppressive therapy

ANSWERS

555. a) The organism most commonly associated with otitis externa is Pseudomonas aeruginosa. Streptococcus pneumoniae is the most frequent cause of acute otitis media. Mycoplasma pneumoniae is the organism most frequently implicated in bullous myringitis. Haemophilus influenzae is next in frequency to Streptococcus pneumoniae as a cause of acute otitis media. Actinomyces, a fungus, is usually seen in mixed infections.

556. c) The most frequent direct cause of otitis externa is interference with the self-cleaning mechanism of the ear canal by insertion of a finger, cotton-tipped applicator, facial tissue, or other object in an attempt to clean the canal. This frequently causes the keratin layer to turn 180 degrees and migrate toward the drumhead, carrying with it cerumen, wisps of cotton, and hair. The resulting double layer of keratin leads to increased moisture, which sooner or later provides an ideal environment for pathogenic organisms.

557. d) Otitis externa most frequently occurs in swimmers. Usually, this begins as cyclic episodes of increased itching, increased use of cotton-tipped applicators, and increased epithelial reactions, which may continue for weeks, months, or years. With invasion of Pseudomonas aeruginosa, the ear canal becomes painful quickly, sometimes within a few hours. There is no increase in otitis externa in any of the other groups mentioned.

558. a) The treatment of otitis externa involves: (1) thoroughly cleansing the ear with a suction apparatus through an operating microscope or irrigating the canal with water containing a few drops of thimerosal (Merthiolate) and (2) applying a topical solution containing an antibacterial, antifungal preparation containing a corticosteroid (Lococorten-Vioform). Generally, such "topical" shotgun therapy is not a good idea, but in this case the infections are often mixed and the epithelium is markedly inflamed.

   If the external canal is on the verge of closure, a wick should be inserted and the topical antibiotic-antiinflammatory agent should be transported medially by this mechanism.

   Normal saline irrigation four times/day would quite probably make the problem worse, as it could provide a moist culture medium for pathogenic microorganisms.

559. c) "Malignant" external otitis was first reported in 1968. The mortality still approaches 50%. The disease occurs mostly in diabetics and persons taking immunosuppressive medications. It begins as an insidious, rather benign indolent infection that is refractory to usual treatment. Granulation tissue soon appears, and deep spaces are seen in the external canal. Pain becomes steady in nature, and the cellulitis and chondritis lead to an avascular osteitis. Without aggressive, appropriate therapy, the infection can progress through the temporal bone and cause facial nerve paralysis, involve the skull base and tha cranial nerves IX through XII, spread to the opposite side, or cause meningitis, brain abscess, and death.

Reference

Bell D. Otitis externa. Postgraduate Medicine 1985; 78(3): 101-106.

PROBLEM #87: A PATIENT COMPLAINING OF DIZZINESS

Questions 560-571 consist of a matching question related to the dizzy patient. Choose the lettered option that most closely fits the numbered description. Each lettered option may be used once, more than once, or not at all.

560. The most common brain stem vascular disorder with vertigo as a prominent symptom.

561. A 35 year old patient with vertigo, blurred vision, transient weakness of both legs, hyperreflexia and inco-ordination of gait.

562. A 20 year old patient with vertigo, loss of consciousness and amnesia for the attack.

563. A 25 year old patient with vertigo, dysphagia, a throbbing occipital headache, and nausea and vomiting.

564. A 30 year old patient with a respiratory tract infection, vertigo, and nausea and vomiting.

565. A 25 year old patient who experiences vertigo when he turns his head to the right.

566. A middle-aged patient with episodic vertigo, fluctuating sensorineural hearing loss and tinnitus.

567. A 30 year old patient with a respiratory tract infection, vertigo, tinnitus and hearing loss.

568. A 55 year old patient with pneumonia who develops vertigo, tinnitus and hearing loss when he is placed on intravenous penicillin and gentamicin.

569. A 70 year old patient who feels faint and develops a dimness of vision and a roaring in the ears when she gets out of bed in the morning.

570. An elderly male with a shuffling gait, disequilibrium and impaired balance.

571. A 20 year old male who experiences vague light-headedness when he gets anxious.

   a) vertebral-basilar migraine
   b) benign paroxsymal positional vertigo
   c) labyrinthine apoplexy
   d) Meniere's disease
   e) vertebro-basilar insufficiency
   f) orthostatic hypotension
   g) hyperventilation syndrome
   h) viral labyrinthitis
   i) vestibular neuronitis
   j) Parkinson's disease
   k) cerebellar hemorrhage
   l) epilepsy
   m) toxic labyrinthitis
   n) Wallenberg's syndrome
   o) multiple sclerosis

ANSWERS

The purpose of this series of questions is to appreciate how to classify the complaint of dizziness and to realize the number of different disorders that may have true vertigo as a symptom. When a patient presents to the office with a complaint of dizziness, the first thing to do is to have him (her) describe the symptoms without using the word "dizzy". The description at this time will usually classify dizziness as:

   1) Vague light-headedness
   2) Vertigo (a definite rotational sensation or hallucination of motion)
   3) Faintness (snycope)
   4) Disequilibrium (impaired balance)

The differential diagnosis of true vertigo involves most of the syndromes described below.

560. n) The most common brain stem vascular disorder with vertigo as a pro-
     minent symptom is Wallenberg's syndrome (the lateral medullary syndrome).
     Wallenberg's syndrome results from obstruction of the posterior inferior
     cerebellar artery or the vertebral artery itself. Suspect this disorder when a
     patient presents with the following constellation of symptoms:

   a) vertigo, nausea, vomiting and nystagmus resulting from involvement of
      vestibular nuclei.
   b) ataxia and falling to the side of the body in which the lesion is located
   c) loss of facial sensation to pain and temperature on the side of the lesion
      and also over the opposite side of the body

d) dysphagia and ipsilateral paralysis of the palate and vocal cords

e) Horner's syndrome — ipsilateral ptosis, miosis, and decreased facial sweating due to involvement of the descending sympathetic tract

561. o) Vertigo is the initial complaint in about 7-10% of patients with multiple sclerosis; eventually vertigo appears in approximately one-third of those with the disease. Commonly the patient complains of vague unsteadiness or mild vertigo, which may be exacerbated by head movement.

562. l) Epilepsy should come to mind when a patient loses consciousness during an attack of vertigo. This is most commonly encountered with temperal lobe epilepsy. A history of brief absence or staring spells, automatism and belligerent behavior, amnesia for the attack, failure to respond when addressed though apparently aware, an unusual sense of familiarity (deja vu), a sense of strangeness or remoteness (jamais vu), facial grimacing, lip smacking and chewing movements may all indicate temporal lobe epilepsy.

563. a) When vertigo is followed by a throbbing occipital headache, nausea and vomiting, suspect vertebral-basilar migraine. Typically, the patient reports an aura-most commonly diffuse scintillating scotomas or homonymous hemianopsia, although dysphagia, hemiparesis, paresthesias and visual blurring may occur.

564. i) A patient with a recent history of a bacterial or viral infection and the sudden onset of severe vertigo and gastrointestinal symptoms point to vestibular neuronitis. Episodes of vertigo in the patient with vestibular neuronitis generally are more severe than vertigo due to benign positional vertigo; in addition, the person with vestibular neuronitis almost always has nausea and vomiting. Vestibular neuronitis differs from Meniere's disease in that tinnitus and deafness are absent, and the single episode of severe vertigo generally endures for 3-6 days rather than 30 minutes to 3 hours.

565. b) A patient who experiences vertigo when he turns his head or changes position probably has benign paroxsymal positional vertigo. In this case the vertigo occurs only when the head is in a "critical position", as opposed to occurring when the patient rises from a sitting or recumbent position, which is indicative of orthostatic hypotension caused by cerebral ischemia. In benign paroxsymal positional vertigo, symptoms may occur when the patient lays down, turns over in bed, moves his head quickly to the right or left or tilts it back. The vertigo typically begins after a latent period of 2-20 seconds (no more than 1 minute) and then completely subsides. The patient may also become pale and experience nausea and vomiting.

566. d) A patient between the age of 30 and 60 who presents with the symptom triad of episodic vertigo, fluctuating sensorineural hearing loss and tinnitus probably has Meniere's diasease. The patient may also report pressure or fullness in the involved ear. Although the patient's chief complaint is often that of violent rotatory vertigo accompanied by nausea and vomiting, the other symptoms of Meniere's disease may precede vertigo by months or years. In patients with early Meniere's disease deafness is primarly for low tones. As the disease progresses and fluctuation in deafness decreases, hearing loss most often is for high tones.

567. h) A patient with a recent history of a viral infection and the sudden onset of severe vertigo and gastrointestinal symptoms accompanied by tinnitus and hearing loss probably has acute viral labyrinthisits. The differientation between this condition and vestibular neuronitis is made on the presence or absence of tinnitus and hearing loss.

568. m) Any patient who experiences vertigo with nausea, vomiting, tinnitus and hearing loss and who is presently or has recently been on any of the ototoxic substances including aminoglycoside antibiotics; tetracycline antibiotics; anticonvulsants such as phenytoin; barbiturates; diuretics such as furosemide or ethacrynic acid; quinidine; salicylates or sedative hypnotics should be suspected of having acute toxic labyrinthitis. The appropriate substance should immediately be discontinued.

569. f) A patient who complains of faintness, especially when they assume the upright position or who have been in the upright position for some time and who complain of dimness of vision, a roaring in the ear and diaphoresis with recovery when they assume the recumbent position probably has orthostatic hypotension. Orthostatic hypotension is often caused by medication including many of the antihypertensive agents, the major tranquillizers and the tricyclic antidepressants.

570. j) An elderly patient who complains of disequilibrium and impaired balance and who in addition has any of a shuffling gait, cog-wheel rigidity, bradykinesia, or a resting tremor should be suspected of having Parkinson's disease.

571. g) A patient who experiences vague lightheadedness when he is anxious is probably hyperventilating. Asking him to place a paper bag over his head will probably abolish the symptoms.

Reference

Burton R, Frederic M, Pulec J and Rubin W. Evaluating Complaints of Dizziness. Patient Care 1981; 15(10): 23-61.

PROBLEM #88: A 20 YEAR OLD MALE WITH A RED EYE

572. A 20 year old male presents with a localized, solidly bloody red eye. You make a diagnosis of subconjunctival hemorrhage. You should now:

    a) hospitalize the patient for 7-10 days
    b) refer the patient to an opthalmologist for immediate surgery
    c) begin oral amoxicillin 500 mg. q.i.d.
    d) begin topical sulfacetamide 10% solution q.i.d.
    e) reassure the patient that it will resolve in 1-3 weeks on its own

573. The most frequent cause of conjunctivitis is:

    a) bacterial infection
    b) viral infection
    c) allergy
    d) exposure to toxin
    e) autoimmune reaction

CODE: (a:1, 2 and 3; b: 1 and 3; c: 2 and 4; d: 4 only; e: all of the above)

574. Which of the following symptoms is/are usually seen in acute iridocyclitis?

    1) blurred vision
    2) pain
    3) photophobia
    4) discharge

575. In which of the following conditions is the hyperemia of a red eye most prominent around the cornea (ciliary or circumcorneal flush)?

    1) conjunctivitis
    2) keratitis
    3) acute narrow-angle glaucoma
    4) iridocyclitis

576. Which of the following symptoms is/are commonly seen with conjunctivitis?

    1) blurred vision
    2) intense pain
    3) photophobia
    4) discharge

577. Which of the following statements is/are TRUE about episcleritis and scleritis?

   1) episcleritis is an acute inflammation of the subconjunctival episcleral tissues
   2) pain is a prominent feature and may be incapacitating in episcleritis
   3) scleritis is usually associated with systemic diseases such as rheumatoid arthritis and other connective tissue disorders
   4) scleritis causes a severe inflammation, and the affected area usually has a bluish-violaceous discoloration

ANSWERS

572. e) Rupture of a conjunctival vessel causes a localized, solidly bloody red eye. This hemorrhage is benign, although its appearance often alarms the patient. It requires no treatment and resolves spontaneously in one-three weeks.

573. b) Viral infection is the most frequent cause of conjunctivitis. A number of viruses have been implicated as etiologic agents. They include adenovirus types 3, 7, 8, 11, and 19 and herpesviruses and enteroviruses. The disease is often preceeded by an upper respiratory tract infection or flu-like illness. Conjunctival hyperemia, eyelid edema and a serous or seropurulent discharge are usually present. A palpable preauricular node, usually present in viral conjunctivitis, is an important sign in differientating this disease from bacterial infection. Viral conjunctivitis, though self-limited, may be treated with the same agents recommended for bacterial conjunctivitis to prevent superinfection. The treatment of choice is 10-15% sulfacetamide or gentamicin drops q.i.d.

   Bacterial infections, allergies and exposure to toxic agents are also common causes of conjunctivitis. An autoimmune reaction will rarely cause conjunctivitis; usually autoimmune reactions are associated with more serious eye pathology.

574. a) See critique of question #575.

575. c) A ciliary or circumcorneal flush occurs in both keratitis and acute iridocyclitis. Keratitis, an inflammation of the cornea is generally a very painful condition, and causes significant blurring of vision and photophobia. The corneal epithelial surface is irregular and lacks its normal luster. This lack of luster is easy to detect on inspection of the cornea with oblique illumination from a slit-lamp or pen light. Epithelial disruption may also be detected by staining the cornea with a sterile fluorescene strip and then illuminating it with a cobalt-blue light. Corneal ulcers may be associated with keratitis. These ulcers may be bacterial, viral or fungal. Viral and fungal corneal ulcers generally worsen with the administration of topical corticosteroids. There-

fore, if the diagnosis is uncertain the use of medications containing topical corticosteroids should be avoided. A broad-spectrum topical antibiotic should be administered until specific sensitivity studies are received.

Acute iridocyclitis is a serious but uncommon cause of the red eye. Most forms of iridocyclitis are thought to be immune-related reactions, and they may accompany systemic diseases such as juvenile rheumatoid arthritis and many of the collagen vascular disorders. Iridocyclitis is typically unilateral. The patient complains of pain, severe photophobia and blurred vision. The hyperemia is most often circumcorneal. The pupil is often small or irregular. Fine, white, cellular deposits (keratitic precipitates) may be seen on the posterior surface of the cornea with a slit lamp. Management of iridocyclitis includes the administration of topical cycloplegics and topical and/or systemic corticosteroids. When acute iridocyclitis is neglected, complications include posterior synechiae, secondary glaucoma, cataracts and corneal decompensation.

Acute angle closure glaucoma occurs when the root of the iris closes off the anterior chamber angle, obstructing aqueous outflow from the eye. The patient notes sudden onset of blurred vision due to corneal edema, severe ocular or periorbital pain and frequently nausea and vomiting. On examination, the eye appears red and the pupil is moderately dilated and not light reactive. A shallow anterior chamber and a red eye should always alert the physician to the possibility of acute narrow-angle glaucoma. The hallmark of glaucoma is increased intraocular pressure which can be easily measured with a Schiotz tonometer. Narrow-angle glaucoma is a serious disease, and an untreated attack may quickly lead to blindness in the affected eye. Treatment is directed toward lowering the intraocular pressure, which may be accomplished by intravenous mannitol and the administration of a topical miotic. Patients resistant to medical treatment require emergency surgical intervention in order to restore normal aqueous outflow.

576. d) Conjunctivitis rarely causes significant blurred vision, intense pain or photophobia. Patients may complain of scratchiness or mild irritation, but never severe pain. The presence of severe pain almost always indicates a more serious eye disease. Discharge with both viral and bacterial conjunctivitis is common. Ideally, this discharge whould be cultured and treatment based on the result of this culture.

577. e) Episcleritis is an acute inflammation of the subconjunctival episcleral tissues. It causes localized conjunctival hyperemia, and the patient complains of photophobia, tearing and exquisite tenderness to palpation. Episcleritis may also be accompanied by iritis. Although it is usually self-limited, episcleritis may become very painful and incapacitating. Treatment consists mainly of topical corticosteroids and management of any accompanying iritis.

Scleritis is usually associated with systemic diseases such as rheumatoid arthritis and other connective tissue diseases. It causes a severe inflammation, and the affected eye usually has a bluish-red violaceous discoloration. The pain is severe and increases with eye movement. Both corticosteroids and non-steroidal anti-inflammatory agents have been used to decrease the inflammation. Scleral grafts are sometimes necessary if the scleral coat becomes thin.

Reference

Whitman J, Cunningham R. The Red Eye. Postgraduate Medicin 1983; 74(5): 65-71.

PROBLEM #89: A 31 YEAR OLD PHYSICIAN WITH A LACERATION

577. A 31 year old physician presents to the emergency room with a laceration to his left hand. As a physician he is interested in the healing of his laceration. He asks you which event is the FIRST to occur in the healing of a laceration by primary intention. You reply:

   a) epithelialization
   b) binding of the wound by red and white blood cells
   c) fibroblastic proliferation and capillary ingrowth
   d) collagen synthesis
   e) collagen remodeling

578. At what time interval after initial repair is the tensile strength or resistance to lengthwise stress sufficient to hold the edges of a wound together without sutures?

   a) 3 days
   b) 5 days
   c) 7 days
   d) 10 days
   e) 14 days

579. Which of the following is an ABSOLUTE CONTRAINDICATION to closure of a laceration with sutures?

   a) signs of inflammation (rubor, calor, tumor and dolor)
   b) time interval since injury of greater than 12 hours
   c) a contaminated wound
   d) allergy to lidocaine
   e) diabetes mellitus

580. Which of the following sutures will produce the LEAST amount of cellular reaction?

   a) nonabsorbable silk
   b) nonabsorbable cotton
   c) absorbable polyglycolic acid
   d) nonabsorbable polypropylene
   e) absorbable polygalactin 9-10

581. Which of the following is the MOST IMPORTANT factor contributing to the formation of suture marks?

    a) quantity and type of dermal appendages at the site of injury
    b) formation of micro-stitch abscesses by low-grade skin contaminants
    c) intrinsic tension
    d) extrinsic tension
    e) needle size

ANSWERS

577. b) The healing process has three confluent phases. In the initial, or lag phase, a fibrous network of red and white blood cells is established. These cells bind the wound edges together during the first two days after injury. Epithelialization, which is the first true evidence of repair, begins about 12 hours after injury. During days three to five, fibroplasia, the second phase of healing, results in fibroblastic proliferation and capillary ingrowth. Coverage of the narrow gap between the wound edges is accomplished by means of epithelial proliferation and migration. The final, or maturation phase, involves collagen synthesis and remodeling. Although biochemical studies show that collagen synthesis occurs between days 3 and 4, the physical evidence of this synthesis does not appear until the fourth to sixth day. Collagen content increases rapidly between the 6th and 17th days and ceases after about 42 days. Therefore, except for a very short period at the beginning of healing, the gain in wound strength is due primarily to remodeling of collagen rather than to total collagen content.

578. c) At one week, tensile strength or resistance to lengthwise stress is sufficient to hold the edges of the wound together without sutures. Tensile strength is gained rapidly for the next 17 days and then more slowly for an additional 10 days. Thereafter, the gain is constant, although almost imperceptible, for several years.

579. a) Any sign of inflammation (rubor, calor, tumor and dolor) is an ABSO-LUTE CONTRAINDICATION to closure of a laceration with sutures. Closure in the presence of inflammation will result in non-healing of the wound in addition to an increase in the inflammation itself.

    Time interval greater than 12 hours since injury is a relative contraindication to wound closure with sutures.

    In patients allergic to lidocaine another local anaesthetic can be used.

    A contaminated wound should be cleaned thoroughly before closure but when clean does not present a contraindication to closure.

    Although diabetes mellitus impairs wound healing and results in a longer period of time necessary for complete healing, it is not in itself a contraindication to surgical closure.

580. d) The type of suture used greatly influences the amount of tissue reaction. All absorbable sutures produce a cellular reaction and therefore are not appropriate for skin closure.

Nonabsorbable sutures vary considerably in the amount of cellular reaction that they induce. Silk and cotton produce the greatest reaction; whereas polypropylene and steel create the least. In uninfected wounds the reaction is microscopic and is important only in areas close to or within the skin. In the presence of infection, however, the reaction is significant, and the sutures should be removed.

581. c) Suture marks are actually areas of scar tissue that show all the histologic features of incisional scars. Several factors may contribute to their formation including the quantity and type of dermal appendages at the site of injury, the formation of micro-stitch abscesses and an inherited tendency toward keloid formation. Cleansing the sutures of blood and fibrous debris during the first 24 hours and applying a water-soluble emollient may minimize microstitch abscesses. Generally, nonabsorbable suture materials produce less in the way of suture marks than absorbable materials.

Intrinsic tension, or the relationship between a suture's tightness and the masses of tissue it encompasses, appears to be the major cause of suture marks. Scar formation is the result of increased local pressure and ischemia. Suture tightness is caused by local edema and by the application of excessive force during suturing. The farther from the skin edge the suture is placed, or the larger the mass included within the suture, the greater the force required to approximate the tissue edges. Larger gauge sutures have more tensile strength; this allows for the application of greater pressure during wound closure and thus a greater tendency to suture marks. Instead, fine, nonabsorbable monofilament sutures with a low reactivity should be used for epidermal alignment approximation.

Extrinsic tension, or the force applied to the cut edges of the wound is greatly influenced by the tension on the wound edges, the size of the tissue gap and the relationship of the wound to the relaxed skin tension lines. Undermining wound edges releases edge tension and allows for more relaxed wounds. Wounds that parallel relaxed skin tension lines result in less obvious scars than those that lie at right angles to the same lines.

Except for tension, the previously mentioned factors that contribute to suture marks are not always controllable. Of the factors that are directly under the surgeon's control-namely needle size, suture size and the length of time the sutures remain in the wound needle size and suture size have no effect. However, the length of time that the sutures remain in place is very important. Sutures that remain in place for more than 14 days will produce the most severe marks, whereas those that are removed within seven days will leave no appreciable marks.

Reference

Rappaport N. Laceration repair. American Family Physician 1985; 30(4): 115-123.

PROBLEM #90: A 57 YEAR OLD MALE WITH A DECREASED URINARY STREAM

582. A 57 year old male presents with a 6 month history of nocturia, hesitancy, and slow stream. On rectal examination the prostate gland is enlarged, feels "rubbery" and has lost it's median sulcus. The most likely diagnosis is:

a) benign prostatic hypertrophy
b) low grade carcinoma of the prostate
c) high grade carcinoma of the prostate
d) carcinoma of the bladder with posterior extension
e) chronic prostatitis

583. The treatment of choice for a patient with symptomatic benign prostatic hypertrophy is:

a) urethral dilatation
b) suprapubic prostatectomy
c) radical prostatectomy
d) transurethral prostatectomy
e) urecholine by mouth

584. The major complication of benign prostatic hypertrophy is:

a) carcinoma of the prostate
b) chronic prostatitis
c) obstruction to the outflow of the bladder
d) chronic pyelonephritis
e) bladder calculi

585. A 69 year old patient presents to the office with a 6 month history of frequency, hestitancy, and nocturia. On physical examination the prostate is enlarged, firm and irregular. The next step in the investigation should be:

a) cystoscopy
b) transurethral resection of the prostate
c) observation and reassessment in 6 months
d) needle biopsy of the prostate
e) radical prostatectomy

586. A 73 year old patient with a biopsy proven adenocarcinoma of the prostate appears to be stage B-2. Investigations including liver function tests, bone scan and CT scan of the pelvis are normal. The next step should be:

a) lymphangiography
b) external radiotherapy to the prostate and pelvis
c) staging lymphadenectomy
d) total body monoclonal antibody scan
e) radical prostatectomy

587. The most important screening test for carcinoma of the prostate is:

    a) acid phosphatase level
    b) monoclonal antibody scan
    c) bone scan
    d) cystoscopy and biopsy
    e) digital rectal exam

CODE: (a:1, 2 and 3; b: 1 and 3; c: 2 and 4; d: 4 only; e: all of the above)

588. Which of the following statements about carcinoma of the prostate is/are CORRECT?

    1) carcinoma of the prostate is the second leading cause of cancer-related deaths in men
    2) carcinoma of the prostate is the most common cause of death in men over the age of 60 years
    3) in clinical stage A-1, no treatment is necessary
    4) 10-30% of all males over the age of 50 years have prostatic carcinoma

ANSWERS

582. a) In men older than age 50, benign adenomatous hyperplasia of the prostate is common and causes different degrees of frequency, urgency and nocturia. Findings on rectal examination can at times be misleading — for example, a prostate that seems small on digital examination may be large enough to cause urethral obstruction. Usually the gland is enlarged, feels "rubbery", and may have lost the median sulcus, or "furrow". Benign prostatic hypertrophy is usually graded on a scale from 1-4. Grade 1 enlargement is slight hyperplasia and grade 4 enlargement is extreme hyperplasia. Although carcinoma of the prostate may be found in any prostate gland, there is no cause and effect relationship between benign prostatic hypertrophy and prostatic carcinoma. In chronic prostatitis, the prostate gland will be slightly tender, and soft and boggy to the touch. Carcinoma of the bladder with posterior extension will not present as an enlarged prostate gland, but rather with irritative bladder symptoms and hematuria.

583. d) The treatment of choice for a patient with benign prostatic hypertrophy is transurethral resection. Transurethral resection is well accepted by patients because it requires no incision and has a low morbidity and mortality rate. Greater degrees of benign hypertrophy may be treated with open surgery via a suprapubic approach. Urethral dilatation and urecholine will not relieve the obstructive symptoms of benign prostatic hypertrophy.

584. c) Obstruction of the outflow of urine from the bladder is the major complication of benign prostatic hypertrophy. Obstruction is manifested by such symptoms as slow stream, dribbling, hesitancy and nocturia. This can lead to acute urinary retention. Bladder calculi and chronic urinary tract infection can result from prostatic hypertrophy and obstruction. Chronic pyelonephritis may result from chronic urinary tract infection. Chronic prostatitis and carcinoma of the prostate are not associated with benign prostatic hypertrophy.

585. d) The patient with an enlarged, firm and irregular prostate has adenocarcinoma of the prostate until proven otherwise. A needle biopsy of the prostate is the diagnostic procedure of choice. Neither transurethral resection or radical prostatectomy should be undertaken until a specific diagnosis is made. Although cystoscopy will show the degree of anterior prostatic enlargement, it will not make a specific diagnosis. Observation and reassessment in 6 months would result in needless delay if the patient has prostatic carcinoma.

586. c) Stage B-2 carcinoma of the prostate is defined as tumor that is confined to the prostrate but involving more than one lobe, or a tumor greater than 1.5 cm in diameter. However, even with CT scanning, lymphangiography and sonography occult lymph node deposits will not be detected. It has been shown that 35% of patients with stage B-2 carcinoma will have lymph node metastasis at the time of surgery. Therefore, the acceptable method of diagnosing nodal metastasis is pelvic lymphadenectomy.

    Monoclonal antibody scans are being developed. This may prove to be a very useful screening test. The treatment of choice for stage A-2, B-1 and B-2 adenocarcinoma of the prostate is external beam radiation to the pelvis and prostate. Some authorities are also treating stage C (cancer extending outside the capsule) and stage D-1 (regional lymph node metastasis) by external radiation. Stage D-2 (distant metastasis) is treated by estrogens or anti-gonadotrophic agents and orchidectomy on a palliative basis.

587. e) Digital rectal examination remains the most important screening test for carcinoma of the prostate. All men over the age of 45 years should have an annual rectal examination. Studies have shown that fewer than 50% of men undergoing annual physical examinations have their prostates palpated. With earlier diagnosis, many tumors could be detected in the B-1 stage, in which a tumor involves only one lobe and which is less than 1.5 cm in diameter.

    The acid phosphatase level will only be elevated and the bone scan positive when the patient has metastic disease and thus these are not good screening tests for early disease. The monoclonal antibody scan may in the future become an important screening test.

    Cystoscopy and biopsy are invasive and very cost-ineffective as a screening test.

588.   e) Cancer of the prostate is the second leading cause of cancer-related deaths in men overall, and the most common cause of cancer death in men over age 60. Clinical stage A-1 disease is disease that is detected on routine transurethral resection for benign prostatic hypertrophy. It carries an excellent prognosis and usually does not require any treatment, unless the focus is poorly differientiated. Ten to thirty percent of all males over the age of 50 years in the United States have prostatic carcinoma. Most of these have asymptomatic stage A-1 disease that does not require treatment.

References

Ahmann, F. Dilemmas in managing prostate carcinoma: localized disease. Modern Medicine of Canada 1985; 40(12): 1156-1162.
Chesley A. Prostatic cancer: The neglected diagnosis. Diagnosis 1985; 2(2): 46-57.

PROBLEM #91: A 25 YEAR OLD MALE WITH FLANK PAIN

589. A 25 year old male presents to the emergency room with an abrupt onset of right sided flank pain. You suspect renal colic. The most common kidney stone causing renal colic is composed of:

a) calcium oxalate
b) mixed calcium oxalate/calcium phosphate
c) calcium phosphate
d) struvite
e) uric acid

590. The most important component of the diagnostic workup in a patient with a kidney stone is:

a) serum calcium/serum uric acid
b) serum creatinine
c) intravenous pyelogram
d) 24-hour urine for creatinine clearance, volume, calcium, uric acid, oxalate and sodium
e) serum parathyroid hormone

591. The upper limits of normal for the excretion of calcium and uric acid in the urine/24 hours in men are:

a) 300 mg calcium, 300 mg uric acid
b) 800 mg calcium, 300 mg uric acid
c) 300 mg calcium, 800 mg uric acid
d) 150 mg calcium, 500 mg uric acid
e) 1000 mg calcium, 500 mg uric acid

592. The drug of choice for idiopathic hypercalciuria is:

a) cellulose sodium phosphate
b) orthophosphates
c) potassium citrate
d) a thiazide diuretic
e) pyridoxine

593. Substances that cause urinary alkalization such as sodium bicarbonate and/or sodium citrate are helpful in the treatment of which of the following urinary stones?

a) calcium oxalate
b) mixed calcium oxalate/calcium phosphate
c) uric acid
d) calcium phosphate
e) struvite

CODE: (a:1, 2 and 3; b: 1 and 3; c: 2 and 4; d: 4 only; e: all of the above)

594. A 25 year old male presents with acute renal colic. The IVP shows blockage just distal to the renal calcyx. Large doses of narcotic analgesics are necesary to control the pain. The treatment(s) of choice if this stone does not pass spontaneously is:

   1) percutaneous ultrasonic lithotripsy
   2) nephrolithotomy
   3) electrohydraulic disintegration
   4) extracorporeal shock wave lithotripsy

595. Which of the following is/are indications for a complete metabolic workup in a patient with renal colic?

   1) recurrent stone formation
   2) positive family history of stones
   3) age of onset < 20 years
   4) single episode of renal colic

596. A 45 year old male is found to have significant hypercalciuria after two episodes of renal colic. Which of the following general measures would be appropriate in this patient?

   1) increase fluid intake to 2 litres/day
   2) restriction of oxalate containing foods
   3) avoidance of supplementary vitamin D
   4) severe restriction of calcium containing foods

ANSWERS

589. a) Calcium oxalate stones are the most common type of kidney stones; they comprise 60%. Other stones in order of frequency are mixed calcium oxalate and calcium phosphate, uric acid, struvite, and cystine.

590. d) The 24-hour urine collection is the most informative and critical part of the workup for kidney stones. The 24-hour urine should include creatinine clearance, volume, calcium, uric acid, oxalate, sodium, and perhaps cystine. Serum levels of electrolytes, calcium, phosphorus, uric acid, creatinine, urea nitrogen and parathyroid hormone should be determined, but abnormalities in the values are much less common than an abnormal 24 hour urine.

   Intravenous pyelography is important in evaluation of stone passage in an acute episode or to document the presence of radiolucent stones or obstruction, but otherwise is of little use in following formers of non-uric acid stones. Analysis of a second-voided morning specimen should be done to check concentrating ability and pH. Low specific gravity suggests a renal disorder or renal damage. A pH greater than 6 or 7 may either indicate lack of normal renal acidification or be a clue to infection with urea-splitting organisms. The urine should also be examined for crystals, including calcium oxalate, uric acid, cystine and triple phosphate.

591. c) The upper limits of calcium and uric acid in males and females respectively in a 24-hour urine are:
calcium 300 mg, uric acid 800 mg (male)
calcium 250 mg, uric acid 750 mg (female)

592. d) Thiazide diuretics are the agents of choice for the treatment of idiopathic hypercalciuria not responsive to conservative measures such as avoidance of calcium gluttony. They are effective and safe when used judiciously. Average daily dose is usually in the range of 50 mg./day of hydrochlorothiazide.
Cellulose sodium phosphate may be used in patients with hyperabsorptive hypercalciuria; however it tends to bind magnesium and other trace elements and interfere with their absorption. Orthophosphates may be used in hypercalciuria associated with a low phosphorus level but diarrhea is a limiting factor. Potassium citrate and pyridoxine are not indicated in the treatment of hypercalciuria.

593. c) Substances that cause urinary alkalinization such as sodium bicarbonate and/or sodium citrate and citric acid are helpful in formers of uric acid stones, particularly during acute episodes of stone passage when a high urine pH may actually dissolve such stones. The drug of choice in patients with hyperuricouria is allopurinol, which is an inhibitor of xanthine oxidase.

594. c) If available, the treatment of choice is extracorporeal shock wave lithotripsy. This technique is especially useful for the primary management of kidney stone disease in the upper urinary tract. In this technique, two shock wave generators are focused on the calculus by means of two separate X-ray monitors. The shock wave is conducted through a water bath in which the patient is immersed and through the water in the body tissues themselves. The energy released by a series of pulsed shocks disintegrates the calculus. Seventy percent of stones in the upper urinary tract can be removed by this method.
Nephrolithotomy can be carried out if extracorporeal shock wave lithotripsy is not available. Electrohydraulic disintegration in which an electric shock wave is conducted through a dilute saline medium is accomplished with a fexible nephroscope passed through a percutaneous nephrostomy tract. It can be performed if a calculi is not readily accessible in the upper ureter or calyx.
Percutaneous ultrasonic lithotripsy, in which ultrasonic energy is placed in direct contact with the stone, again through a nephroscope, can also be used in this situation.

595. a) Since 40% of stone formers never have a second episode and since stone passage is rarely life-threatening, persuing a metabolic workup in all cases does not make good medical sense. The criteria for a selective approach to metabolic investigation of stone formers are listed below:

1) recurrent stone formers
2) positive family history of kidney stones
3) history of major stone complication
4) solitary kidney
5) age of onset < 20 years
6) an associated disorder predisposing to stone formation
   a) renal tubular acidosis
   b) infection with urea-splitting bacteria
   c) malabsorption syndrome

A single episode of renal colic does not warrant a metabolic workup.

596. a) Recommended general measures for recurrent stone formers or patients with idiopathic hypercalciuria include increased fluid intake (aimed at 2 litres/day); restriction of foods high in oxalate such as spinach, colas, brewed tea and rhubarb; and avoidance of supplemental vitamin D.

Decreased calcium intake cannot be recommended except in cases of calcium gluttony. Calcium normally binds to oxalate in the intestines, and decreased availability of intestinal calcium can result in increased oxalate absorption. Therefore, in theory, calcium restriction may paradoxically exacerbate a tendency toward calcium oxalate stone formation.

Reference

Kanig S, Conn R. Kidney Stones. Postgraduate Medicine 1985; 78(6): 38-51.

PROBLEM #92: A 28 YEAR OLD MALE WITH CHRONIC BACK PAIN

A 28 year old male with chronic low back pain presents to the office. He has previously been seen by a chiropractor, a physiotherapist, a hypnotist, 3 family physicians and 2 orthopedic surgeons.

Questions 597-600 are TRUE and FALSE questions about chronic low back pain. If the statement is TRUE mark (a), if it is FALSE, mark (b).

597. Chronic low back pain ranks second to alcoholism as a reason for absenteeism from work.

598. Chronic low back pain can be defined as back pain lasting for a period longer than 1 year.

599. Psychological methods are important in treating patients with chronic low back pain.

600. The single most important ingredient in determining a successful treatment program for chronic low back patients is patient education.

Select the single best answer to the following question:

601. The most common cause of chronic low back pain is:

    a) trauma
    b) degenerative processes
    c) congenital deformity
    d) inflammatory disease
    e) emotional disturbances

CODE: (a:1, 2 and 3; b: 1 and 3; c: 2 and 4; d: 4 only; e: all of the above)

602. Which of the following laboratory investigations should be done on every patient that presents with chronic low back pain?

    1) urinalysis
    2) serum calcium and phosphorus
    3) erythrocyte sedimentation rate
    4) serum alkaline phosphatase

603. Which of the following medications is/are appropriate for use in patients with chronic low back pain?

   1) acetaminophen
   2) acetaminophen with codeine
   3) amitriptyline
   4) pentazocine

604. Which of the following treatment has a role in the treatment of patients with chronic low back pain?

   1) back supports
   2) physical therapy
   3) injection therapy
   4) transcutaneous nerve stimulation

605. Which of the following is/are characteristic of chronic low back pain?

   1) a single treatment will rarely cure it
   2) the patient often has unrealistic expectations of treatment
   3) the doctor often has unrealistic goals of treatment
   4) medications are often taken inappropriately by the patient

ANSWERS

597. a) (TRUE) Chronic low back pain is a major cause of absenteeism. In 1980, the National Safety Council in the United States established chronic low back pain (CLO-BAP) as the second most frequent reason for missed work days. It ranks next to alcoholism in this regard.

598. b) (FALSE) Chronic low back pain can be defined as back pain lasting for a period of time longer than 3 months; as a recurrence of previous back pain; or as a result of a complication of treatment.

599. a) (TRUE) Psychological methods are important in treating patients with chronic low back pain. The use of the Minnesota Multiphasic Inventory test has indicated that there is a typical "triad" of hypochondriasis, depression and hysteria in many chronic back pain patients.

600. a) (TRUE) The most important ingredient in determining a successful treatment program for chronic low back patients is patient education. When patients begin to comprehend the anatomical and physiological aspects of pain, the treatment is enhanced and prognosis improves. Commonly, the patients have had little insight into the problem and have indulged for long periods in a wide variety of treatments, medications, and devices without any understanding of what these pain therapies are supposed to accomplish.

601. b) The most common cause of chronic low back pain is degenerative disease such as osteoarthritis of the spine and hip joints, spinal stenosis, and disc degeneration.

Other causes include (1) congenital problems such as spondylolysis and spondylolisthesis; (2) trauma such as ligamentous muscle and joints strains, dislocations and fractures; (3) inflammatory conditions such as ankylosing spondylitis and rheumatoid arthritis; (4) tumors; (5) metabolic problems such as osteoporosis, gout, and Paget's disease; (6) endocrine problems such as hyperparathyroidism; (7) neurologic nerve root compression; (8) ischemia of neural elements; (9) scar formation from previous surgery; (10) emotional problems such as psychoneurosis; (11) scoliosis; and (12) visceral problems such as pelvic inflammatory disease and aortic aneursym.

602. e) Urinalysis may show Bence-Jones protein, indicative of multiple myeloma. The following blood chemistry determinations should be done to rule out these conditions: calcium and phosphorus for hyperparathyroidism, human leukocyte antigen-B27 for ankylosing spondylitis, erythrocyte sedimentation rate for inflammatory or infectious processes, uric acid for gout, and alkaline phosphatase for metastatic bone disease.

603. b) Acetaminophen, aspirin, other non-steroidal anti-inflammatory agents and tricyclic antidepressants such as amitriptyline are appropriate agents for the treatment of chronic pain. Narcotic agents such as codeine and pentazocine should generally not be used.

Those patients who are taking narcotic agents should be detoxified. Experience suggests that chronic pain patients are easily detoxified because they are psychologically addicted rather than physically addicted. Subsequent use of amitriptyline or doxepin has proven to be a good substitute for past indiscriminate use of narcotic drugs for pain.

604. e) The treatment of chronic low back pain is multidisciplinary. The goal of treatment of chronic low back pain is to treat all physical, emotional and socioecomonic elements at the same time. The treatment regime may involve (1) analgesic and antidepressant medications; (2) physical therapy emphasizing both flexion and extension exercises; (3) steroid injection therapy; (4) back support devices; (5) psychological therapies including behavior modification, relaxation techniques, hypnotherapy, biofeedback, and desensitization; and (6) vogue therapies such as transcutaneous nerve stimulation, acupuncture and facet denervation by thermocoagulation.

605. e) The characteristics of chronic low back pain can best be explained as a series of rules. If it is chronic low back pain:

a) it is rare that a single treatment will cure it
b) there is usually a psychological factor involved
c) that has not responded to appropriate treatment, there is seldom a "certain" cause for it
d) and a spinal surgical procedure has been performed previously, there is only a 30% chance that additional spinal surgery will be of major help
e) and two or more surgical spinal procedures have been performed, there is only a 5% chance of success if additional surgery is performed
f) the patient will almost certainly have taken medications inappropriately
g) the patient will usually have unrealistic expectations of treatment results
h) the doctor will usually have unrealistic goals of treatment results

Reference

Addison R. Chronic Low Back Pain (CLO-BAP). The Clinical Journal of Pain 1985; 1: 50-59.

PROBLEM #93: A 79 YEAR OLD FEMALE WITH A SORE FOOT

606. A 79 year old female presents to the office with a sore right foot. On examination, you diagnose a bunion deformity. The most common cause of bunion deformity is:

   a) trauma
   b) neurovascular disease
   c) hypermobility of the first metatarsal-phalangeal unit in an adducted forefoot
   d) osteoarthritis
   e) pes planus

607. The initial treatment for bunions is:

   a) stiff-sole shoes
   b) padding between the first and second toes
   c) low-heeled broad-toe shoes with pads for the first metatarsalphalangeal joint
   d) osteotomy
   e) surgical removal of the first metatarsal head

608. The most common cause of onychocryptosis (ingrown toenail) is:

   a) a narrow shoe
   b) a bunion on the big toe
   c) neurovascular disease
   d) improper trimming of the toenail
   e) onychomycosis

609. The most common cause of plantar foot pain is:

   a) plantar callus
   b) Morton's neuroma
   c) metatarsal stress fracture
   d) plantar warts
   e) plantar fasciitis

CODE: (a:1, 2 and 3; b: 1 and 3; c: 2 and 4; d: 4 only; e: all of the above)

610. Which of the following statements regarding fungal infections of the feet is/are CORRECT?

   1) salicylic acid preparations may be used to reduce the scales of Trichophyton rubrum infections
   2) removal of the toenail may be indicated
   3) local antifungal agents are often helpful in treating the infection
   4) systemic griseofulvin therapy is recommended for tinea infections of the nails

611. Plantar warts are usually adequately treated by:

    1) carbon dioxide laser therapy
    2) trichloroacetic acid
    3) liquid nitrogen
    4) salicyclic acid

612. Effective treatment of an ingrown toenail includes:

    1) removal of all or a portion of the nail
    2) ablation of part of the nail bed with 89% phenol or 10% sodium hydroxide
    3) education regarding proper cutting of the nail
    4) oral antibiotics

613. Which of the following statements concerning the care of the diabetic patient's foot is/are CORRECT:

    1) daily inspection of the foot is essential
    2) topical moisturizing agents should be avoided to prevent maceration
    3) decreased sensitivity may result in the wearing of successively tighter shoes
    4) ischemic necrotic changes may occur in a matter of hours

ANSWERS

606. c) Hallux abducto valgus, or bunion deformity, is characterized by adduction and a valgus displacement of the great toe. The etiology of the deformity is primarily hypermobility of the first ray in an adducted forefoot.

    Rheumatoid arthritis, neuromuscular disease and trauma can also cause the deformity. There is little doubt that shoes are an important factor in the development of bunions. However, it is the abnormal mechanics of the foot that cause a bunion to develop in the first place.

    Osteoarthritis and pes planus are not implicated in the etiology of bunions.

607. c) Treatment for bunions should be directed toward reducing the mechanical pressure at the first metatarsal head. This can be accomplished by modifying the shoe, wearing a low-heeled broad-toe shoe and applying pads to protect the first MTP joint.

    Simple bunionectomy, or removal of the medial eminence of the first metatarsal head will not correct the deformity. Osteotomy of the metatarsal and/or proximal phalanx with capsule tendon balancing procedures is effective but probably should be reserved for situations in which conservative measures fail.

    Stiff-toed shoes and padding between the 1st and 2nd toes do not decrease pressure on the metatarsal head and thus are not indicated.

608. d) Onychocryptosis, or ingrown toenail, is most commonly caused by improper trimming of the toenail. Toenails should be cut straight across, following the general contour of the distal aspect of the toe. The nail should never be cut so short that the corner of the nail is proximal to the distal end of the groove.

Other causes of ingrown toenails include trauma and digital deformity. Neurovascular disease secondary to trauma may produce ingrown toenails. Narrow shoes could aggravate the pain associated with ingrown toenails but are unlikely to cause the deformity.

Bunions and onychomycosis are not associated with ingrown toenails.

609. a) The most common cause of plantar foot pain is a plantar callus. This results from abnormal pressures and mechanical stress exerted on the skin in an intermittent fashion. Plantar calluses can best be thought of as a symptom of an ill-fitting shoe, a mechanical fault in the foot or abnormal gait rather than a disorder or abnormality itself.

Morton's neuroma, which is a disorder arising from trauma to the common digital nerve running between the 3rd and 4th metatarsals produces pain in the forefoot.

Metatarsal stress fractures, usually of the second and third metatarsals and secondary to activities such as jogging, also produce pain in the forefoot.

Plantar warts may produce pain on walking underneath the bony surfaces. They are easily differentiated from plantar calluses.

Plantar fasciitis usually produces pain in the region of the heel.

Plantar calluses are best treated by changing the shoe to a low-heeled, thick soled shoe with a broad forefoot. Applications of salicyclic acid and pearing of the callus with a #10 or #20 scalpel blade are helpful in removing the hyper-keratotic tissue.

610. a) Tinea rubrum is the most common fungal organism producing the chronic type of dermatophytosis seen in onychomycosis. Tinea rubrum infections are chronic. Treatment is symptomatic because a cure is not likely. Keratolytics (salicyclic acid preparations) and local antifungals are useful in reducing the scales and any exacerbation which may occur.

Fungal nails are treated by debridement of the nail as it becomes thick. This can be most easily accomplished by having the patient file the nails. If the nail growth results in pain which is not resolved by debriding, a partial or complete nail ablation procedure is indicated.

Griseofulvin is not recommended for the treatment of chronic tinea of the feet or involved toenails because it is usually not possible to alter the suscepti-bility of the patient to the fungus.

611. e) Plantar warts are caused by a viral infection which creates a hyperkeratotic growth on the sole of the foot. When pared, a circuscribed lesion with pinpoint bleeding is noted, unlike a callus.

Treatments available for verrucae are varied, attesting to the difficulty in resolving them. Common treatments include 60% salicyclic acid and trichloroacetic acid followed by moleskin application; carbon dioxide laser; liquid nitrogen; 4% formalin and 5-fluorouracil.

Electrocautery is generally not recommended as it may result in scarring.

612. a) Ingrown toenails are prevented by patient education. Patients should be encouraged to cut the nails straight across, following the general contour of the distal aspect of the toe.

In a relatively flat nail that has been improperly cut, packing cotton beneath the advancing edge of the nail may afford relief of pain as the nail grows forward. If this technique is unsuccessful or the toe is infected, the margin of the nail must be removed. This is easily accomplished under local anaesthesia. The nail will grow back after such a procedure and will most likely assume the same shape and cause the same difficulty as the nail that was removed. In order to prevent this occurrence, the matrix should be cauterized by the application of 89% phenol (carbolic acid), or 10% sodium hydroxide.

Oral antibiotics are not indicated unless there is an accompanying cellulitis.

613. e) The most important aspect of diabetic foot care is prevention. By daily inspection of the feet and the avoidance of tight-fitting shoes, especially in a patient with peripheral neuropathy, the development of significant ulcers can be decreased. Also, if an area of redness or ulceration does occur, and this can be in a matter of hours, the avoidance of weight bearing and agents that encourage maceration should be encouraged.

Reference

Siwek J, ed. Common Foot Problems in Office Practice (Monograph 77). American Academy of Family Physicians. Kansas City: 1985, pages 5-46.

PROBLEM #94: A 63 YEAR OLD MALE WITH A WORK RELATED INJURY

614. A 63 year old male slipped in a hole while carrying a beam at a worksite. He presents to the emergency department with an acutely swollen, discolored left ankle, with more swelling on the lateral side. X-ray studies reveal no fracture, but a significant varus instability of the ankle is seen on a stress view. The patient has sustained no previous ankle injuries. The most likely diagnosis is:

a) Grade I sprain
b) Grade II sprain
c) Grade III sprain
d) Grade IV sprain
e) Grade V sprain

615. The preferred treatment of the injury described in the question above is:

a) operative repair
b) tensor bandage and elevation
c) splinting and elevation
d) below knee cast
e) crutches and elevation

616. The patient described in question #614 is treated appropriately for his injury. Six months later, he still complains of chronic ankle pain. Mortise views of the ankle show no varus instability. He states that he doubts very much if he will ever be able to go back to work, and requests that you place him on permanent compensation. When asked about his work he states that "it's probably all for the best, I never did like my job". The most likely explanation for the discrepancy between physical findings and his pain is:

a) acute situational anxiety
b) a secondary gain from the injury incurred
c) reactive depression
d) the early retirement syndrome
e) a chronic instability of the ankle that cannot be seen radiologically

617. A 16-year old high school basketball player sustained an injury while playing in the championship game. He recalls a "pop" in his knee and feeling some instability while walking off the court. Before examining this patient, you suspect damage to which one of the following structures?

a) lateral collateral ligament
b) anterior cruciate ligament
c) medial meniscus
d) lateral meniscus
e) medial collateral ligament

CODE: (a:1, 2 and 3; b: 1 and 3; c: 2 and 4; d: 4 only; e: all of the above)

618. The ligaments most commonly injured in an inversion injury of the ankle include:

    1) talofibular
    2) calcaneofibular
    3) anterior tibiofibular
    4) talonavicular

619. The ligaments most commonly injured in a ligamentous knee injury include:

    1) lateral collateral
    2) medial collateral
    3) posterior cruciate
    4) anterior cruciate

ANSWERS

614. c) Sprains are classified as Grade I, II, or III. Grade I sprain refers to an injury in which the ligament is partially torn but no instability occurs as a result of the injury. Grade II sprain refers to an injury in which the ligament is partially torn but significantly enough to produce some instability of the joint. Grade III sprain refers to a complete disruption of the ligament with accompanying instability.

    The patient described in this question most probably has a Grade III sprain.

615. d) The proper treatment for this patient is complete immobilization. This is best accomplished by a below-knee cast for 6 weeks. As well, the patient should be instructed to keep his leg elevated during the acute phase to reduce the swelling.

    A much younger patient, especially an athlete, would be a candidate for operative repair. However, the age of this patient would probably dictate conservative management as the treatment of choice.

    Tensor bandages and splints will not properly immobilize the ankle and therefore are not reasonable treatments. Crutches without immobilization are not appropriate.

616. b) Workman's compensation injuries are notorious for lengthy, drawn-out recuperations. Many workers find that their compensation packages, considering the benefits are non-taxable, are just as good as their regular salaries. This lends itself to a "secondary gain" from the injury. Although these attitudes are by no means universal, they are encountered more frequently than we would like to believe.

The situation described is not an acute situational anxiety or reactive depression as the patient does not manifest any of the symptoms associated with those conditions.

Although there is no entity that is defined as "the early retirement syndrome", this patient may very well be hoping for just that.

Assuming that the ankle injury was treated appropriately, six months is more than adequate time for complete healing. There is unlikely to be an associated injury that cannot be identified radiologically.

617. b) Anterior cruciate ligament tears have become recognized as a major problem in athletes. Typically, the athlete hears or feels a "pop" in his knee and is immediately aware of the accompanying instability. These injuries are often accompanied by significant hemarthrosis. Physical examination with the knee flexed at 20 degrees reveals anterior movement of the tibia on the femur. This is known as the "anterior drawer" sign or "Lachman's test".

The treatment of choice in this patient, considering he is a young athlete, is surgical repair of the ligament.

618. a) The ligaments most commonly injured in an inversion sprain of the ankle include the anterior tibiofibular, the calcaneofibular and the talofibular. The talonavicular is situated more centrally in the forefoot and is not often injured in an inversion injury.

619. c) The ligaments most commonly injured in a ligamentous knee injury are the anterior cruciate and the medial collateral either singly or in combination. Injury to these ligaments is confirmed clinically by the valgus stress test for the medial collateral and the Lachman test for the anterior cruciate.

   . Treatment will vary depending on the patient and his age, but operative repair is the treatment of choice in a young, physically active individual.

Reference

Moyer R. Is it a sprain, a tear or a rupture? Diagnosis 1985; 2(2): 78-93.

Geriatric Medicine

PROBLEM #95: AN 86 YEAR OLD FEMALE WITH MULTIPLE BRUISES

620. An 86 year old female presents to the emergency room with multiple bruises. You determine that she has recently been abused by her son with whom she lives. Current estimates indicate that up to what percentage of the elderly who live with their families may suffer from abuse or neglect at some time?

    a) 1%
    b) 5%
    c) 10%
    d) 25%
    e) 50%

621. The most common expression of elder abuse is:

    a) financial exploitation
    b) abandonment
    c) passive neglect
    d) verbal or emotional abuse
    e) physical abuse

622. People who commit acts of elder abuse:

    a) are usually related to the victim
    b) have usually had a short association with the abused
    c) are usually under age 50
    d) usually have a psychotic depression
    e) do not tend to have a common profile

CODE: (a:1, 2 and 3; b: 1 and 3; c: 2 and 4; d: 4 only; e: all of the above)

623. The following characteristics is/are risk factors for the victims of elder abuse:

    1) female sex
    2) age greater than 75
    3) lack of financial independence
    4) physically healthy

624. Which of the following is/are objectives for the family physician in dealing with elder abuse:

    1) to provide information about the disorder to the caregiver
    2) to move the elder away from all contact with the abuser as soon as possible
    3) to give the caregiver permission to meet his or her own needs
    4) to report the abuse to the authorities and ensure that legal action is taken against the caregiver

ANSWERS

620. d) Some authorities believe that as many as one-fourth of the elderly who live with their families may suffer from abuse or neglect at some time. The United States House of Representatives have prepared a report that has documented abuse in at least one million persons.

    The term "abuse" should be broadly defined as: the willful infliction of injury, unreasonable confinement, intimidation, or cruel punishment with resulting physical harm or pain or mental anguish; or the willful deprivation by a caretaker of goods or services which are necessary to avoid physical harm, mental anguish, or mental illness. The term 'exploitation' means the illegal or improper act or process of a caretaker using the resources of an elder for monetary or personal benefit, profit, or gain. The term 'neglect' means the failure to provide the goods or services which are necessary to avoid physical harm, mental anguish or mental illness or the failure of a caregiver to provide such goods or services. The term 'physical harm' means bodily pain, injury, impairment or disease.

621. c) Results of a recent survey indicated that neglect of a passive nature (inattention or isolation) is by far the most common form of elder abuse. Verbal or emotional abuse, active neglect (e.g. abandonment, financial exploitation, or malicious withholding) are less common.

622. a) Several characteristics are common to the abuser of elders. The perpetrator of elder abuse is most often a relative of the victim and has taken care of that person for a number of years. The average length of time is 9.5 years.

The caregiver is often burdened with stressors, including mental or physical deterioration in the elderly person, troublesome financial demands and social isolation. The caregiver may be overwhelmed by what seems to be an inextricable situation.

Studies have shown that 75% of principal caregivers are over the age of 50 years, and nearly 20% are over the age of 70 years. About 40% of abusers are spouses of victims, and 50% are children or grandchildren.

As the emotional status of the elder deteriorates, so does that of the caregiver. In one study, 91% of the caregivers were clinically depressed, and in 63% the abuser was suffering from alcoholism, drug addiction or psychosocial stress at the time of the abusive act. Psychotic depression is not a characteristic of the caregiver.

623. a) The vast majority of the victims of elder abuse are women. Typically, they are over age 75, widowed and without sufficient income to live independently. Economic dependency usually prompts them to move in with their families. Generally, victims have at least one physical or mental impairment that prevents them from caring for themselves.

624. b) The family physician should have five objectives when dealing with a situation of elder abuse. These are (1) to provide information about the disorder; (2) to give the caregiver permission to meet his or her own needs; (3) to respond to the major behavioral problems of the impaired person; (4) to arrange for respite or alternative care if the caregiver's burden becomes too great, and (5) to help the caregiver maximize the elderly individual's abilities.

The family physician may be faced with a situation in which the elder should be removed from the environment. In this case it is his responsibility to see that it is done. Fortunately, this is not necessary in the majority of cases.

Likewise, the family physician may be faced with a situation in which the elder abuse should be reported to the authorities. This is especially true in physical abuse. It is the responsibility of the physician to see that this is done.

Reference

Taler G, Ansello E. Elder Abuse. American Family Physician 1985; 32(2): 34-36, 107-114.

PROBLEM #96: AN 85 YEAR OLD FEMALE WITH URINARY INCONTINENCE

625. You are called to the nursing home to see an 85 year old female with urinary incontinence. You recall that the most common type of *established* incontinence in the elderly is:

   a) stress incontinence
   b) reflex incontinence
   c) overflow incontinence
   d) urge incontinence
   e) transient incontinence

626. Transient incontinence is responsible for what percentage of cases of incontinence in elderly patients?

   a) 10%
   b) 50%
   c) 20%
   d) 30%
   e) 80%

627. Which of the following agents HAVE NOT been implicated as a cause of transient incontinence in the elderly?

   a) antibiotics
   b) calcium channel entry blockers
   c) antipsychotics
   d) opiates
   e) loop diuretics

CODE: (a:1, 2 and 3; b: 1 and 3; c: 2 and 4; d: 4 only; e: all of the above)

628. Which of the following is/are causes of transient incontinence in the elderly?

   1) urinary tract infections
   2) atrophic vaginitis and urethritis
   3) delirium or confusional states
   4) depression

629. Reflex incontinence:

   1) is present when no stress or warning precedes periodic voiding
   2) may be associated with a suprasacral spinal cord lesion
   3) is amenable to treatment with alpha-adrenoceptor agonists
   4) should be treated with an indwelling urinary catheter

ANSWERS

625. d) The most common cause of established incontinence in the elderly patient is urge incontinence. Urge incontinence occurs when involuntary voiding is preceeded by a warning of a few seconds to several minutes. Leakage is periodic but frequent, the volume leaked is moderate to large, and nocturnal frequency and incontinence are common. The usual cause is detrusor over-activity. Treatment is composed of simple measures such as provision of a bedside urinal or commode and more frequent voiding. Pharmacological agents include anticholingerics, smooth-muscle relaxants, and antidepressants.

Stress incontinence, as the name implies, is the involuntary leakage of urine during periods of increased intraabdominal pressure. Typical stress inconti-nence is characterized by the daytime loss of small to moderate amounts of urine, infrequent nocturnal incontinence, and a low post-voiding residual volume. The usual cause is urethral hypermobility due to pelvic floor laxity. Treatment includes weight loss if obesity is present, pelvic floor exercises, and locally or topically administered estrogens. The definative treatment is surgi-cal correction and bladder elevation.

Reflex incontinence is present when no stress or warning preceeds periodic involuntary voiding. Voiding is frequent, moderate in volume, and occurs equally during the day and night. Classically, reflex incontinence is due to a suprasacral spinal-cord lesion (spondylosis or tumor). In the elderly, however, severe cortical damage may cause detrusor hyperreflexia and may also dimin-ish awareness of bladder filling, thereby mimicking symptomatically the effect of a spinal cord lesion on the bladder. Treatments include alpha-adrenoceptor antagonists such as prazosin, striated muscle relaxants, and intermittant catheterization.

Overflow incontinence occurs when the weight of urine in a distended bladder overcomes outlet resistance. In this condition, leakage of small amounts of urine is frequent throughout the day and night. The bladder is often palpable. Overflow incontinence is caused by either outlet obstruction or an underreactive detrusor attributable to myogenic or neurogenic factors. If obstruction is the cause it should be relieved. If no obstruction is present, the use of prazosin, bethanechol, phenoxybenzamine, or intermittant catheteriza-tion is often helpful.

Transient incontinence is not *established* incontinence and can often be cured by removal of the offending agent or treatment of the underlying condition.

626. b) Transient incontinence is responsible for up to 50% of all causes of incontinence in the elderly. Of the remainder, as many as 2/3 can be cured or markedly improved.

627. a) The pharmacologic agents that have been implicated as causes of transient incontinence in the elderly include sedatives or hypnotics, loop diuretics, anticholinergic agents (including antipsychotics, antidepressants, antihistamines, antiarrhythmics, antispasmodics, opiates, and antidiarrheal agents), alpha-adrenoreceptor agonists and antagonists, and calcium-channel blockers. Antibiotics are not usually associated with incontinence.

628. e) Transient incontinence, as well as being associated with pharmacologic agents is common in the following conditions: (1) delirium or confusional states, (2) urinary and other infections, (3) atrophic urethritis or vaginitis, (4) psychological disorders, especially depression, (5) endocrine disorders including hypercalcemia and hyperglycemia, (6) restricted mobility, and (7) stool impaction.

629. a) Reflex incontinence is present when no stress or warning precedes involuntary voiding. It may be associated with a suprasacral spinal cord lesion, and it is amenable to treatment with alpha-adrenoreceptor antagonists, striated muscle relaxants, or intermittant catherization. An indwelling urinary catheter will make the dyssynergia worse.

Reference

Resnick N, Subbarao V. Management of urinary incontinence in the elderly. New England Journal of Medicine 1985; 313(13): 799-804.

PROBLEM #97: A DAUGHTER WHO WANTS HER FATHER CONFINED TO A NURSING HOME

The following questions are based on this case history:

Mr. Jones is a 68 year old widower. He is being treated in hospital for a broken hip resulting from an accident. His injury has now healed and he is ready to be discharged. Mr. Jones lives by himself in an apartment and occasionally receives assistance from a cleaning woman and a friendly neighbor.

Mr. Jones also has periods of confusion, during which he has been found wandering downtown without purpose and at some risk to himself. His children believe that he should not be discharged from hospital to live on his own. They want him kept under supervision, either in hospital or in a nursing home.

During periods of apparent rationality, Mr. Jones indicates that he is aware of his problem and the risks it poses to his health and well being. He prefers to accept these risks rather than be confined to an institution. The medical team and Mr. Jone's family have decided that Mr. Jones will be confined to hospital until a vacancy in a suitable nursing home becomes available. His request to be discharged is refused. When he protests aggressively he is sedated to a level that ensures his compliance.

630. Based on the facts presented above, the decision of this medical team is:

a) medically sound
b) legally sound
c) ethically sound
d) all of the above
e) none of the above

631. Which of the following statements with regard to the correlation between the state of the brain and the legal criterion for competency is CORRECT?

a) there is a direct correlation
b) there is an indirect correlation
c) some correlation exists but it is as yet defined
d) there is no reliable correlation

CODE: (a:1, 2 and 3; b: 1 and 3; c: 2 and 4; d: 4 only; e: all of the above)

632. When considering the use of restraints in any patient, which of the following must be strongly considered?

1) the risk of the patient to himself
2) the risk of the patient to other patients
3) the risk of the patient to staff
4) the risk of the patient to the community

633. When considering the administration of neurotropic agents to patients with dementia, which of the following statements is/are CORRECT?

1) as the patient has dementia, he is unable to give an informed consent, and thus he may be given the drugs as the medical staff sees fit
2) if the neurotropic drugs will keep the patient compliant, and the rest of the ward quiet, they are problably indicated
3) the neurotropic drugs are indicated if the patient poses any risk to himself, regardless of whether or not he wants them
4) a patient who exhibits symptoms of dementia is not necessarily incompetent to give or withhold informed consent

ANSWERS

630. e) Based on the facts presented, the decision of the medical staff is neither medically, legally nor ethically sound.

On medical grounds, the fact that he is confused does not prove that he has a chronic, progressive form of brain failure that will eventually make him incapable of making rational decisions.

On legal grounds, the patient has not been found incompetent by a court of law. Even a mentally ill person who is subjected to restraint, pursuant to the provisions of a provincial or state mental health act, is entitled to all the rights and privileges of a citizen, unless those rights have been specifically curtailed.

On ethical grounds, when an elderly patient is labelled as incapable of rational choice, those who apply the label, as well as others, view the patient as not fully a person. Frequently the patient comes to view him-or herself as less than unworthy of respect. In other words, the stigma associated with restraints tends to become internalized and so produces a diminution of the patient's sense of self-worth.

631. d) There is no reliable correlation between the state of the brain and the legal criteria for competency. There is often severely advanced cerebral arteriosclerosis present on post-mortem examinations in individuals who exhibit no striking intellectual or behavioral abnormalities. On the other hand, the brain of an elderly person who appears to be intellectual impaired may appear pathologically to be perfectly normal!

632. e) When considering the use of restraints in the elderly, the risk of the patient to himself, to other patients, to the staff, and to the community must be considered. As well, the magnitude of risk must be assessed in each case. It is medically, legally, and ethically unsound to restrain a patient against his will unless the risks have been assessed and found to be substantial.

633. d) Neurotropic drugs, used as a method of restraint are not indicated unless the risks to the patient and others have been assessed and found to be substantial (see critique of question 632). In a recent landmark court decision, it was ruled that one cannot automatically assume that demented patients or patients thought to be insane cease to be competent to give or withhold consent for medication. One ought not to assume that a patient who exhibits symptoms of dementia is necessarily incompetent to give or withhold informed constent to restrictions of liberty.

Reference

Schafer A. Restraints and the elderly: when safety and autonomy conflict. Canadian Medical Association Journal 1985; 132: 1257-1260.

PROBLEM #98: AN 80 YEAR OLD MALE WITH INCREASING CONFUSION AND MEMORY LOSS

634. An 80 year old male presents to your office with his daughter. His daughter states that he is becoming increasing forgetful. You recall that the most common cause of dementia in the elderly population is:

a) Alzheimer's disease
b) multi-infarct dementia
c) depressive dementia
d) hypothyroidism
e) mixed dementia (Alzheimer plus multi-infarct)

635. Which of the following statements concerning Alzheimer's disease is CORRECT?

a) Alzheimer's disease is present to some degree in all persons over the age of 80 years
b) Alzheimer's disease is a pathological diagnosis
c) Alzheimer's disease is a rapidly progressive dementia
d) Alzheimer's disease is easy to differentiate from other dementias.
e) Alzheimer's disease usually has a sudden onset

636. Which of the following diseases is the MOST COMMON disease usually confused with Alzheimer's disease?

a) hypothyroidism
b) alcoholism
c) congestive cardiac failure
d) depression
e) normal pressure hydrocephalus

637. Which of the following treatments have been shown to be of benefit in Alzheimer's disease?

a) amitriptyline
b) nicotinic acid
c) vasopressin
d) dihydroergotoxin (Hydergine)
e) none of the above

CODE: (a:1, 2 and 3; b: 1 and 3; c: 2 and 4; d: 4 only; e: all of the above)

638. Which of the following drugs have been shown to result in confusion in elderly patients, thereby producing a syndrome that is often indistinguishable from dementia?

    1) cimetidine
    2) propranolol
    3) haloperidol
    4) pyridoxine

639. Which of the following laboratory investigations should be ordered in a patient with dementia, to rule out the possibility of an underlying, reversible cause?

    1) complete blood count
    2) chest X-ray
    3) CAT scan
    4) electroencephalogram

ANSWERS

634. a) The most common cause of dementia in the elderly population is Alzheimer's disease. In a recent survey, 50% of patients with dementia had Alzheimer's disease, 18% had multi-infarct dementia, 18% has a mixed Alzheimer/multi-infarct dementia, 15% had depressive dementia (pseudodementia), and 10% were unclassified. Four percent of patients had other causes, including hypothyroidism.

635. b) The diagnosis of Alzheimer's disease is established at necropsy. The two characteristic pathological lesions are an Alzheimer "plaque" around a centre of protein, and neurofibrillary degeneration of neurons.

    Although the incidence of Alzheimer's disease increases with age it is not part of the normal aging process. Only 25% of patients over the age of 80 will show cognitive dysfunction characteristic of Alzheimer's disease.

    Alzheimer's disease has a slowly progressive, deteriorating course, and it's onset, likewise, is slow and often unnoticed by both family and family physician.

    Alzheimer's disease can be extremely difficult to differentiate from other dementias, and requires careful investigation.

636. d) The disease most commonly confused with Alzheimer's disease is depression. Up to 15% of patients that are labelled as "Alzheimer's" actually have a depression. This has been referred to as "pseudodementia". This depression responds rapidly and often completely to tricyclic antidepressants or MAO inhibitors.

637. e) None of the treatments listed in the question has been shown to be of benefit in patients with Alzheimer's disease.

Amitripyline is only beneficial in patients with depressive dementia (pseudodementia). Nicotinic acid, vasopressin and dihydroergotoxin (Hydergine) have not been shown to be beneficial in improving cognitive function in controlled trials.

638. a) Cimetidine is now considered to be the most common pharmacological cause of confusion in the elderly.

Propranolol is probably the most common cause of hallucinations in the elderly.

All psychotropics, including haloperidol, and all benzodiazepines are potential causes of a dementia syndrome.

Pyridoxine (Vitamin B-6) has not been implicated as a cause of reversible dementia in elderly patients. It's main neurological manifestations are confined to the peripheral nervous system, where it is a potent cause of peripheral neuropathy if taken in doses greater than 500 mg./day.

639. e) To rule out a potentially reversible cause of dementia all patients should have a complete blood count; a complete urinalysis; electrolytes; a biochemical battery that includes calcium, phosphorus, blood urea nitrogen, and creatinine; vitamine B_{12}; and electrocardiogram; a chest film; a CAT scan; and an electroencephalogram.

Reference

Blass J. Dementia. The Medical Clinics of North America 1982; 66(5): 1143-1160.

PROBLEM #99: A 75 YEAR OLD FEMALE WITH THE SUDDEN ONSET OF DEMENTIA

640. A 75-year old female develops rapidly progressive dementia. Her family is concerned that she be looked after appropriately, and ask you to arrange her nursing home admission. Before doing this, you order a number of investigations, but find them to all be within normal limits. Your next step should be:

   a) arrange for the patient to be admitted to the chronic care facility and placate the family
   b) prescribe diazepam for the family and haloperidol for the patient
   c) refuse to return the calls from the family
   d) begin a trial of a tricyclic antidepressant in the patient

641. Recent studies have suggested that some patients originally diagnosed as having dementia are not demented but rather depressed. This syndrome has become known as "pseudodementia". What percentage of all patients with diagnosis of dementia does this represent?

   a) 40-50%
   b) 8-15%
   c) 4-5%
   d) 1-2%
   e) less than 1%

642. In contrast to dementia, the cognitive impairment associated with pseudodementia often:

   a) comes on more slowly
   b) comes on more rapidly
   c) is usually only a minor impairment
   d) is not improved with tricyclic antidepressants

643. In contrast to dementia, patients with pseudodementia often:

   a) complain about their cognitive deficits
   b) deny that their cognitive deficits exists
   c) try to conceal their cognitive deficits
   d) usually try to answer questions even if they don't know the answers
   e) perform consistently on tasks of equal difficulty

CODE: (a:1, 2 and 3; b: 1 and 3; c: 2 and 4; d: 4 only; e: all of the above)

644. Pseudodementia has certain characteristics that distinguish it from dementia. Which of the following are PARTICULARLY IMPORTANT in differientating dementia from pseudodementia?

    1) a history of psychiatric illness
    2) a history of an affective prodrome
    3) the duration of illness
    4) the rapidity of progression

645. Which of the following laboratory investigations should be performed to help distinguish a patient with dementia from one with pseudodementia?

    1) complete blood count
    2) electroencephalogram
    3) CT scan of the brain
    4) NMR imaging of the brain

ANSWERS

640. d) Before labeling this patient as "demented" and relegating her to a nursing home, it is prudent to perform the definitive diagnostic test; a trial of anti-depressant medication. The results are often dramatic and take both the family and the family physician by surprise. The drug of choice is probably one with a low incidence of anticholingeric side effects such as desipramine. Dosage should probably be started at 25-50 mg. h.s. and increased as necessary if a response seems to be starting. At least a 4-week trial of therapy is indicated.

641. b) The diagnosis of dementia is usually made on clinical grounds, without the benefit of specific, sensitive laboratory tests. Reliance on the clinical picture results in a certain amount of diagnostic error, which has been documented in several studies. In these studies, 8 to 15% of the patients initially given a diagnosis of dementia were later judged to be suffering from depressive illness.

642. c) One of the most important clinical differences between dementia and pseudodementia associated with a psychiatric disorder relates to the onset of symptoms and the rapidity of their progression. In the dementing disorders, particularly the degenerative dementias, the onset of cognitive impairment is insidious, with a slow progression of symptoms. Thus, there may be an interval of several years between the time that the patient or family members first notice the symptoms and the time that they initially seek health care. This time interval is commonly 3-5 years.

   In pseudodementia, particularly that associated with depressive illness in the elderly the onset of symptoms is more rapid. Impairment often progresses to the point of incapacitation over a period of several months, although it is occasionally as long as a year. Thus, medical attention is sought much sooner.

643. a) Patients with pseudodementia often complain vociferously of their cognitive deficits, frequently to an extent that is disproportionate to any observable or measurable defect. In some instances, observers may notice a discrepancy between these patients' preceived impairment and their actual level of functioning.

   In contrast, patients with dementing disorders characteristically deny the extent of their cognitive decline and attempt to make light of it or conceal it. This leads to another helpful sign: While pseudodemented patients often respond to questions with "I don't know" answers demented patients usually try to answer questions. As a result, they often respond to "near miss" answers.

   Patients with pseudodementia often perform inconsistently on tasks of equal difficulty, whereas demented patients demonstrate a consistently poor performance on similar tasks.

   Nocturnal worsening is common in dementia, whereas patients with pseudodementia are, if anything worse in the morning.

644. e) A careful history will often give a clue as to the liklehood of a pseudodementia masquerading as a dementia. The most relevant points in the history which favor pseudodementia include:

   a) past history of psychiatric illness
   b) history of affective prodrome prior to the onset of dementia
   c) short duration of illness
   d) rapid progression of illness

   A Mini-Mental State Assessment is also often helpful. The one following has been developed by the Toronto Western Hospital. The maximum score is 30 points. Individuals with cognitive impairment will generally score less than 24 points. In this test, 4 areas of psychometric evaluation are tested: memory, attention, language, and visuospatial ability.

ORIENTATION

   What is the year, season, month, date, and day? (5 points)
   Where are we? (country, province, city, hosptial and floor) (5 points)

REGISTRATION

   Name 3 objects: 1 second to say each. Then ask the patient to repeat all three after you have said them. 1 point for each correct. Then repeat them until he learns them. Count trials and record. (3 points)

ATTENTION AND CALCULATION

Serial 7's. 1 point for each correct. Stop at 5 answers. (5 points)

RECALL

Ask for the objects above. 1 point for each correct.

LANGUAGE TESTS

Name: pencil, watch (2 points)

Repeat: no ifs, ands, or buts (1 point)
Follow a 3 stage command: "Take the paper in your right hand, fold it in half, and put it on the floor." (3 points)
Read and obey the following:
    CLOSE YOUR EYES. (1 point)
Write a sentence spontaneously below. (1 point)
Copy the design below: (1 point)

645. a) Certain laboratory investigations may reveal an abnormality that tends to exclude pseudodementia unless a patient has elements of both dementia and pseudodementia. The baseline laboratory investigations include a complete blood count; urinalysis; electrolytes; a biochemical battery including calcium, phosphorus, blood urea nitrogen, and creatinine; vitamin B-12 and folate levels; a VDRL; serum thyroxine; an electrocardiogram; a chest film; a CAT scan; and an electroencephalogram. In a patient with pseudodementia all of these investigations will be normal. In a patient with dementia, they may or may not be normal.

NMR imaging at this time offers no therapeutic advantage over CT scanning in looking for cortical atrophy and the cost of the procedure is prohibitive.

References

McAllister T. Recognition of Pseudodementia. American Family Physician 1985; 32(4): 175-181.
Lautenschlaeger, E, Meier R. Cognitive Assessment: Indispensable in Evaluation of Elderly Patients. Geriatric Medicine 1986; 1: 151.

PROBLEM #100: AN 81 YEAR OLD FEMALE WITH CONSTIPATION

646. An 81 year old female presents to the office with a one year history of constipation. In elderly patients, the major complication of constipation is:

    a) confusion
    b) fecal incontinence
    c) idiopathic megacolon
    d) sigmoid volvulus
    e) chronic abdominal pain

647. Which of the following agents SHOULD NOT be used in elderly patients with constipation?

    a) docusate sodium
    b) docusate calcium
    c) phenolphthalein
    d) senokot
    e) psyllium

648. Ingestion of large amounts of bulking agents may result in failure to absorb *ALL BUT* which one of the following?

    a) calcium
    b) magnesium
    c) glucose
    d) zinc
    e) iron

CODE: (a:1, 2 and 3; b: 1 and 3; c: 2 and 4; d: 4 only; e: all of the above)

649. Which of the following is/are possible etiologic factors for constipation in the elderly?

    1) carcinoma of the colon or rectum
    2) diverticulitis
    3) immobility
    4) diabetes

650. Regarding constipation in the elderly, which of the following statements is/are TRUE?

    1) frequency of bowel evacuation decreases as aging occurs
    2) laxative consumption is more prevalent in elderly patients than in younger ones
    3) transit time in elderly patients is usually decreased compared to younger patients
    4) a decreased intake of food and fluids may be an etiologic factor for constipation in the elderly

651. Which of the following medications is/are common causes of constipation in the elderly?

    1) amitriptyline
    2) digoxin
    3) verapamil
    4) nitroglycerin

ANSWERS

646. b) Fecal incontinence is the major complication of constipation, especially chronic constipation. Fecal incontinence in elderly patients not only is a frequent reason for institutionalization, but also is responsible for a great deal of the indignity with which the elderly are treated, especially when dementia coexists. Incontinence is usually due to impacted stool which causes mucosal irritation of the rectum and sigmoid colon, leading to increased mucus production. The mucus bypasses the impaction, dissolves a portion of the surface stool and results in leakage of liquid or semi-solid stool whenever intraabdominal pressure increases, as with coughing or movement.

Confusion, idiopathic megacolon, sigmoid volvulus and chronic abdominal pain are all recognized complications of constipation in elderly patients but are not as frequent as fecal incontinence.

647. c) Phenolphthalein is usually not recommended for use in elderly patients because it is excreted in the bile and can be reabsorbed via the intestine, leading to prolonged action and potential depletion of fluids and electrolytes. The treatment of constipation in the elderly should follow an orderly progression once a thorough evaluation of possible etiologic factors has been undertaken. The progression includes: 1) increase in fluid intake, activity and correction of toilet habits; 2) addition of bran 2-4 grams/day; 3) addition of bulking agents such as psyllium; 4) addition of stool softeners such as docusate sodium and docusate calcium; 5) addition of standardized senna preparation; and 6) addition of fleet or tap water enema PRN.

Emollient laxatives such as mineral oil (which may inhibit the absorption of fat soluble vitamins); stimulant cathartics (which may result in dehydration and excessive electrolyte loss); and saline cathartics should not be used.

648. c) Addition of natural bran or other bulking agents may interfere with the absorption of minerals, especially calcium, magnesium, iron and zinc. Because of the risk of osteoporosis and its sequelae from calcium lack, especially in elderly women, a calcium supplement should be added.

649. e) Three general categories of dysfunction are typically reported by patients with the complaint of constipation: 1) that defecation is less frequent than in the past; 2) that the amount of stool passed is less than what the patient considers normal and 3) that bowel movements are either painful or difficult to initiate. Many etiologic factors contribute to these symptoms in elderly patients. They include factors associated with:

1) intrinsic pathology — such as carcinoma of the colon or rectum; diverticulitis; ulcerative colitis; granulomatous colitis; spastic colitis; and anal pathology such as fissure, stricture or hemorrhoids.
2) neurologic disease — including the autonomic neuropathy associated with diabetes; multiple sclerosis; and cerebrovascular disease (eg. — stroke)
3) collagen vascular diseases
4) endocrine disorders such as hypothyroidism, hyperparathyroidism and adrenal and pituitary dysfunction
5) electrolyte disorders including hypokalemia and hypercalemia
6) drugs such as antihypertensives; diuretics (potassium and water depletion); anticholinergic agents including antihistamines; narcoleptics; tricyclics and antiparkinsonian agents; hematinics; aluminum containing antacids and analgesics
7) depression
8) miscellaneous factors such as immobility, dietary abnormalities, deficient fiber and water intake and poor mastication

650. c) The frequency of bowel evacuation and the transit time in elderly patients not confined to bed is not significantly different from their younger counterparts; however their consumption of laxatives is much higher. This appears in many cases to be because of habit. A decreased intake of food and/ or fluids is often an important etiologic factor in individual patients.

651. b) Amitriptyline, with its potent anticholingeric properties and verapamil are important iatrogenic causes of constipation in the elderly. Digoxin usually produces nausea, vomiting and diarrhea. Nitroglycerine is not usually associated with constipation.

Reference

Kallman H. Constipation in the Elderly. American Family Physician 1983; 27(1): 179-184.

PROBLEM #101: A 75 YEAR OLD FEMALE WITH A BAGFULL OF PILLS

652. A 75 year old female presents to your office with her daughter. Her daughter complains that her mother began seeing "pink rats coming out of the walls" 3 days ago. The daughter brings in her mother's medications in a bag. From the history you ascertain that the mother went to her local doctor 1 week ago for assessment of high blood pressure, arthritis, a nervous stomach and back pain. The doctor prescribed propranolol, hydrochlorothiazide, ibuprofen, cimetidine, and maalox. Knowing that medications in the elderly can often produce significant side effects you conclude that there probably is a connection between the pink rats and a medication. The most likely medication to produce this side effect is:

   a) propranolol
   b) hydrochlorothiazide
   c) ibuprofen
   d) cimetidine
   e) maalox

653. The medication producing the problem described in question #652 is discontinued. One week later the mother again presents to your office with her daughter. From the history you ascertain that within 24 hours of stopping the medication the pink rats disappeared. However, 2 days later the mother became confused and incoherent. On examination and laboratory evaluation there appears to be no discernable cause for the confusion. Again, you conclude that it may be related to one of the medications that she was recently prescribed. The most likely pharmacologic cause of the mother's confusion is:

   a) propranolol
   b) hydrochlorothiazide
   c) ibuprofen
   d) cimetidine
   e) maalox

654. A recent survey indicated that four out of five elderly Americans living independently received at least how many prescriptions a year for chronic diseases?

   a) 3
   b) 5
   c) 10
   d) 15
   e) 20

655. The most common side effect of antihypertensive medication in the elderly is:

   a) confusion
   b) orthostatic hypotension
   c) dizziness
   d) fatigue
   e) skin rash

CODE: (a:1, 2 and 3; b: 1 and 3; c: 2 and 4; d: 4 only; e: all of the above)

656. Which of the following is/are important risk factors for undesirable side effects of medication in the elderly?

   1) multiple drugs
   2) multiple physicians
   3) multiple pharmacies
   4) living alone

657. Which of the following is/are important variables in increasing the incidence of adverse drug reactions in the elderly?

   1) altered free concentration of drug in serum
   2) altered volume of distribution
   3) altered renal drug clearance
   4) altered tissue sensitivity

ANSWERS

652. a) The most common iatrogenic cause of hallucination in elderly patients is propranolol. Many patients who are started on this medication develop visual or auditory hallucinations. Unfortunately, many of these patients are then started on antipsychotics to treat the hallucinations. Although other medications may produce this side effect, propranolol is by far the most common medication implicated.

653. d) Cimetidine is currently the most common iatrogenic cause of confusion in the elderly. It is important to realize that any medication can cause confusion in the elderly. Thus, when a patient becomes acutely confused, a medication should be the number one suspect.

654. e) Four out of five elderly Americans living independently receive 20 or more prescriptions a year for chronic diseases. The most commonly prescribed medications are: cardiovascular drugs (digitalis, diuretics, vasodilators, other antihypertensivies); psychotropic drugs including sedatives, hypnotics, anti-depressants and antipsychotics); laxatives; antibiotics; anti-inflammatory agents and analgesics. The elderly use twice as many nonprescription preparations as drugs that are prescribed for them, and this practice increases with age. The most common non-prescription drugs are for pain, colds, indigestion or constipation, or as dietary supplements (vitamins and minerals).

655. b) Antihypertensive medication produces many side effects in the elderly. The most significant side effect is orthostatic hypotension. Orthostatic hypotension is due to impaired cardiovascular homeostasis and may result in dizziness, falls, and hip fractures. Therefore, any patient on antihypertensive medication should have their blood pressure taken in both the sitting and the standing position. Confusion, fatigue, and impotence are other common side effects.

656. e) Many factors increase the risk of undesirable drug effects in the elderly. They are (1) a physician with no knowledge of pharmacogeriatrics; (2) multiple drugs; (3) history of a tendency to adverse drug reactions; (4) concurrent diseases, especially renal disease and severe liver insufficiency; (5) impairments: mental, visual, auditory, locomotive; (6) late senescence: very limited homeostasis; (7) self-medication; (8) multiple physicians; (9) multiple pharmacies; (10) lower lean body mass; (11) living alone; (12) lack of community support services; and (13) soci-economic problems resulting in inadequate follow-up.

657. e) Many physiological and social variables increase the incidence of adverse drug reactions in the elderly. They include:

1) number of drugs: in the elderly there is a threefold increase both in the number of products used and in adverse reactions produced
2) compliance: compliance is decreased because of confusion, side effects, psychosocial factors and visual impairment
3) absorption: active diffusion (with calcium and ferrous ions as well as thiamine) may be slowed
4) free drug in serum: the amount of free drug in serum is generally increased due to decreased binding with reduced serum albumin, reduced number of receptors on the albumin molecule and displacement from albumin of one drug by another
5) volume of distribution: this is decreased because of decreased body size, body water and lean body mass; increased body fat/lean-mass ratio affects fat-soluble drugs
6) tissue sensitivity: elderly patients have increased sensitivity to many drugs, with a tendency to ototoxicity, dementia, depression and nephrotoxicity

7) metabolic clearance: clearance is decreased because of a decrease in liver mass, blood flow and microsomal enzyme activity
8) renal drug clearance: glomerular and tubular function decreases — the most important clearance factor for most drugs
9) general homeostasis: senescence is a process of gradual reduction in homeostatic reserves. Thus, a combination of pathophysiologic changes plus untoward pharmacologic effects may determine the clinical presentation.

Reference

Jennigan J. Update on drugs and the elderly. American Family Physician 1984; 29(4): 338-247.

PROBLEM #102: AN 80 YEAR OLD NURSING HOME RESIDENT WITH A BED SORE

658. An 80 year old female residing in a nursing home is hospitalized with a fever of 40 degrees Celcius. On examination, you notice a 10×5 cm. pressure sore on the sacrum that is oozing pus. You suspect septicemia. Which of the following statements concerning the prevention and etiology of pressure sores is FALSE?

a) pressure sores are very difficult to prevent in immobilized elderly patients
b) good nutrition in the elderly will often help prevent pressure sores
c) anemia in the elderly will often help prevent pressure sores
d) incontinence in the elderly increases the risk of pressure sores by a factor of five
e) patients who sit for long periods of time are just as likely to develop pressure sores as bed-ridden patients

659. Concerning the patient described in question #658, how long would it take the large ulcer described to develop from a small untreated ulcer?

a) > 28 days
b) 21-28 days
c) 14-21 days
d) 7-10 days
e) 1-2 days

660. An elderly immobilized male is seen with a small 1 cm. area of erthyema and bruising on his left heel. Which of the following is the MOST IMPORTANT aspect of treatment of a pressure sore at this stage?

a) application of a full-thickness skin graft
b) extensive debridement of the lesion and cleansing with an iodine-based solution
c) application of a foam pad to protect the heel from further damage
d) application of microscopic beads of dextran to the lesion
e) elevation of the left leg by 30 degrees

CODE: (a:1, 2 and 3; b: 1 and 3; c: 2 and 4; d: 4 only; e: all of the above)

661. Pressure higher than normal capillary pressure exerted for a sufficient time may cause which of the following pathological changes?

1) local edema
2) local thrombosis in small vessels and the microcirculation
3) occulsion of vessels by platelets
4) an aseptic mass of necrosis beneath the skin

662. Which of the following have been found useful in the treatment of pressure sores?

    1) unna paste dressings
    2) antibiotic lotions and povidine-iodine
    3) a gel of mixed streptokinase and streptodornase
    4) absorbable gelfoam

ANSWERS

658. a) Pressure sores are a common problem in elderly, immobilized patients. The primary causal factor is the pressure created when a major part of the body weight is transmitted between a bony prominence and a relatively hard surface below, compressing the skin and adjacent soft tissues. The most vulnerable points are the sacrum, the heels, the greater trochanters, the knees, the iliac crest and the shoulders. The bed-fast state puts these pressure points at risk, but equally problematic is the unrelieved sitting position in which the area under the ischial tuberosities is subjected to pressure. A skin tear or minimal break in any area subject to pressure, maceration of the skin, or repeated incontinence resulting in a patch of erythema or "urine rash" will predispose to an ulcer. Incontinence multiplies the risk five-fold.

Good nutrition including a high protein diet will prevent anemia and hypoproteinemia which both substantially increase the risk of pressure sores. Pressure sores can be prevented by observing the following principles:

    1) use old soft sheets, processed sheep skin and deerskin; segmented pressure mattresses; or a sponge rubber or air filled rubber for the bed or wheelchair
    2) rotate the patient every 1-2 hours
    3) check all pressure points twice/day in good light
    4) avoid alcohol rubs
    5) avoid complete bathing every day; use corn oil, mineral oil or cold cream for gentle massage and cleaning
    6) use hydrotherapy and exercises (both active and passive) daily
    7) consider the addition of sawdust to a bed in which a patient is incontinent
    8) ensure a high-protein, high-vitamin diet

659. e) Erythema may progress to ulceration very quickly. A small ulcer can progress to a large one within 24-48 hours. Essentially the progression is due to local edema and/or infection, the former being the most important factor. As in the patient presented in question #658, severe infections can lead to **septicemia, which must be recognized and treated with appropriate systemic antibiotic therapy.**

660. c) Early lesions, as evidenced by erythema and mild bruising should be treated by the application of a foam pad to protect the area from further damage. Use of a hydrofloat device will help reverse the early changes and help fully developed lesions heal more quickly. Extensive debridement of the lesion and application of a full-thickness skin graft, and application of microscopic beads of dextran are not indicated for a lesion at the early stage described. Elevation of the leg to an angle of 30 degrees will not enhance the healing of the ulcer.

The following therapy is recommended for definite ulcerations:

a) debridement with forceps and scissors after compressing with saline soaks. (Some authorities prefer the enzymatic debridement with streptokinase or streptodornase.

b) use of an antibiotic lotion or organic iodide solution on the affected area (eg. — neomycin-polymyxin B, povidone-iodine

c) application of an absorbable gelfoam into the ulcer

d) overlay of the gelfoam with a "pressure-sandwich", which consists of an inner layer of gauze, a middle layer consisting of four to eight thickness of gauze 1-2 cm. larger than the periphery of the ulcer, and an outer layer of gauze.

e) an "unna paste dressing" gently applied over the "pressure sandwich" followed by a double layer of tubular gauze (especially for elbows, heels, knees, trochanteric and sacral areas).

661. e) Pressure higher than normal capillary pressure exerted for a sufficient time causes edema, local thrombosis in small vessels and the microcirculation, and damages vacular endothelium. Just beyond the site of greatest pressure there is also occulsion of vessels by platelets and a further area of risk to tissue. Tissue death then results in an open ulcer of epidermal depth, full thickness depth, or worse. Pressure persisting over a region where thick muscle, fat or fascia underlies the skin may lead to a huge "blind" aseptic mass of necrosis which bursts through the skin, sometimes without apparent warning, leaving a cavity with undermined edges often several inches across.

662. e) See critique of question #660.

References

Agnate J. Pressure sores. In: Principles and Practice of Geriatric Medicine. Patly M, editor. Chichester: 1985; John Wiley and Sons, pages 899-905.

Beninson J. Decubitus ulcer. In Current Therapy; Conn H, editor. Philadelphia: 1983; W.B. Saunders Co., pages 613-615.